Dietary Supplements and Functional Foods: Processing Effects and Health Benefits

Dietary Supplements and Functional Foods: Processing Effects and Health Benefits

Edited by Winston Ford

SYRAWOOD
PUBLISHING HOUSE
New York

Published by Syrawood Publishing House,
750 Third Avenue, 9th Floor,
New York, NY 10017, USA
www.syrawoodpublishinghouse.com

Dietary Supplements and Functional Foods: Processing Effects and Health Benefits
Edited by Winston Ford

International Standard Book Number: 978-1-64740-372-0 (Hardback)

Cataloging-in-publication Data

Dietary supplements and functional foods : processing effects and health benefits / edited by Winston Ford.
p. cm.
Includes bibliographical references and index.
ISBN 978-1-64740-372-0
1. Dietary supplements. 2. Functional foods. 3. Nutrition. 4. Health. I. Ford, Winston.
RM258.5 .D54 2023
615.1--dc23

TABLE OF CONTENTS

PREFACE

This book has been a concerted effort by a group of academicians, researchers and scientists, who have contributed their research works for the realization of the book. This book has materialized in the wake of emerging advancements and innovations in this field. Therefore, the need of the hour was to compile all the required researches and disseminate the knowledge to a broad spectrum of people comprising of students, researchers and specialists of the field.

Functional foods and dietary supplements are classified as nutraceuticals, which is an umbrella term used to describe food products that have purported health or medical benefits. These benefits might include improving cardiovascular health, and prevention or treatment of diseases. Functional foods are ingredients that offer health benefits that extend beyond their nutritional value. They may be enriched or fortified to restore preprocessed nutrient levels such as in the case of enriched flour. The primary purpose of functional foods may be to improve the nutritional quality of otherwise nutrient-deficient foods or to resolve public health issues such as deficiency of vitamin D in milk or iodine in regular salt. Food supplements are concentrated sources of nutrients such as minerals and vitamins, or other substances, with a nutritional or physiological effect. These are marketed in dose form that includes pills, tablets, capsules, and liquids in measured doses. The book aims to shed light on some of the unexplored aspects of functional foods and dietary supplements and the recent researches on them. A number of latest researches have been included to keep the readers up-to-date with the global concepts in this area of study.

At the end of the preface, I would like to thank the authors for their brilliant chapters and the publisher for guiding us all-through the making of the book till its final stage. Also, I would like to thank my family for providing the support and encouragement throughout my academic career and research projects.

Editor

1

Cyanobacteria and Microalgae as Sources of Functional Foods to Improve Human General and Oral Health

Gianmaria Fabrizio Ferrazzano [1,2,*], Cristina Papa [1], Antonino Pollio [3], Aniello Ingenito [1], Giancarla Sangianantoni [1] and Tiziana Cantile [1]

1 Department of Neurosciences, Reproductive Sciences and Oral Sciences, School of Paediatric Dentistry, University of Naples "Federico II", 80131 Naples, Italy; cristina.papa95@gmail.com (C.P.); ingenito@unina.it (A.I.); giancarla.sangia@yahoo.com (G.S.); tizianacantile@yahoo.it (T.C.)
2 Unesco Chair on Health Education and Sustainable Development, University of Naples, "Federico II", 80121 Naples, Italy
3 Department of Biology, University of Naples "Federico II", 80126 Naples, Italy; antonino.pollio@unina.it
* Correspondence: gianmariafabrizio@yahoo.it.

Abstract: In the scenario of promising sources of functional foods and preventive drugs, microalgae and cyanobacteria are attracting global attention. In this review, the current and future role of microalgae as natural sources of functional foods for human health and, in particular, for oral health has been reported and discussed in order to provide an overview on the state of art on microalgal effects on human oral health. It is well known that due to their richness in high-valuable products, microalgae offer good anti-inflammatory, antioxidant, antitumoral, anti-glycemic, cholesterol-lowering, and antimicrobial activity. Moreover, the findings of the present research show that microalgae could also have a significant impact on oral health: several studies agree on the potential application of microalgae for oral cancer prevention as well as for the treatment of chronic periodontitis and different oral diseases with microbial origin. Thus, beneficial effects of microalgae could be implemented in different medical fields. Microalgae and cyanobacteria could represent a potential natural alternative to antibiotic, antiviral, or antimycotic therapies, as well as a good supplement for the prevention and co-adjuvant treatment of different oral diseases. Nevertheless, more studies are required to identify strains of interest, increase overall functioning, and make safe, effective products available for the whole population.

Keywords: microalgae; *Spirulina platensis*; *Chlorella vulgaris*; oral health; antimicrobial activity; *Streptococcus mutans*

---

1. Introduction

Today, the majority of the bioactive peptides added in well-being promoting aliments, food supplements, pharmaceutic, and cosmetic formulations are realized by chemical production or by the partial digestion of proteins derived from animals. Therefore, they are not always well-regarded by the users due to the risks related to solvent contamination or the utilization of animal-derived ingredients. Alternatively, plant and microalgae-resulting peptides are recognized as selective, useful, nontoxic and well accepted when consumed, having a significant potentiality for utilization in functional aliments, drugs, and cosmetic products. Furthermore, due to the increasing issue of the antibiotic resistance against pathogenic bacteria, research has been targeted to exploring new antibacterial compounds derived from different natural environments [1–4]. Consequently, in recent years, growing scientific interest has been centered on the study of the bioactivity of extracts derived from plant species. In particular, the focus is on food plants included in the so-called traditional medicine [5–8]. For example, polyphenols derived from some edible plants drew attention as potential sources of agents that, among the wide range of health benefits, were shown to inhibit the bacterial growth of some oral pathogens [9,10]. A recent study on a large sample of vulnerary plants from Italian areas has identified a small number of extracts that could find application for the prevention of dental caries [11]: extracts of *Camelia sinensis* and *Plantago lanceolata*, rich in flavonoids, showed inhibitory activity against the species of cariogenic Streptococci [11,12].

Functional foods are arising as a dietary resource for preventing diseases. They can be defined as technologically developed ingredients explicating specific actions on human health. In the scenario of growing promising sources of functional foods and preventive drugs, cyanobacteria and microalgae are drawing global interest, due to their content of highly valuable substances [13,14].

Cyanobacteria and microalgae are respectively prokaryotic or eukaryotic microorganisms growing through oxygenic photosynthesis. Their energetic intake requires light, carbon dioxide, water, and nutrients with phosphorus and nitrogen as major nutrients, whereas the products of metabolic activity are primarily carbohydrates, along with a surprisingly high number of chemicals, some of which are known to be useful for humans [13].

Both cyanobacteria and microalgae are widely spread in freshwater and marine ecosystems as well as on terrestrial habitats and in a wide range of extreme environments, from hot springs to barren rocks of deserts. This flexibility makes them the major producers of biomass under sustainable conditions, since they do not deprive agriculture of sources, while allowing water recycling and lowering polluting gas emissions [15]. Moreover, cyanobacteria and microalgae bring the potential to be converted into a wide range of products of economic interest, such as biofuels, cosmetics, renewable chemicals and other valuable compounds [15], animal and human food, especially as sources of proteins, lipids, and phytochemicals (Figure 1) [16].

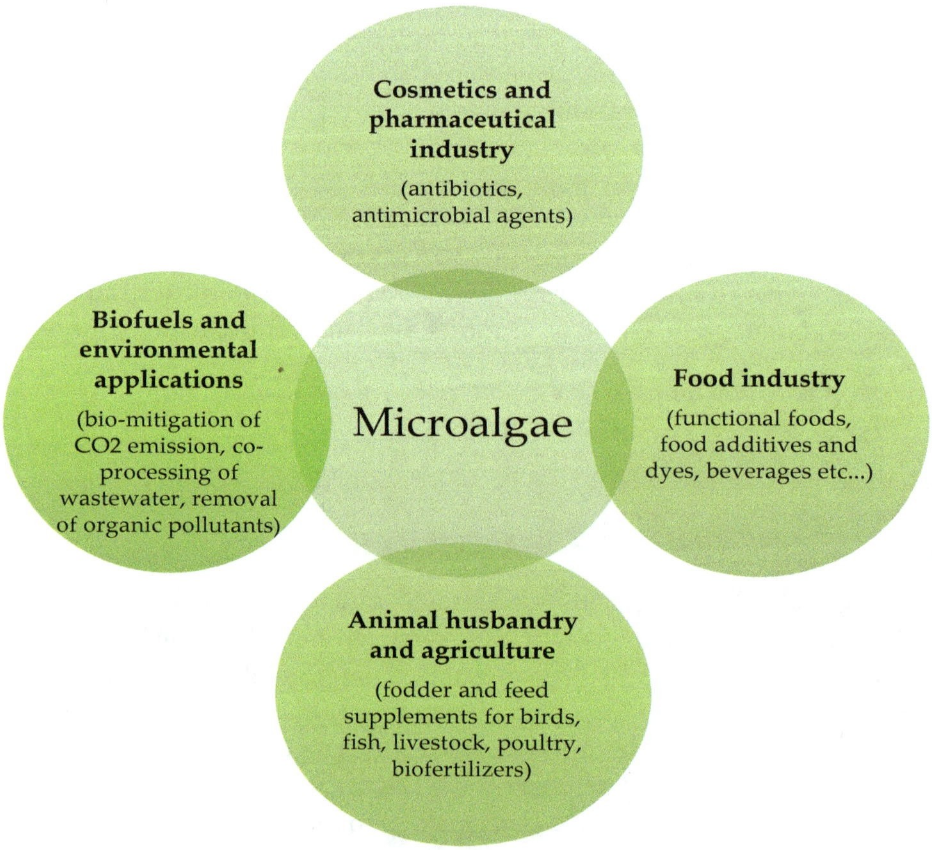

Figure 1. Application of microalgae in different fields.

In this review, the present and future role of cyanobacteria and microalgae as sources of drugs and food supplements useful for human well-being and, in particular, for oral health has been reported and discussed, focusing on the main classes of microalgal compounds with health implications. The aim is to offer a view on the state of art on the microalgal role and potential benefits to human well-being and, in particular, to oral health.

2. Health Beneficial Effects of Cyanobacteria and Microalgae Crude Extracts and Fractions

2.1. A Taxonomic Controversy: *Arthrospira* vs. *Spirulina*

Spirulina platensis and *Spirulina maxima* are the most frequently utilized names to designate the strains of filamentous cyanobacteria worldwide cultivated as food or to produce fine chemicals. However, both names are incorrect from a taxonomical point of view and have generated confusion on the identification of the most promising strains. The genera *Spirulina* and *Arthrospira* were erected respectively by Turpin in 1829 and Stitzenberger in 1852; this latter author proposed including in the new genus *Arthrospira* helical-shaped Oscillatoriaceae, which were previously included in *Spirulina*. Since then, the two genera have been reunited and separated several times, until in 1989, Castenholtz proposed distinguishing *Arthrospira* from *Spirulina* based on selected morphological features such as a degree of inclination of the trichome axis, the presence of cross walls in the filament, and the cell wall pore pattern. Molecular analysis confirmed the separation of the two genera and evidenced difficulties in the circumscription of the species generally accepted [17]. However, most of the strains worldwide cultivated belong to the genus *Arthrospira*, even though they are commonly sold as *Spirulina*. Unfortunately, also, many studies refer to *Arthrospira* strains as "*Spirulina*", engendering further confusion. To avoid misunderstandings, in this review, we have maintained the names adopted by the authors of each study independently of their taxonomical consistency.

With its high nutritional value, *Arthrospira*/*Spirulina* has been consumed as food for centuries in Central Africa [18]. Thanks to its high content of important proteins, amino acids, vitamins, carotenoids and other pigments, mineral substances, indispensable fatty acids, and polysaccharides, *S. plantensis* has found application as bioactive additive, and it is now widely used as a nutraceutical food supplement worldwide [19].

S. platensis causes an immunostimulating action, improving the resistance of humans, mammals, chickens, and fish to infections, thanks to the ability of affecting hemopoiesis, stimulating the production of antibodies and cytokines [20]. Under the effect of *S. platensis*, macrophages, T and B cells are activated. *S. platensis* sulfolipids have shown to be valid against HIV. Moreover, *S. platensis* biomass supplementations have appeared to be effective against herpes virus, cytomegalovirus, influenza virus, etc. *S. platensis* extracts are capable of impeding cancerogenesis [18] (Table 1).

S. platensis preparations are known as functional products playing a role in preserving the resident intestinal microflora, principally lactic acid bacilli and bifidobacteria, and in decreasing the level of *Candida albicans* [18]. In particular, in 2017, in vitro experiments assessed the impact of a fully characterized water extract of *S. platensis* against 22 varieties of *Candida* spp. The natural waves pattern of uterine myometrium and the major health-promoting bacteria of the vaginal flora were not affected by *S. platensis*, which was administered at the concentrations active against *Candida* [21].

S. platensis stimulates cellular antioxidant enzymes, reduces lipid peroxidation and DNA damage, scavenges free radicals, and increases the effect of superoxide dismutase and catalase. According to clinical studies conducted in 2016, *S. platensis* protects skeletal muscle from injury under exercise-generated oxidative stress and can induce the production of antibodies and up- or downregulate the expression of cytokine-encoding genes involved in the immunomodulatory and anti-inflammatory processes. Although the molecular mechanism(s) by which *S. platensis* makes these actions is still partially unknown, phycocyanin and β-carotene are likely to give a crucial contribution [22].

The Paracas strain of *S. platensis* is renowned as a potential source of precious skin-beneficial substances and recently, it has been applied in skincare products. Gunes et al. (2017) developed and analyzed skin creams enriched with bioactive *S. platensis Paracas* extract. Collagen 1 immunoreactivity was notably ameliorated along with the increase of extract concentration, as demonstrated by immunohistochemical analysis. The cell viability, wound curative action, and genotoxicity results indicated that *S. platensis* strain *Paracas*-enriched skin cream can bring highly valuable benefits in cosmeceutical and biomedical applications [23].

Eventually, it is worth mentioning the case study conducted by Kiziltan et al. in 2015, intending to evaluate the advantages of combining therapy with *S. platensis* and metronidazole with radiotherapy to ameliorate the treatment response of relapsed verrucous vulvar cancer. After the adjunction of conventional therapy with microalgae assumption, the tumor regressed, and there were no adverse effects involving the woman's dermatological or general health [24].

Table 1. Different actions of *S. platensis* on human health and related bibliographical references.

S. platensis's **Medicinal Properties**	**Ref.**
Highly nutrient	[19]
Immunostimulating	[20]
Antiviral	[18]
Antimicotic	[18]
Anti-cancer	[18,24]
Antioxidant	[22]
Skin-beneficial	[23]

2.2. Chlorella sp.: A Multifunctional Dietary Supplement with Diverse Medical Properties

Chlorella is a unicellular microalgae genus belonging to the class Treouxiophyceae (Chlorophyta) with biological and pharmacological potential important for human well-being. "*Chlorella* growth factor", the hot water extract of *Chlorella*, appeared to be active in the growth promotion and immunoregulation [25]. At the present moment, no systematic analysis has assessed the state of research of *Chlorella* sp. and its bioactivity. However, according to the growing scientific literature, *Chlorella* sp. not only has great importance in immunoregulation and cancer inhibition, but it is also effective in ameliorating metabolic syndrome, scavenging for free radicals, protecting from ultraviolet damage, chelating heavy metals, and preventing liver and bowel disease [25]. Nevertheless, not all scientific literature is consistent with these findings: for example, a randomized, double-blind, placebo-controlled trial in 2003 showed that *Chlorella*-derived dietary supplement did not exhibit any action in increasing the antibody response to influenza vaccine in the whole study population [26].

According to clinical studies conducted in 2016, integration with *Chlorella vulgaris* can ameliorate hyperlipidemia and hyperglycemia and protect from oxidative stress, cancer, and chronic obstructive pulmonary disease [27]. In 2013, Panahi et al. investigated the effect of supplementation with *C. vulgaris* on the burden of oxidative stress in Iranian smokers. After six weeks of supplementation, this integrator significantly enhanced the antioxidant status and reduced lipid peroxidation in chronic cigarette smokers. Therefore, *C. vulgaris* could impede the disease burden and mortality rate connected with smoking [28]. In another study carried out in 2015, the same author assessed the medicinal beneficial effect of an antioxidant-rich *C. vulgaris* ethanolic extract administered as a supplement of standard therapy in subjects with major depressive disorder (MDD), as oxidative stress has been reported to contribute significantly in the pathophysiology of MDD. This pilot study gives the first scientific evidence on the effectiveness and safety of supplementary therapy with *C. vulgaris* ethanolic extract in enhancing physical and cognitive symptoms of depression and anxiety in subjects undergoing standard antidepressant treatment [29].

In 2017, an interventional trial studied the consequences of *C. vulgaris* supplementation on glucose homeostasis, insulin resistance, and inflammatory biomarkers in subjects with non-alcoholic fatty liver disease [30]. This condition, representing a hepatic symptom of metabolic syndrome, is highly related to insulin resistance and inflammation. Weight decrease (mean values) was significantly higher in the *C. vulgaris*-treated group with respect to the placebo group. Serum concentrations of liver enzymes also significantly diminished, and serum insulin concentration significantly improved only in the group that had undergone *C. vulgaris* therapy. According to these findings, *C. vulgaris* supplementation could be considered as an adjunctive therapy to reduce weight and improve glycemic status as well as to ameliorate liver function in subjects with non-alcoholic fatty liver disease [30].

An in vitro study in 2016 compared the antibacterial activity of the methanolic extracts of five cyanobacteria and microalgal species, namely *Nostoc caeruleum*, *S. platensis*, *Cylindrospermum majus*, *Oscillatoria formosa*, and *C. vulgaris* against six bacteria (*Staphylococcus aureus*, *Staphylococcus epidermidis*, *Streptococcus pyogenes*, *Klebsiella pneumoniae*, *Pseudomonas aeruginosa*, and *Escherichia coli*) and four fungi strains (*Aspergillus fumigatus*, *C. albicans*, *Geotrichum candidum*, and *Trichophyton mentagrophytes*). The results suggested that the extract of *C. vulgaris* was the most effective agent against the tested bacteria and fungi strains, followed by *S. platensis* [31]. Other studies, conducted respectively in 1988 and 2015, agree that antibacterial and antimicotic effects are prevalent from *Chlorella* sp. [32,33]. Furthermore, according to chemical analyses, *C. vulgaris* showed the highest percentages of total phenolic and total flavonoid contents, which are identified as mainly responsible for antioxidant potential. *C. vulgaris* extract was also tested for its antitumor activity against specific cancer cell lines: the obtained data indicate that liver cancer cells HepG-2 were the most sensitive, followed by colon cancer cells HCT-116, and then breast cancer cells MCF-7 [25].

In 2017, Lin et al. studied for the first time the anti-cancer properties of *Chlorella sorokiniana* in two human non-small lung cancer cell lines (A549 and CL1–5 human lung adenocarcinoma cells), and its action on cancer growth in a subcutaneous xenograft tumor model. The results proved that exposure of the two cell lines to *C. sorokiniana* determined a concentration-dependent decrease in cell viability and a dose-dependent increase in the number of apoptotic cells. In addition, it was detected that the tumor growth of the subcutaneous xenograft in vivo was notably reduced after oral administration of *C. sorokiniana* [34].

These promising results suggest that *Chlorella* sp. extracts could represent a source of antitumor, anti-inflammatory, antioxidant, and antimicrobial bioactive compounds (Table 2). However, more studies are needed to investigate all the clinical effects of *Chlorella*-derived dietary supplements on human health.

Table 2. Different actions of *Chlorella* sp. on human health and related bibliographical references.

***Chlorella* sp. Medicinal Properties**	**Ref.**
Anti-cancer	[25,27,34]
Antioxidant	[27–29]
Anti-inflammatory	[30]
Antibacterial, antimicotic	[31–33]

3. Microalgal Effects on Oral Health

In the current scientific literature, there is still a lack of evidence about benefits derived from microalgal use in terms of treatment and the prevention of oral diseases. The collected studies mainly claim the potential role of *Spirulina* sp. in improving oral health.

3.1. Antiviral Activity

Herpes virus is a double-stranded DNA virus from the family of Herpesviridae. As its peculiarity, this virus does not leave the host after the first contact, settling in neural ganglion and causing a latent infection. This can take place in a variable time, depending on the type of virus and the host susceptibility. The causes that induce the reactivation of the viral activity can be temperature changes (hot/cold), traumas, fever, stress, and, above all, reduction of the host immunological response [35].

A study carried out in 2016 examined the antiviral activity of a defined *S. platensis* microalgal extract and of purified calcium spirulan (Ca-SP), which is a sulfated polysaccharide contained therein. Ca-SP inhibited HSV-1 infection in vitro with an effectiveness similar to that of acyclovir by blocking viral attachment and penetration into host cells. Ca-SP also impeded the entry of Kaposi sarcoma-associated herpesvirus/human herpes virus 8. Actually, in the experimental model of herpes exacerbation, the prophylactic activity of a cream containing Ca-SP and microalgae extract was greater than that of acyclovir cream. These results highlight a possible clinical use of Ca-SP containing *Spirulina* sp. extract for the prophylactic management of *herpes labialis* and indicate promising effects of Ca-SP against infections caused by other herpes viruses [36].

3.2. Oral Cancer Chemoprevention

Another interesting application for *Spirulina* sp. and, in particular, for the blue-green microalga *S. platensis* might be in oral cancer chemoprevention. Oral cancer represents 3% of all human carcinomas. Squamous cell carcinoma accounts for over 90% of the oral cancers, and others include adenocarcinoma derived from minor salivary gland, sarcoma, malignant lymphoma, and metastatic cancer. It shows a survival rate at 5 years of 51%, which is mainly due to late diagnosis in a clinical advanced stage. It is localized most frequently on the tongue, on the floor of the mouth, and on the cheek mucous, and it is mainly related to alcohol, smoking, and Human Papilloma Virus (HPV) infection [37]. Especially, smoke-related cancer is often preceded by some typical preneoplastic lesions, such as oral leucoplakia, erytroplakia, lichen planus, or persistent ulcers. Today, conventional therapy of potential pre-neoplastic conditions is mostly limited to mouth washes with antibacterial and antimycotic products in order to remove any superinfections, along with the elimination of risk factors, patient follow-up, and eventually, biopsy. On the other hand, the first choice for oral cancer treatment is still the surgical approach, causing inevitable esthetic and functional impairments [38]. Hence, there is a huge need to develop specific and less invasive strategies for oral cancer prevention and therapy.

Mathew et al. in 1995 evaluated the chemopreventive activity of *Spirulina fusiformis* (1 g/day for 12 months) in reversing oral leukoplakia in pan tobacco chewers in Kerala, India. Complete regression of lesions was documented in 20 of 44 (45%) evaluable patients supplemented with *S. fusiformis*, as opposed to three of 43 (7%) in the placebo arm. When stratified by type of leukoplakia, the response was more significant in homogeneous lesions: complete regression was observed in 16 of 28 (57%) patients with homogeneous leukoplakia, two of eight with erythroplakia, two of four with verrucous leukoplakia, and zero of four with ulcerated and nodular lesions. During one year of discontinuing supplements, nine of 20 (45%) complete responders with *S. fusiformis* developed recurrent lesions. Supplementation with *S. fusiformis* did not provoke any adverse effect [39]. This was the first human study assessing the chemopreventive potential of *S. fusiformis*.

Another study conducted in 2015 estimated if astaxanthin could be applied to ameliorate the symptoms of oral lichen planus by decreasing inflammation. Following astaxanthin treatment, the level of inflammatory cytokines (interleukin-6, tumor necrosis factor-α) tended to decrease, and cell proliferation significantly increased in human gingival keratinocytes in vitro. These results indicate that astaxanthin could be beneficial for improving chronic inflammation such as that associated with oral lichen planus [40].

Several experimental studies in animal models have demonstrated an inhibitory effect of *S. platensis* microalgae on oral carcinogenesis process. Some studies conducted on rats sustain that astaxanthin has significant preventive activities on 4-nitroquinoline-1-oxide (4-NQO)-induced tongue carcinogenesis [41]. In particular, after 8 weeks of treatment, the incidence of oral preneoplastic lesions and cell proliferation activity decreased significantly, and no oral neoplasms developed in rats fed with astaxanthin [42]. Grawish and his team carried out two experimental studies on hamsters (2008 and 2010) both aiming to investigate oral chemopreventive strategies using astaxanthin. In the first work, 30 male golden Syrian hamsters were divided into three groups: the first group had the right buccal pouch painted with 0.5% solution of 7,12-dimethylbenz[a]anthracene (DMBA), to the second group, 10 mg/daily *S. platensis* extract was administered, in addition to the same painting, and the last was a control group, not having painting nor *S. platensis* treatment. They observed moderate dysplastic changes extending into the midspinous layer in group one 7 weeks after DMBA painting, which reached half the thickness of the hyperplastic epithelium after 14 weeks. However, in group two, mild dysplastic changes were observed after 7 weeks, which were restricted to the basilar and parabasilar layers of the epithelium after 14 weeks of treatment. An overall significant difference among the three groups ($p < 0.01$) was indicated with one-way analysis of variance [43]. The second study from the same author confirmed these results. In particular, it focused on the proliferating cell nuclear antigen expression, showing that it was directly related to the severity of pathological alterations from normal epithelium to dysplasia and from dysplasia to squamous cell carcinoma in the study groups at the different extended periods of DMBA application and *S. platensis* extract administration [44].

S. platensis extracts, especially astaxanthin carotenoid, might have a big potential not only on precancerous lesions, but even on proper oral cancer. As in 1988, it was already proven that an extract of *S. platensis–Dunaliella* could inhibit tumor development in hamster buccal pouch [45], more recent data provided extensive evidence that dietary astaxanthin avoids the development and progression of hamster buccal pouch carcinomas through the inhibition of JAK-2/STAT-3 signaling and its downstream events [46].

Many scientists investigated the mechanisms behind *S. platensis* potent anti-cancer activity. Their results are summarized as follows.

In 2019, Sannasimuthu et al. identified an RNA sequence encoding the glutathione oxido-reductase (GR) enzyme from *S. platensis*, and the modifications in its gene expression profile were investigated throughout H_2O_2 stress. GR is a primary antioxidant enzyme of many organisms that prevents cellular oxidative stress by reducing glutathione from its oxidized form. Overall, the study demonstrates that the GM15 peptide (a short antioxidant peptide from *S. platensis* glutathione oxido-reductase) scavenges superoxide, hydroxyl radicals, reduces intracellular oxidative stress, and has antitumor activity in oral cancer cells [47]. According to Kavitha et al. (2013), astaxanthin exerts chemopreventive effects by concurrently inhibiting the phosphorylation of transcription factors and signaling kinases, and inducing intrinsic apoptosis. In fact, they found that the microalgal carotenoid inhibits NF-κB (nuclear factor kappa-light-chain-enhancer of activated B cells) and Wnt (wingless/integrated) signaling by downregulating the key regulatory enzymes IKKβ and GSK-3β [48]. Eventually, in a recent investigation, Kowshik et al. (2019) reported that astaxanthin prevents cancer hallmarks by inhibiting PI3K/Akt and the associated downstream NF-κB and STAT-3 signaling pathways in SCC131 and SCC4 oral cancer cells as well as in the hamster buccal pouch carcinogenesis model. Additionally, astaxanthin downregulated the noncoding RNAs (ncRNAs), miR-21 and HOTAIR, which influence PI3K/Akt signaling, emphasizing their modulatory effects on epigenetic regulation [49].

Taking into account all these promising results, it can be concluded that *S. platensis* and, particularly, its most potent pigment, astaxanthin, plays a beneficial role in oral cancer regression and prevention, representing a potential valuable candidate for anti-cancer drug development.

3.3. Oral Antimicrobial Activity

Another property of cyanobacteria and microalgae that appears to be worthy of note for oral health implications is their antimicrobial activity. Among oral bacteria, *Streptococcus mutans* is a Gram-positive bacteria that is frequently found in the oral cavity's normal flora and involved in the pathogenesis of caries [50,51]. Caries is the most common infective pathology worldwide, affecting especially that part of the population with a lower socio-economic status. It has a multifactorial pathogenesis, including diet and host susceptibility as co-factors together with the over-growing of *S. mutans*. *S. aureus* is also an abundant Gram-positive bacterium that has a strong connection with dental implant infections [52]. *Enterococcus faecalis* has been connected to oral infections, such as caries, endodontic infections, periodontitis, and peri-implantitis [53].

Fatty acid methyl esters (FAME) derived from lipids of microalgae are recognized as a suitable super-curator and superior anti-pathogenic. Experiments in 2018 assessed the effectiveness of FAME extracted from the microalga *Scenedesmus intermedius* as an antimicrobial agent against Gram-positive bacteria (*S. aureus*, *S. mutans*, and *Bacillus cereus*), Gram-negative bacteria (*E. coli* and *P. aeruginosa*), and fungi (*Aspergillus parasiticus* and *C. albicans*). FAME here analyzed displayed a solid antimicrobial effect at a lower MIC than those of recent reports. This result claimed that the FAME of *S. intermedius* has a potent antimicrobial and antioxidant activity and that it could find application as a powerful source against microbial diseases [54].

Microalgal extracts screened for their antimicrobial activities could be more effective than antibiotics and fungicides. An in vitro study in 2011 demonstrated the antimicrobial properties of *Chaetoceros calcitrans*, *Skeletonema costatum*, *Chroococcus turgidus*, and *Nannochloropsis oceanica*. Extracts exhibited inhibitory effects against *S. aureus*, *S. pyogenes*, and *Bacillus subtilis*. Antifungal activity was identified only in *S. costatum* and *C. turgidus*, but *Aspergillus flavus* and *A. niger* showed resistance to all the four microalgae. The highest in vitro inhibition zone was observed in acetone extract of *Chlorococcum* sp. against *S. aureus* and *E. coli* compared to other dried green microalgae extracts [55].

Another in vitro study in 2011 collected 46 species of freshwater cyanobacteria and selected five strains based on their growth characteristics, namely *Oscillatoria latevirens*, *Phormidium corium*, *Lyngbya martensiana*, *Chrococcus minor*, and *Microcystis aeruginosa*. The results clearly indicated that the acetone extracts of *O. latevirens* and ethanol extracts of *P. corium* gave the highest antimicrobial activity against *S. aureus*, *S. mutans*, and *Micrococcus mutans* and *S. aureus*, respectively. At the same time, the extract of *L. martensiana* had an antibacterial effect toward *B. subtilis*, *S. aureus*, and *E. coli* but negative effect toward *S. mutans*, *M. mutans*, and *K. pneumoniae*. In addition, *O. latevirens*, *C. minor*, and *M. aeruginosa* were shown to have antifungal activity on *C. albicans*. It was found that the effect of standard antibiotics was more than that of algal extracts on *B. subtilis* and *E. coli*. Meanwhile, the antibacterial potential of algal extracts on *S. aureus*, *S. mutans*, and *M. mutans* were even higher than those of standard antibiotics. The antimicrobial activity of these microalgae could be explained by presence of cyclic peptides, alkaloids, and lipopolysaccharides [56].

An investigation carried out in 2016 used *S. platensis* extract as a biomaterial for the biosynthesis of silver nanoparticles. Nanoparticles have unique biological and optical properties, which make them considered as efficient materials of the next technology generation with therapeutic and diagnostic applications. Metal nanoparticles are highly employed in a broad number of biomedical applications, especially as antimicrobials [57]. Silver ions and silver-based compounds are known bactericides, due to their large surface area that comes into contact with the microbial cells [58,59]. The application of nanoparticles in dentistry is of interest, as the oral cavity frequently comes across a superfluity of microorganisms. The results of the study suggest that the silver nanoparticles biosynthesized using *S. platensis* extract have good antibacterial activity against the three Gram-positive oral pathogens *S. mutans*, *E. faecalis*, and *S. aureus* [60].

3.4. Potential Effects in the Treatment of Periodontitis

Oral periodontitis is an inflammatory pathology affecting the supporting gum and bone tissues of the tooth. It is characterized by a cyclical evolution, alternating phases of quiescence with acute phases, which determines an irreversible loss of the clinical epithelium-connective attachment around the tooth and, as a consequence, progressive bone resorption [61]. Today, chronic periodontitis mostly requires three conventional treatment modalities: non-surgical techniques as scaling and root plaining, surgical conservative approaches for more compromised teeth and, ultimately, the extraction of hopeless teeth [62].

Several studies claim the potential clinical effectiveness of *S. platensis* for the treatment of oral periodontitis, which is probably due to its anti-inflammatory and antioxidant effects. Mahendra et al. in 2013 demonstrated that locally delivered *S. platensis* gel, along with scaling and root plaining, caused a beneficial impact in the treatment of chronic periodontitis. The efficacy of the product as a local drug delivery system in the non-surgical management of periodontitis without any side effects has been tested [63]. According to these findings, a recent pre-clinical study evaluated the effects of astaxanthin on alveolar bone loss and histopathological changes in ligature-induced periodontitis in rats. It can be suggested that astaxanthin administration may reduce alveolar bone loss by enhancing osteoblastic activity and decreasing osteoclastic action in an experimental periodontitis model [64]. The suppression effect of astaxanthin on bone loss is confirmed by Hwang et al. (2018), who studied the anti-osteoporotic effect of astaxanthin on bone mass in ovariectomized mice and its possible mechanism of action. The administration of astaxanthin (5, 10 mg/kg) for six weeks suppressed the enhancement of serum calcium, inorganic phosphorus, alkaline phosphatase, total cholesterol, and tartrate-resistant acid phosphatase activity. The bone mineral density and bone microarchitecture were improved by astaxanthin exposure [65].

Furthermore, in 2016, a study evaluated the effects of another microalgal carotenoid, fucoxanthin, on alveolar bone resorption in rats with periodontitis. Systemic fucoxanthin treatment resulted in a small reduction in tumor necrosis factor-α, interleukin-1β, and interleukin-6 levels and a significant reduction in oxidative stress index. It was noted that fucoxanthin induced a significant decrease in receptor activator of nuclear factor kappa-β ligand (RANKL) levels and a statistically non-significant elevation in osteoprotegerin and bone–alkaline phosphatase levels. There were no significant differences in alveolar bone loss levels between the case and control groups. Hence, according to this experimental study, fucoxanthin determines a limited decrease in alveolar bone resorption in rats with periodontitis [66].

Eventually, a recent work in 2018 analyzed the effects of a cyanobacterial component on the inflammation process induced by *Phorphyromonas gingivalis*, which is a Gram-negative bacterium co-responsible for oral periodontitis. Lipopolysaccharide (LPS) from *P. gingivalis* (Pg-LPS) is a key bacterial structure involved in the maintenance of a chronic pro-inflammatory environment during periodontitis. Similar to other Gram-negative LPS, Pg-LPS induces the release of pro-inflammatory cytokines through interaction with Toll-Like Receptor 4 (TLR4) and is able to stimulate negative TLR4 regulatory pathways, such as those involving microRNA (miRNA). In this work, the authors employed CyP, an LPS with TLR4-MD2 antagonist activity obtained from the cyanobacterium *Oscillatoria planktothrix* FP1, to study the effects on pro-inflammatory cytokine production and miRNA expression in human monocytic THP-1 cells stimulated with Pg-LPS. The results showed that CyP inhibited TNF-α, IL-1β, and IL-8 expression [67]. These outcomes could open new perspectives for innovative therapeutic approaches based on microalgal and cyanobacterial extracts for the treatment of oral periodontitis.

3.5. Control of Oral Submucous Fibrosis

A new horizon in *S. platensis* use can be in the management of an insidious and disabling disease affecting oral mucosa, such as Oral Submucous Fibrosis (OSMF). OSMF is a chronic progressive pathology that alters the flexibility of oral mucosa, ending in lockjaw and a higher risk of developing squamous oral cancer. It is a common condition in India and southeastern Asia, while it is infrequent in other parts of the world [68]. The results of trials of many treatment options, such as medical, physical, or surgical interventions, have suggested that combined therapies give better outcomes. A study conducted in 2019 intended to assess the effectiveness of *S. platensis* together with different physiotherapeutic approaches in the treatment of OSMF. After administration of *S. platensis* 500 mg twice a day for 3 months, all subjects have reported statistically significant amelioration in burning perception, mouth opening, tongue protrusion, and cheek flexibility. Moreover, *S. platensis* did not cause any considerable adverse effect [69]. Another experimental work carried out in 2013 evaluated the efficacy of the same *S. platensis* treatment in addition to corticosteroid injections in the treatment of oral submucous fibrosis symptoms. After 3 months of therapy, highly significant clinical improvements in mouth opening and reduction in burning perception were recorded in favor of the *S. platensis* group [70]. The reported effects indicate that *S. platensis* could be applied as an adjuvant therapy in the treatment of initial symptoms in subjects with OSF. Nevertheless, studies involving larger samples and longer follow-up are recommended in the future [71].

3.6. Salivary Secretion Improving

Salivary secretion is fundamental for the oral well-being, considering that hyposalivation compromises food chewing and swallowing, reduces mucosal immune function, increases the risk for oral diseases such as dental caries and candidiasis, and causes dysphagia, dysgeusia, and prosthetical inadaptation. Oral dryness is normally associated to aging or menopause, but it can also be caused by some pharmacological therapies, radio- and chemotherapy, or Sjogren's syndrome. In any case, oxidative stress clearly plays a role in decreasing saliva secretion. Then, treatment with antioxidant agents, such as astaxanthin, may be beneficial [72].

Kuraji et al. (2015) estimated the effects of astaxanthin on the saliva secretory function of aging mice. The saliva flow increased in the case group 72 weeks after treatment, while that of the control decreased by half. Moreover, the submandibular glands of astaxanthin-treated mice had fewer inflammatory cells than the control did [72]. These results were corroborated by the work carried out by Yamada et al. (2010), which was structured in three parts. First, they evaluated the reactive oxygen species (ROS) scavenging capacity of astaxanthin on a human salivary gland epithelial cell line and obtained that the carotenoid partially suppressed hydrogen peroxide-induced ROS in salivary gland cells. Secondly, they examined the effects of astaxanthin on salivary secretion in a mouse model of irradiation-induced salivary gland dysfunction, resulting in the inhibition of oral dryness. Lastly, they tested astaxanthin treatment in six patients affected by Sjogren's syndrome compared to a control group: an increase in salivary flow was detected in both groups of patients, and the level of oxidative stress marker, hexanoyil-lysine, in the saliva was decreased after astaxanthin administration [73].

According to Otsuki et al. (2016), *Chlorella* sp.-derived multicomponent supplementation, as well, is able to increase saliva production in subjects with lower levels of saliva secretion [74].

These results suggest that therapy with extracts derived from *Spirulina* sp. or *Chlorella* sp. has a good potential for the prevention and treatment of different clinical conditions of hyposalivation.

3.7. More Oral Benefits from Chlorella sp. and Other Algal Extracts

The long-term microalgal extract supplementation can bring several unexpected benefits to oral health.

C. vulgaris extract in conjunction with aminosulphurate (nutraceuticals) supplementation has determined a detoxification from heavy metals in subjects with long-term titanium dental implants and/or amalgam fillings compared to baseline levels and untreated controls. It is known how the accumulation of heavy metals represents a serious risk for human health. In particular, mercury toxicity can end in kidney dysfunction and neurologic anomalies. The administration of microalgae and nutraceutical supplements for 90 consecutive days reduced Hg^{2+}, Ag, Sn, and Pb with respect to baseline levels and did not have any side effects [75].

Finally, another interesting application for microalgal-derived components might be as drug carriers for bisphosphonates. Bisphosphonates are a class of drugs widely used in the clinical treatment of disorders of bone metabolism, such as osteoporosis, fibrous dysplasia, myeloma, and bone metastases. As a result of the negative side effects caused by the oral administration of bisphosphonates, various silica mesoporous materials have been investigated for a confined and controlled release of these drugs. Following a novel strategy, sodium alendronate can be in vivo incorporated into biosilica shells of the diatom *Thalassiosira weissflogii* by feeding the algae with an aqueous solution of the drug. According to a recent study conducted in 2019, the loading percentage of sodium alendronate into biosilica was able to decrease the metabolic activity of J774 osteoclasts-like cells until 5% over glass control. Osteoclasts inhibition of the functionalized biosilica opens the way to interesting applications for diatom microalgae as a bioinspired mesoporous material for tissue engineering [76].

A summary of the main sources of bioactive compounds reviewed in the current study, bringing benefits for oral health, is provided in the following table (Table 3).

Table 3. Effects of cyanobacteria and microalgae on oral health: outcomes of the examined in vitro/in vivo studies, potential therapeutic applications, and related bibliographic references.

Species/Source	Type of Study	Results	Potential Application	Ref.
S. platensis extract containing Calcium spirulan (Ca-SP)	In vitro	Inhibition of HSV-1, Kaposi sarcoma-associated herpes virus, and human herpes virus 8.	Prophylactic treatment of herpes viruses infections.	[36]
S. fusiformis	In vivo	Complete regression of precancerous lesions in 45% of subjects.	Chemopreventive therapy for tobacco-induced oral leucoplakia.	[39]
Astaxanthin	In vitro	Decrease of IL-6 and TNF-α and increase of cell proliferation in oral lichen planus.	Anti-inflammatory treatment for oral lichen planus.	[40]
Astaxanthin	In vivo	Decrease of the incidence of oral pre-neoplastic lesions and cell proliferation activity in rats after 8 weeks of treatment.	Prevention of 4-NQO-induced tongue carcinogenesis.	[41,42]
S. platensis	In vivo	Decrease of dysplastic changes on hamsters' buccal pouch after 14 weeks of treatment.	Oral cancer preventive therapy.	[43,44]
Spirulina-Dunaliella extract containing astaxanthin	In vivo	Inhibition of JAK-2/STAT-3 downstream events in hamster buccal pouch tumor progression.	Oral cancer therapy.	[45,46]
GM15 peptide from *Spirulina Arthrospira platensis*	In vitro	Scavenge of superoxide and hydroxyl radicals and reduction of intracellular oxidative stress.	Antioxidant treatment for oral cancer.	[47]
FAME extracted from *S. intermedius*	In vitro	Inhibition of *S. aureus, S. mutans, B. cereus, E. coli, P. aeruginosa, A. parasiticus,* and *C. albicans.*	Antimicrobial therapy against Gram-positive bacteria, Gram-negative bacteria, and fungi.	[54]
C. calcitrans, S. costatum, C. turgidus, and *N. oceanica*	In vitro	Inhibition of *S. aureus, S. pyogenes, B. subtilis, S. costatum,* and *C. turgidus* showed also antimycotic action.	Antibiotics and fungicides.	[55]
Acetone extracts of *O. latevirens*	In vitro	Inhibition *of S. aureus, S. mutans,* and *C. albicans.*	Antibiotic and fungicide.	[56]
Ethanol extracts of *Phormidium corium*	In vitro	Inhibition of *M. mutans* and *S. aureus.*	Antibiotic.	[56]
Extract of *L. martensiana*	In vitro	Inhibition of *B. subtilis, S. aureus, E. coli.*	Antibiotic.	[56]
Extract of *C. minor* and *M. aeruginosa*	In vitro	Inhibition of *C. albicans.*	Fungicides.	[56]
Silver nanoparticles biosynthesized from *S. platensis* extract	In vitro	Inhibition of *S. mutans, E. faecalis,* and *S. aureus.*	Antibiotic.	[60]
Locally derived *S. platensis* gel	In vivo	Beneficials in the treatment of chronic periodontitis.	Co-adjuvant in the non-surgical treatment of periodontitis.	[63]
Systemic astaxanthin administration	In vivo	Reduction of alveolar bone loss in ligature-induced periodontitis in rats.	Treatment of periodontitis.	[64]

Table 3. *Cont.*

Species/Source	Type of Study	Results	Potential Application	Ref.
Cyp, an *Oscillatoria planktothrix FP1*-derived lipopolysaccharide	In vitro	Inhibition of TNF-α, IL-1β, and IL-8 expression.	Treatment of periodontitis.	[67]
Systemic *S. platensis* administration	In vivo	Significant improvement in oral submucous fibrosis symptoms after 3 months of therapy.	Adjuvant therapy in the management of oral submucous fibrosis.	[69]
Systemic *S. platensis* administration in addition to corticosteroid injections	In vivo	Highly significant clinical improvements in oral submucous fibrosis after 3 months of therapy.	Adjuvant therapy in the management of oral submucous fibrosis.	[70]
Astaxanthin	In vivo	Increase of saliva flow after 72 weeks of treatment.	Hyposalivation treatment.	[72]
Astaxanthin	In vitro and in vivo	Increase of saliva flow and decrease of oxidative stress markers.	Hyposalivation treatment.	[73]
Chlorella-derived multicomponent supplementation	In vivo	Increase of saliva flow in subjects with lower levels of saliva secretion.	Hyposalivation treatment.	[74]
C. vulgaris extract in conjunction with amminosulphurate supplementation	In vivo	Reduction of Hg++, Ag, Sn, and Pb in subjects with long-term titanium dental implants and/or amalgam fillings.	Heavy metal detoxyfing agents.	[75]
Sodium alendronate incorporated into biosilica shells of cultured *Thalassiosira weissflogii* diatoms	In vitro	Decrease of metabolic activity of J774 osteoclast-like cells.	Drug-carrier for bifosphonates.	[76]

4. Conclusions

Cyanobacteria and microalgae are attracting global attention as promising sources of functional foods and preventive drugs, because of their richness in high-valuable products, comprising carotenoids, proteins, vitamins, essential amino acids, and omega-rich oils. They represent an almost untapped resource of natural anti-inflammatory and antioxidant compounds due to their enormous biodiversity, and a growing number of experiments suggests that the positive effects of microalgae on human well-being could be extended to the prevention or delay of cancer and cardiovascular diseases, as well as the management of diabetes, hypercholesterolemia, and inflammatory chronic diseases. Shifting the focus to oral health, several studies agree on the potential application of microalgae in the field of oral cancer prevention, in the treatment of a disabling condition as Oral Submucosal Fibrosis, and the management of chronic periodontitis complications. Moreover, due to their antiviral, antibacterial, and antifungal properties, microalgae could have a significant impact on oral health, acting as protective agents against *H. labialis*, *S. mutans*, and *C. albicans*.

Probably, one of the major constraints to a larger use of algal extracts and products is due to the erratic use of botanic nomenclature to designate the strains considered promising for biotechnological applications. Taking into account the two most studied and commercialized phototrophic microorganisms, *Arthrospira*/*Spirulina platensis* and *Chlorella*, a nomenclatural reassessment of the most frequently used strains is required, in light of the profound taxonomic changes that both genera have undergone in the last decade. This is the first important step needed in order to identify new strains of clinical interest, increase overall functioning, and make safe, effective products available for the whole population.

Cyanobacteria and microalgae cultivation can allow a high rate of biomass production, also achieving the synthesis of fine chemicals, as protein, carbohydrates, lipids, and pigments, that are used as components of human and animal feeds, biofuels, pharmaceuticals, and nutraceuticals. Moreover, phototrophic microorganisms can be grown on soils not suitable for agriculture, also using wastewater as a source of water. However, these promising economical perspectives are hindered by several difficulties; in particular, the need for large-scale facilities requires relevant investments that are not balanced by adequate revenues. At the moment, cyanobacteria and microalgae can be successfully grown in different kinds of bioreactors, but only open ponds are economically convenient. Therefore, in temperate zones, phototrophic microorganisms must face severe climatic conditions related to fall and winter seasons, with a consequent dramatic drop of production. There is an urgent necessity of identifying strains that are able to endure these constraints, ensuring adequate growth rates.

The possibility of using cyanobacteria and microalgae in the health market is appealing, but more stringent data are necessary to expand this possibility. The bottleneck is the scaling up of cultivation from laboratory-controlled conditions to the industrial production: the ability of strains to resist predation pressures and to co-grow with other microorganisms, such as bacteria, is a key aspect. In addition, the presence of both predators and commensal prokaryotes can induce relevant physiologic changes, leading to a decrease of fine chemical production and/or a shift toward the synthesis of unwanted metabolites. Experiments designed to overwhelm these constraints should focus on innovative biotechnology approaches, based on the activation or deactivation of specific genes to attain higher biomass production and synthesis of bioactive compounds [77].

Author Contributions: Conceptualization, G.F.F.; methodology, T.C.; software, G.S.; validation, A.I.; formal analysis, T.C.; investigation, A.P.; resources, C.P.; data curation, G.S.; writing—original draft preparation, C.P.; writing—review and editing, A.P.; visualization, G.F.F.; supervision, A.I.; project administration, G.F.F. All authors have read and agreed to the published version of the manuscript.

Acknowledgments: www.unescochairnapoli.it for any other detail on chair objectives, programs and staff organization.

References

1. Mundt, S.; Kreitlow, S.; Nowotny, A.; Effmert, U. Biochemical and pharmacological investigations of selected cyanobacteria. *Int. J. Hyg. Environ. Health* **2001**, *203*, 327–334. [CrossRef] [PubMed]
2. Safonova, E.; Kvitko, K.; Kuschk, P.; Möder, M.; Reisser, W. Biodegradation of Phenanthrene by the Green Alga Scenedesmus obliquus ES-55. *Eng. Life Sci.* **2005**, *5*, 234–239. [CrossRef]
3. Ghasemi, Y.; Mohagheghzadeh, A.; Mohammad, H.M.; Moradian, A.; Shadman, S. Antifungal and Antibacterial Activity of the Microalgae Collected from Paddy Fields of Iran: Characterization of Antimicrobial Activity of Chroococcus disperses. *J. Biol. Sci.* **2007**, *7*, 904–910.
4. Prakash, O.; Hussain, K.; Aneja, K.R.; Sharma, C. Synthesis and Antimicrobial Activity of Some New 2-(3-(4-Aryl)-1-phenyl-1H-pyrazol-4-yl) Chroman-4-ones. *Indian J. Pharm. Sci.* **2011**, *73*, 586–590. [CrossRef] [PubMed]
5. De Natale, A.; Pollio, A. Plants species in the folk medicine of Montecorvino Rovella (inland Campania, Italy). *J. Ethnopharmacol.* **2007**, *109*, 295–303. [CrossRef]
6. Perrin, S.; Fougnies, C.; Grill, J.P.; Jacobs, H.; Schneider, F. Fermentation of chicory fructo-oligosaccharides in mixtures of different degrees of polymerization by three strains of bifidobacteria. *Can. J. Microbiol.* **2002**, *48*, 759–763. [CrossRef]
7. Lee, M.H.; Kwon, H.A.; Kwon, D.Y.; Park, H.; Sohn, D.H.; Kim, Y.C.; Eo, S.K.; Kang, H.Y.; Kim, S.W.; Lee, J.H. Antibacterial activity of medicinal herb extracts against Salmonella. *Int. J. Food Microbiol.* **2006**, *111*, 270–275. [CrossRef] [PubMed]
8. Mazzanti, G. Pharmacological considerations on herbal medicine use. *Ann. Ist. Super. Sanita* **2005**, *41*, 23–26.
9. Taguri, T.; Tanaka, T.; Kouno, I. Antimicrobial activity of 10 different plant polyphenols against bacteria causing food-borne disease. *Biol. Pharm. Bull.* **2004**, *27*, 1965–1969. [CrossRef]

10. Ferrazzano, G.F.; Cantile, T.; Roberto, L.; Ingenito, A.; Catania, M.R.; Roscetto, E.; Palumbo, G.; Zarrelli, A.; Pollio, A. Determination of the in vitro and in vivo antimicrobial activity on salivary Streptococci and Lactobacilli and chemical characterisation of the phenolic content of a Plantago lanceolata infusion. *Biomed. Res. Int.* **2015**, *2015*, 286817. [CrossRef]
11. Ferrazzano, G.F.; Roberto, L.; Catania, M.R.; Chiaviello, A.; De Natale, A.; Roscetto, E.; Pinto, G.; Pollio, A.; Ingenito, A.; Palumbo, G. Screening and Scoring of Antimicrobial and Biological Activities of Italian Vulnerary Plants against Major Oral Pathogenic Bacteria. *Evid. Based Complement. Altern. Med.* **2013**, 316280. [CrossRef] [PubMed]
12. Ferrazzano, G.F.; Amato, I.; Ingenito, A.; Zarrelli, A.; Pinto, G.; Pollio, A. Plant polyphenols and their anti-cariogenic properties: A review. *Molecules* **2011**, *16*, 1486–1507. [CrossRef]
13. Galasso, C.; Gentile, A.; Orefice, I.; Ianora, A.; Bruno, A.; Noonan, D.M.; Sansone, C.; Albini, A.; Brunet, C. Microalgal Derivatives as Potential Nutraceutical and Food Supplements for Human Health: A Focus on Cancer Prevention and Interception. *Nutrients* **2019**, *11*, 1226. [CrossRef]
14. Apone, F.; Barbulova, A.; Colucci, M.G. Plant and Microalgae Derived Peptides Are Advantageously Employed as Bioactive Compounds in Cosmetics. *Front. Plant Sci.* **2019**, *10*, 756. [CrossRef] [PubMed]
15. Camacho, F.; Macedo, A.; Malcata, F. Potential Industrial Applications and Commercialization of Microalgae in the Functional Food and Feed Industries: A Short Review. *Mar. Drugs* **2019**, *17*, 312. [CrossRef]
16. Langi, P.; Kiokias, S.; Varzakas, T.; Proestos, C. Carotenoids: From Plants to Food and Feed Industries. *Methods Mol. Biol.* **2018**, *1852*, 57–71.
17. Papapanagiotou, G.; Gkelis, S. Taxonomic revision of commercially used Arthrospira (Cyanobacteria) strains: A polyphasic approach. *Eur. J. Phycol.* **2019**, *54*, 595–608. [CrossRef]
18. Blinkova, L.P.; Gorobets, O.B.; Baturo, A.P. Biological activity of Spirulina. *Zh Mikrobiol. Epidemiol. Immunobiol.* **2001**, *2*, 114–118.
19. Deng, R.; Chow, T.J. Hypolipidemic, antioxidant, and antiinflammatory activities of microalgae Spirulina. *Cardiovasc. Ther.* **2010**, *28*, 33–45. [CrossRef] [PubMed]
20. Finamore, A.; Palmery, M.; Bensehaila, S.; Peluso, I. Antioxidant, Immunomodulating, and Microbial-Modulating Activities of the Sustainable and Ecofriendly Spirulina. *Oxid. Med. Cell. Longev.* **2017**, *2017*. [CrossRef]
21. Marangoni, A.; Foschi, C.; Micucci, M.; Nahui Palomino, R.A.; Gallina Toschi, T.; Vitali, B.; Camarda, L.; Mandrioli, M.; De Giorgio, M.; Aldini, R.; et al. In vitro activity of Spirulina platensis water extract against different Candida species isolated from vulvo-vaginal candidiasis cases. *PLoS ONE* **2017**, *12*, 11. [CrossRef]
22. Wu, Q.; Liu, L.; Miron, A.; Klímová, B.; Wan, D.; Kuča, K. The antioxidant, immunomodulatory, and anti-inflammatory activities of Spirulina: An overview. *Arch. Toxicol.* **2016**, *90*, 1817–1840. [CrossRef] [PubMed]
23. Gunes, S.; Tamburaci, S.; Dalay, M.C.; Deliloglu Gurhan, I. In vitro evaluation of Spirulina platensis extract incorporated skin cream with its wound healing and antioxidant activities. *Pharm. Biol.* **2017**, *55*, 1824–1832. [CrossRef] [PubMed]
24. Kiziltan, H.S.; Gunes Bayir, A.; Taspinar, O.; Yucesan, G.; Tastekin, D.; Sonmez, F.C.; Coban, G.; Kilic, G.; Eris, A.H.; Aydin, T.; et al. Radioprotectant and Cytotoxic Effects of Spirulina in Relapsed Verrucous Vulvar Cancer: A Case Report. *Altern. Ther. Health Med.* **2015**, *21*, 68–72.
25. Zhuang, X.; Huang, Y.; Zhang, D.; Tao, L.; Li, Y. Research status and prospect on hot water extract of Chlorella: The high value-added bioactive substance from Chlorella. *Sheng Wu Gong Cheng Xue Bao* **2015**, *31*, 24–42.
26. Halperin, S.A.; Smith, B.; Nolan, C.; Shay, J.; Kralovec, J. Safety and immunoenhancing effect of a Chlorella-derived dietary supplement in healthy adults undergoing influenza vaccination: Randomized, double-blind, placebo-controlled trial. *CMAJ* **2003**, *169*, 111–117.
27. Panahi, Y.; Darvishi, B.; Jowzi, N.; Beiraghdar, F.; Sahebkar, A. Chlorella vulgaris: A Multifunctional Dietary Supplement with Diverse Medicinal Properties. *Curr. Pharm. Des.* **2016**, *22*, 164–173. [CrossRef]
28. Panahi, Y.; Mostafazadeh, B.; Abrishami, A.; Saadat, A.; Beiraghdar, F.; Tavana, S.; Pishgoo, B.; Parvin, S.; Sahebkar, A. Investigation of the effects of Chlorella vulgaris supplementation on the modulation of oxidative stress in apparently healthy smokers. *Clin. Lab.* **2013**, *59*, 579–587. [CrossRef]
29. Panahi, Y.; Badeli, R.; Karami, G.R.; Badeli, Z.; Sahebkar, A. A randomized controlled trial of 6-week Chlorella vulgaris supplementation in patients with major depressive disorder. *Complement. Ther. Med.* **2015**, *23*, 598–602. [CrossRef]

30. Ebrahimi-Mameghani, M.; Sadeghi, Z.; Abbasalizad Farhangi, M.; Vaghef-Mehrabany, E.; Aliashrafi, S. Glucose homeostasis, insulin resistance and inflammatory biomarkers in patients with non-alcoholic fatty liver disease: Beneficial effects of supplementation with microalgae Chlorella vulgaris: A double-blind placebo-controlled randomized clinical trial. *Clin. Nutr.* **2017**, *36*, 1001–1006. [CrossRef] [PubMed]
31. Entesar, A. Antimicrobial activity of microalgal extracts isolated from Baharia Oasis, Egypt. *Glob. Adv. Res. J. Microbiol.* **2016**, *5*, 033–041.
32. Cannell, R.J.; Kellam, S.J.; Owsianka, A.M.; Walker, J.M. Results of a large scale screen of microalgae for the production of protease inhibitors. *Planta Med.* **1988**, *54*, 10–14. [CrossRef]
33. Aremu, A.O.; Neményi, M.; Stirk, W.A.; Ördög, V.; van Staden, J. Manipulation of nitrogen levels and mode of cultivation are viable methods to improve the lipid, fatty acids, phytochemical content, and bioactivities in Chlorella minutissima. *J. Phycol.* **2015**, *51*, 659–669. [CrossRef] [PubMed]
34. Lin, P.Y.; Tsai, C.T.; Chuang, W.L.; Chao, Y.H.; Pan, I.H.; Chen, Y.K.; Lin, C.C.; Wang, B.Y. Chlorella sorokiniana induces mitochondrial-mediated apoptosis in human non-small cell lung cancer cells and inhibits xenograft tumor growth in vivo. *BMC Complement. Altern. Med.* **2017**, *17*, 88. [CrossRef] [PubMed]
35. Suzich, J.B.; Cliffe, A.R. Strength in diversity: Understanding the pathways to herpes simplex virus reactivation. *Virology* **2018**, *522*, 81–91. [CrossRef]
36. Mader, J.; Gallo, A.; Schommartz, T.; Handke, W.; Nagel, C.H.; Günther, P.; Brune, W.; Reich, K. Calcium spirulan derived from Spirulina platensis inhibits herpes simplex virus 1 attachment to human keratinocytes and protects against herpes labialis. *J. Allergy Clin. Immunol.* **2016**, *137*, 197–203. [CrossRef]
37. Wong, T.; Wiesenfeld, D. Oral Cancer. *Aust. Dent. J.* **2018**, *1*, 91–99. [CrossRef]
38. Shibahara, T. Oral cancer -diagnosis and therapy-. *Clin. Calcium* **2017**, *27*, 1427–1433.
39. Mathew, B.; Sankaranarayanan, R.; Nair, P.P.; Varghese, C.; Somanathan, T.; Amma, B.P.; Amma, N.S.; Nair, M.K. Evaluation of chemoprevention of oral cancer with Spirulina fusiformis. *Nutr. Cancer* **1995**, *24*, 197–202. [CrossRef] [PubMed]
40. Miyachi, M.; Matsuno, T.; Asano, K.; Mataga, I. Anti-inflammatory effects of astaxanthin in the human gingival keratinocyte line NDUSD-1. *J. Clin. Biochem. Nutr.* **2015**, *56*, 171–178. [CrossRef]
41. Mori, H.; Tanaka, T.; Sugie, S.; Yoshimi, N.; Kawamori, T.; Hirose, Y.; Ohnishi, M. Chemoprevention by naturally occurring and synthetic agents in oral, liver, and large bowel carcinogenesis. *J. Cell. Biochem. Suppl.* **1997**, *27*, 35–41. [CrossRef]
42. Tanaka, T.; Makita, H.; Ohnishi, M.; Mori, H.; Satoh, K.; Hara, A. Chemoprevention of rat oral carcinogenesis by naturally occurring xanthophylls, astaxanthin and canthaxanthin. *Cancer Res.* **1995**, *55*, 4059–4064.
43. Grawish, M.E. Effects of Spirulina platensis extract on Syrian hamster cheek pouch mucosa painted with 7,12-dimethylbenz[a]anthracene. *Oral Oncol.* **2008**, *44*, 956–962. [CrossRef]
44. Grawish, M.E.; Zaher, A.R.; Gaafar, A.I.; Nasif, W.A. Long-term effect of Spirulina platensis extract on DMBA-induced hamster buccal pouch carcinogenesis (immunohistochemical study). *Med. Oncol.* **2010**, *27*, 20–28. [CrossRef] [PubMed]
45. Schwartz, J.; Shklar, G.; Reid, S.; Trickler, D. Prevention of experimental oral cancer by extracts of Spirulina-Dunaliella algae. *Nutr. Cancer* **1988**, *11*, 127–134. [CrossRef]
46. Kowshik, J.; Baba, A.B.; Giri, H.; Deepak Reddy, G.; Dixit, M.; Nagini, S. Astaxanthin inhibits JAK/STAT-3 signaling to abrogate cell proliferation, invasion and angiogenesis in a hamster model of oral cancer. *PLoS ONE* **2014**, *9*, 109–114. [CrossRef] [PubMed]
47. Sannasimuthu, A.; Kumaresan, V.; Anilkumar, S.; Pasupuleti, M.; Ganesh, M.R.; Mala, K.; Paray, B.A.; Al-Sadoon, M.K.; Albeshr, M.F.; Arockiaraj, J. Design and characterization of a novel Arthrospira platensis glutathione oxido-reductase-derived antioxidant peptide GM15 and its potent anti-cancer activity via caspase-9 mediated apoptosis in oral cancer cells. *Free Radic. Biol. Med.* **2019**, *135*, 198–209. [CrossRef]
48. Kavitha, K.; Kowshik, J.; Kishore, T.K.K.; Baba, A.B.; Nagini, S. Astaxanthin inhibits NF-κB and Wnt/β-catenin signaling pathways via inactivation of Erk/MAPK and PI3K/Akt to induce intrinsic apoptosis in a hamster model of oral cancer. *Biochim. Biophys. Acta (BBA)-Gen. Subj.* **2013**, *1830*, 4433–4444. [CrossRef]
49. Kowshik, J.; Nivetha, R.; Ranjani, S.; Venkatesan, P.; Selvamuthukumar, S.; Veeravarmal, V.; Nagini, S. Astaxanthin inhibits hallmarks of cancer by targeting the PI3K/NF-κB/STAT3 signalling axis in oral squamous cell carcinoma models. *IUBMB Life* **2019**, *71*, 1595–1610. [CrossRef]

50. Azizi, A.; Aghayan, S.; Zaker, S.; Shakeri, M.; Entezari, N.; Lawaf, S. In Vitro Effect of Zingiber officinale Extract on Growth of Streptococcus mutans and Streptococcus sanguinis. *Int. J. Dent.* **2015**, *2015*, 489842. [CrossRef]
51. Zhou, Y.; Millhouse, E.; Shaw, T.; Lappin, D.F.; Rajendran, R.; Bagg, J.; Lin, H.; Ramage, G. Evaluating Streptococcus mutans Strain Dependent Characteristics in a Polymicrobial Biofilm Community. *Front. Microbiol.* **2018**, *9*, 1498. [CrossRef]
52. Rakic, M.; Galindo-Moreno, P.; Monje, A.; Radovanovic, S.; Wang, H.L.; Cochran, D.; Sculean, A.; Canullo, L. How frequent does peri-implantitis occur? A systematic review and meta-analysis. *Clin. Oral Investig.* **2018**, *22*, 1805–1816. [CrossRef]
53. Komiyama, E.Y.; Lepesqueur, L.S.; Yassuda, C.G.; Samaranayake, L.P.; Parahitiyawa, N.B.; Balducci, I.; Koga-Ito, C.Y. Enterococcus Species in the Oral Cavity: Prevalence, Virulence Factors and Antimicrobial Susceptibility. *PLoS ONE* **2016**, *11*, e0163001. [CrossRef]
54. Davoodbasha, M.; Edachery, B.; Nooruddin, T.; Lee, S.Y.; Kim, J.W. An evidence of C16 fatty acid methyl esters extracted from microalga for effective antimicrobial and antioxidant property. *Microb. Pathog.* **2018**, *115*, 233–238. [CrossRef]
55. Uma, R.; Sivasubramanian, V.; Niranjali Devaraj, S. Preliminary phycochemical analysis and in vitro antibacterial screening of green microalgae, *Desmococcus Olivaceous, Chlorococcum humicola* and *Chlorella vulgaris*. *J. Algal Biomass Utln.* **2011**, *2*, 74–81.
56. Madhumathi, V.; Deepa, P.; Jeyachandran, S.; Manoharan, C.; Vijayakumar, S. Antimicrobial Activity of Cyanobacteria Isolated from Freshwater Lake. *Int. J. Microbiol. Res.* **2011**, *2*, 213–216.
57. Zarska, M.; Novotny, F.; Havel, F.; Sramek, M.; Babelova, A.; Benada, O.; Novotny, M.; Saran, H.; Kuca, K.; Musilek, K.; et al. Two-Step Mechanism of Cellular Uptake of Cationic Gold Nanoparticles Modified by (16-Mercaptohexadecyl) trimethylammonium Bromide. *Bioconjug. Chem.* **2016**, *27*, 2558–2574. [CrossRef]
58. Wei, L.; Lu, J.; Xu, H.; Patel, A.; Chen, Z.S.; Chen, G. Silver nanoparticles: Synthesis, properties, and therapeutic applications. *Drug Discov. Today* **2015**, *20*, 595–601. [CrossRef]
59. Salaheldin, T.A.; Loutfy, S.A.; Ramadan, M.A.; Youssef, T.; Mousa, S.A. IR-enhanced photothermal therapeutic effect of graphene magnetite nanocomposite on human liver cancer HepG2 cell model. *Int. J. Nanomed.* **2019**, *14*, 4397–4412. [CrossRef] [PubMed]
60. Rashad, S.; El-Chaghaby, G.A.; Elchaghaby, M.A. Antibacterial activity of silver nanoparticles biosynthesized using Spirulina platensis microalgae extract against oral pathogens. *Egypt. J. Aquat. Biol. Fish.* **2019**, *23*, 261–266. [CrossRef]
61. Bosshardt, D.D. The periodontal pocket: Pathogenesis, histopathology and consequences. *Periodontology 2000* **2018**, *76*, 43–50. [CrossRef]
62. Deas, D.E.; Moritz, A.J.; Sagun, R.S., Jr.; Gruwell, S.F.; Powell, C.A. Scaling and root planing vs. conservative surgery in the treatment of chronic periodontitis. *Periodontology 2000* **2016**, *71*, 128–139. [CrossRef] [PubMed]
63. Mahendra, J.; Mahendra, L.; Muthu, J.; John, L.; Romanos, G.E. Clinical effects of subgingivally delivered spirulina gel in chronic periodontitis cases: A placebo controlled clinical trial. *J. Clin. Diagn. Res.* **2013**, *7*, 2330–2333. [CrossRef] [PubMed]
64. Balci Yuce, H.; Lektemur Alpan, A.; Gevrek, F.; Toker, H. Investigation of the effect of astaxanthin on alveolar bone loss in experimental periodontitis. *J. Periodontal Res.* **2018**, *53*, 131–138. [CrossRef]
65. Hwang, Y.; Kwang-Jin, K.; Su-Jin, K.; Seul-Ki, M.; Seong-Gyeol, H.; Young-Jin, S.; Sung-Tae, Y. Suppression Effect of Astaxanthin on Osteoclast Formation In Vitro and Bone Loss In Vivo. *Int. J. Mol. Sci.* **2018**, *19*, 912. [CrossRef]
66. Kose, O.; Arabaci, T.; Yemenoglu, H.; Kara, A.; Ozkanlar, S.; Kayis, S.; Duymus, Z.Y. Influences of Fucoxanthin on Alveolar Bone Resorption in Induced Periodontitis in Rat Molars. *Mar. Drugs* **2016**, *14*, 70. [CrossRef]
67. Molteni, M.; Bosi, A.; Rossetti, C. The Effect of Cyanobacterial LPS Antagonist (CyP) on Cytokines and Micro-RNA Expression Induced by *Porphyromonas gingivalis* LPS. *Toxins* **2018**, *10*, 290. [CrossRef]
68. Orpha.Net. Available online: https://www.orpha.net/consor/cgi-bin/OC_Exp.php?lng=IT&Expert=357154 (accessed on 10 February 2019).
69. Kanjani, V.; Annigeri, R.G.; Revanappa, M.M.; Rani, A. Efficacy of Spirulina along with Different Physiotherapeutic Modalities in the Management of Oral Submucous Fibrosis. *Ann. Maxillofac. Surg.* **2019**, *9*, 23–27. [CrossRef] [PubMed]

70. Shetty, P.; Shenai, P.; Chatra, L.; Rao, P.K. Efficacy of spirulina as an antioxidant adjuvant to corticosteroid injection in management of oral submucous fibrosis. *Indian J. Dent. Res.* **2013**, *24*, 347–350. [CrossRef]
71. Mulk, B.S.; Deshpande, P.; Velpula, N.; Chappidi, V.; Chintamaneni, R.L.; Goyal, S. Spirulina and pentoxyfilline-a novel approach for treatment of oral submucous fibrosis. *J. Clin. Diagn. Res.* **2013**, *7*, 3048–3050.
72. Kuraji, M.; Matsuno, T.; Satoh, T. Astaxanthin affects oxidative stress and hyposalivation in aging mice. *J. Clin. Biochem. Nutr.* **2016**, *59*, 79–85. [CrossRef]
73. Yamada, T.; Ryo, K.; Tai, Y.; Tamaki, Y.; Inoue, H.; Mishima, K.; Tsubota, K.; Saito, I. Evaluation of Therapeutic Effects of Astaxanthin on Impairments in Salivary Secretion. *J. Clin. Biochem. Nutr.* **2010**, *47*, 130–137. [CrossRef]
74. Otsuki, T.; Shimizu, K.; Zempo-Miyaki, A.; Maeda, S. Changes in salivary flow rate following Chlorella-derived multicomponent supplementation. *J. Clin. Biochem. Nutr.* **2016**, *59*, 45–48. [CrossRef] [PubMed]
75. Merino, J.J.; Parmigiani-Izquierdo, J.M.; Toledano Gasca, A.; Cabaña-Muñoz, M.E. The Long-Term Algae Extract (*Chlorella and Fucus* sp.) and Aminosulphurate Supplementation Modulate SOD-1 Activity and Decrease Heavy Metals (Hg^{++}, Sn) Levels in Patients with Long-Term Dental Titanium Implants and Amalgam Fillings Restorations. *Antioxidants* **2019**, *8*, 101. [CrossRef]
76. Cicco, S.R.; Vona, D.; Leone, G.; De Giglio, E.; Bonifacio, M.A.; Cometa, S.; Fiore, S.; Palumbo, F.; Ragni, R.; Farinola, G.M. In vivo functionalization of diatom biosilica with sodium alendronate as osteoactive material. *Mater. Sci. Eng. C Mater. Biol. Appl.* **2019**, *104*, 109897. [CrossRef]
77. Khan, M.I.; Shin, J.H.; Kim, J.D. The promising future of microalgae: Current status, challenges, and optimization of a sustainable and renewable industry for biofuels, feed, and other products. *Microb. Cell Factories* **2018**, *36*. [CrossRef]

2

Nutritional and Functional Properties of Fermented Mixed Grains by Solid-State Fermentation with *Bacillus amyloliquefaciens* 245

Su Jin Heo [1], Ah-Jin Kim [1], Min-Ju Park [2], Kimoon Kang [1] and Do Yu Soung [1,*]

1 Food Research Institute, CJ Cheil Jedang, 42, Gwanggyo-ro, Yeongtong-gu, Suwon-si, Gyeonggi-do 16495, Korea; sujin.heo@cj.net (S.J.H.); ahjin.kim@cj.net (A.-J.K.); kimoon.kang@cj.net (K.K.)

2 BIO Research Institute, CJ Cheil Jedang, 42, Gwanggyo-ro, Yeongtong-gu, Suwon-si, Gyeonggi-do 16495, Korea; minju.park@cj.net

* Correspondence: doyu.soung@cj.net.

Abstract: Fermented foods have several advantages, including increased nutritional value, improved bioavailability, and functional health properties. We examined that these outcomes were also observed in fermented mixed grains (FMG) containing wheat germ, wheat bran, oats, brown rice, barley, quinoa, and lentils following solid-state fermentation (SSF) by *Bacillus amyloliquefaciens* 245. The metabolic profile during fermentation was screened using capillary electrophoresis time-of-flight mass spectrometry (CE-TOF-MS). The amino acids were quantitatively measured for the validation of the changes in metabolites. The activity of enzymes (e.g., amylase, protease, and fibrinolysis) and antioxidant capacity was also assessed to elucidate the functionality of FMG. The essential amino acid contents gradually increased as fermentation progressed. As the metabolites involved in the urea cycle and polyamine pathway were changed by fermentation, arginine was used as a substance to produce citrulline, ornithine, and agmatine. FMG showed dramatic increases in enzyme activity. FMG incubated for 36 h also displayed higher total phenolic contents and free radical scavenging ability than MG. The data suggest that FMG produced by *Bacillus amyloliquefaciens* 245 possess improved nutritional and functional quality, leading to their potential use as dietary supplements.

Keywords: solid-state fermentation; *Bacillus amyloliquefaciens*; grain; metabolites; enzymatic activity

---

1. Introduction

Wheat (*Triticum aesticum* L.) is one of the most consumed grains in the world. The usage of wheat was 760.2 million tonnes from the production of 771.5 million tonnes (USDA) in 2019/20 [1]. Throughout the processing chain of wheat flour, a large quantity of byproducts including the germ and bran is generated. Although wheat bran is rich in dietary fiber, phenolic acids, and proteins, its bioavailability is limited by the insoluble cell layer structure and high content of anti-nutritional factors such as phytate [2]. Similarly, wheat germ has high nutritional value, being a source of vitamin E, B vitamins, protein, dietary fiber, minerals, unsaturated fatty acids, and functional phytochemicals. However, its consumption is also restricted by anti-nutritional substances and existing lipase activity [3].

To overcome these issues, microbial fermentation has been noted for the successful use of wheat and other grain byproducts in the application of functional foods. For example, fermentation has extensively decomposed the cell wall structure of wheat bran, leading to an increase in soluble arabinoxylans and digestible protein [4]. Rizzello et al. demonstrated that lower lipase activity in fermented wheat germ than raw wheat germ effectively reduced the technological obstacles in baking [5]. The fermented quinoa flour also significantly degraded phytate while improving the bioavailability of zinc and iron [6]. Through fermentation, barley and oat bran were used to obtain xylitol and folate which is employed in sugar-free products and maternity dietary supplements, respectively [7]. Additionally, the heat-stabilized defatted rice bran during fermentation released more phenolic compounds such as gentistic, caffeic, syringic, p-coumaric, ferulic, sinapic, and benzoic acids than the control [8].

A choice of microbial bioprocesses and microorganisms suitable for fermentation is an important factor that strengthens the nutritional and functional properties of grain byproducts. Solid-state fermentation (SSF) requires only a small amount of water, close to that found in the natural environment of the microorganisms. This allows SSF to exert a positive economic and environmental impact when used in place of conventional submerged fermentation [9]. Some examples of foods fermented using SSF are cheonggukjang, natto, tempeh, fermented enzyme products, and kimchi. Among the microorganisms that may be used for SSF, *Bacillus amyloliquefaciens* rather than *Lactobacillus* and *Saccharomycess*, decreased the amount of anti-nutritional factors and increased the level of antioxidant activity in fermented soybean meal [10]. *Bacillus amyloliquefaciens* also produced higher levels of amino acids than *Aspergillus oryzae*, in soybeans, wheat, and rice [11]. Thus, SSF with *Bacillus amyloliquefaciens* might be a good candidate for the fermentation of grains.

We have characterized *Bacillus amyloliquefaciens* 245 isolated from Nuruk, a traditional Korean fermentation starter that produces rice-based wine. Its Genbank accession number is KR535604 [12]. We demonstrated that among 1008 *Bacillus* strains from either Nuruk or soybeans, *Bacillus amyloliquefaciens* 245 was one of the best in terms of amylase, protease, and fibrinolytic activity [13]. In particular, the largest amount of amino acids was observed when the mixed grain (MG)—including wheat germ, wheat bran, oats, brown rice, barley, quinoa, and lentils—was used as the substrate for SSF with *Bacillus amyloliquefaciens* 245 compared to when individual grains were used on a same-total basis [13]. We performed scientific metabolic profiling and investigated the nutritional and functional value of MG fermented by *Bacillus amyloliquefaciens* 245 during the different stages of SSF.

2. Materials and Methods

2.1. Materials

The MG consisted of wheat germ, wheat bran, oats, brown rice, barley, quinoa, and lentils at a weight ratio of 40:30:10:5:5:5:5. We used *Bacillus amyloliquefaciens* 245 isolated from Nuruk, a traditional Korean fermentation starter that produces rice-based wine.

2.2. Solid-State Fermentation (SSF)

The MG was steamed at 100 °C for 30 min in an autoclave. After inoculation with a 10% of *Bacillus amyloliquefaciens* 245 in the sterilized mixed grain (*w/w*), the fermented MG (FMG) was incubated for 0, 8, 12, and 36 h at a constant temperature (37 °C) in a chamber under 95% humidity. The concentration of *Bacillus amyloliquefaciens* 245 was 5.0×10^9–1.5×10^{10} CFU/mL. The FMG was dried at 60 °C for 12 h, crushed using a cyclone mill, and then used for analysis.

2.3. Metabolic Profiling Using Capillary Electrophoresis Time of Flight Mass Spectrometry (CE-TOF-MS) Analysis

Samples were mixed with 600 μL of methanol containing internal standards (50 μM) using a homogenizer (1500 rpm for 120 s, three times). After adding chloroform (600 μL) and distilled water (240 μL), the homogenates were thoroughly mixed and centrifuged (2300× *g*, 4 °C, 5 min). The aqueous layer was filtered through a 5-kDa cut-off filter (ULTRAFREE-MC-PLHCC, Human Metabolome Technologies, Yamagata, Japan) to remove macromolecules, and the filtrate was centrifuged and resuspended in 50 μL of distilled water immediately before the measurement. As previously described [14,15], the anionic and cationic metabolites in the samples were analyzed using an Agilent CE-TOF-MS system (Agilent Technologies, Santa Clara, CA, USA) equipped with fused silica capillaries in a 50 μm (i.d.) × 80 cm CE-MS column. Conditions were as follows: buffer solutions were used; MS capillary voltages, 3500 V (anion mode) and 4000 V (cation mode); MS scan range, *m/z* 50–1000; and the Human Metabolome Technologies (HMT) sheath liquid was used. The peaks detected in the CE-TOF-MS analysis were extracted using automatic integration software (Master Hands ver. 2.17.1.11, developed at Keio University, Keio, Japan), and the peak area was converted to a relative peak area. Putative metabolites were assigned using HMT's standard and known–unknown peak libraries on the basis of the *m/z* and migration time. The tolerance was ±0.5 min in MT and ±10 ppm in *m/z*. Hierarchical cluster analysis (HCA) was performed using statistical analysis software.

2.4. *Free Amino Acid Analysis*

Samples (1 g) were extracted with 20 mL of water by shaking for 1 h. The extract was centrifuged at 12,000× *g* for 5 min. The supernatant was then filtered through a 0.22 μm membrane filter and injected into an HPLC (high-performance liquid chromatography) column. Each amino acid was analyzed using two mobile phases as follows [16]. Mobile Phase A was a solution of 10 mM Na_2HPO_4, 10 mM $Na_2B_4O_7$, and 5 mM NaN_3 in 1 L of distilled water at pH 8.2. Mobile Phase B was a mixture of acetonitrile, methanol, and water at a volumetric ratio of 45:45:10. Pre-column derivatization was performed in the autosampler and the programmable injector units. Then, 2.5 μL of 0.1 M borate buffer (Agilent Technologies, Palo Alto, CA, USA) were mixed with 1 μL of sample by drawing air five times. After 0.2 min, 0.5 μL of ortho-phthalaldehyde, 0.4 μL of 9-fluorenylmethyl chloroformate, and 32 μL of injection diluent reagents were added, mixed eight times by drawing air, and injected after 0.1 min of waiting. Separation was carried out using an Agilent ZORBAX Eclipse Plus C18, 4.6 × 150 mm, 3.5 μm particle size i.d. HPLC column with detection at 338 nm. The gradient program started with 2% Phase B at a flow rate of 1.8 mL/min and changed linearly between 0.5 and 18 min to 51.3% Phase B. Next, 100% Phase B was applied from 18.1 to 21.5 min, and then, 98% of Phase A was applied until the end of the program at 25 min.

2.5. *Quantitative Estimation of Targeted Arginine Metabolites Using HPLC*

Arginine metabolites were analyzed using the method described by Caro et al. [17], with modifications. Samples (1 g) were extracted with 20 mL of distilled water by shaking for 1 h. The extract was centrifuged at 12,000× *g* for 5 min. The supernatant was remixed with 20 mL of 0.01 N HCl, filtered through a 0.22 μm membrane filter, and injected into an HPLC column. The HPLC analysis was performed using the autosampler (the Agilent 1200 series, Agilent Technologies, Palo Alto, CA, USA) equipped with a ZORBAX Eclipse Plus C18, 4.6 × 150 mm, 3.5 μm particle size i.d. HPLC column and a UV (DAD) detector at 40 °C with detection at 338 nm. The mobile phase consisted of a mixture of Mobile Phases A (50 mM sodium phosphate buffer, pH 6.8) and B (6:2:2 mixture of methanol, acetonitrile, and water). Separation was obtained at a flow rate of 1 mL/min with a gradient program that allowed for 0 min at 20% Phase B followed by 10 min of increasing Phase B to 80%.

2.6. *Determination of Enzymatic Activity*

2.6.1. Sample Extraction

Each sample (5 g) was extracted with 95 mL of distilled water by shaking at 180 rpm for 5 min. The mixture was centrifuged at 1628× *g* for 5 min, and then, the supernatant was filtered through Whatman No. 2 filter paper.

2.6.2. Amylase Activity Assay

Amylase activity was determined as described by Pfueller and Elliott [18]. One mL of the extracted sample was mixed with 13 mL of 0.1 N sodium phosphate buffer (pH 7.0), 1 mL of 0.1% calcium chloride, and 5 mL of 1% soluble starch solution. The mixture was incubated at 37 °C for 30 min and added to a color reagent solution. Absorbance was measured at 660 nm. One unit (U) of amylase activity is defined as the amount of amylase required to hydrolyze 10 mg of starch per 30 min.

2.6.3. Protease Activity Assay

Protease activity was assayed using the method described by Kum et al. [19], with modifications. One mL of the extracted sample was mixed with 1 mL of 0.6% casein and incubated at 37 °C for 10 min. The reaction was stopped by adding 2 mL of 0.4 M trichloroacetic acid and incubating at 37 °C for 25 min. The mixture was centrifuged at 13,000× *g* for 5 min. An amount of 1 mL of each supernatant was mixed with 5 mL of 0.4 M sodium carbonate, and then 1 mL of thrice-diluted 2 N Folin reagent was added. The mixture was incubated at 37 °C for 20 min. The absorbance was measured at 660 nm. One unit of protease activity is defined as the amount of protease required to release 1 μg of tyrosine per min.

2.6.4. Fibrinolytic Activity Assay

Fibrinolytic activity was measured according to the method described by Chang et al. [20], with modifications. A 100 μL volume of extract mixed with 300 μL of 0.1 M Tris-HCl (pH 7.8) containing 10 mM $CaCl_2$ was incubated in a 30 °C water bath for 5 min. After adding 300 μL of 1.2% fibrin solution (pH 7.8) prepared in 0.5 N NaOH, the mixture was incubated at 30 °C for another 10 min. The reaction was stopped by adding 600 μL of 0.11 M trichloroacetic acid containing 0.22 M sodium acetate and 0.33 M acetic acid. After centrifugation, the absorbance was measured at 275 nm. One fibrinolytic unit is defined as the amount of enzyme that induces an increase in absorbency at 275 nm equivalent to 1 μg of tyrosine per min at 37 °C.

2.7. Antioxidant Activity Assay

2.7.1. Sample Extraction

Each sample (1 g) was extracted twice with 9 mL of 70% ethanol by shaking at 180 rpm for 3 h. After centrifuging the extract at 1628× *g* for 10 min, the supernatant was filtered through Whatman No. 2 filter paper and then freeze-dried.

2.7.2. Total Phenolic Content (TPC)

TPC determination followed a method described by Singleton et al. [21], with modifications. One mL of each sample dissolved in the extracted solvent was mixed with 0.5 mL of 1 N Folin–Ciocalteu reagent and then 2.5 mL of 20% sodium carbonate. The mixture was incubated at room temperature for 40 min in the dark, and the absorbance was measured at 725 nm. The results are presented as gallic acid equivalent (GAE) in mg/g of sample.

2.7.3. 2,2′-Azino-Bis (2-Ethyl Benzothiazoline-6-Sulphonate) (ABTS) Assay

The ABTS assay was conducted using the method described by Puchalska et al. [22], with modifications. An ABTS stock solution made from 7 mM ABTS and 2.45 mM potassium persulfate was incubated at 25 °C for 12–16 h in the dark. For analysis, the solution was diluted in methanol to obtain 0.70 ± 0.02 arbitrary units (AU) at 734 nm. Ten mg of sample was dissolved in 1 mL of extracted solvent. An amount of 10 μL of sample was mixed with 990 μL of diluted ABTS solution and then incubated at room temperature for 10 min in the dark. The absorbance was measured at 734 nm.

3. Results and Discussion

3.1. Comparison of MG (Mixed Grains) Metabolites during Fermentation

The variation of the MG metabolites during fermentation was determined by CE-TOF-MS. Metabolomic analysis revealed a total of 276 peaks (165 metabolites in cation mode and 111 metabolites in anion mode) (File S1), which were annotated on the HMT's standard library. To further classify related units in the analysis, a HCA with heatmap visualization was performed (Figure 1). The data showed that the growth of *Bacillus amyloliquefaciens* 245 in the presence of MG resulted in increased essential amino acids, bioactive polyamines (i.e., spermidine and agmatine), and phenolic compounds (i.e., homovanillic acid, 2.5-dihydroxybenzoic acid, and p-hydroxybenzoic acid).

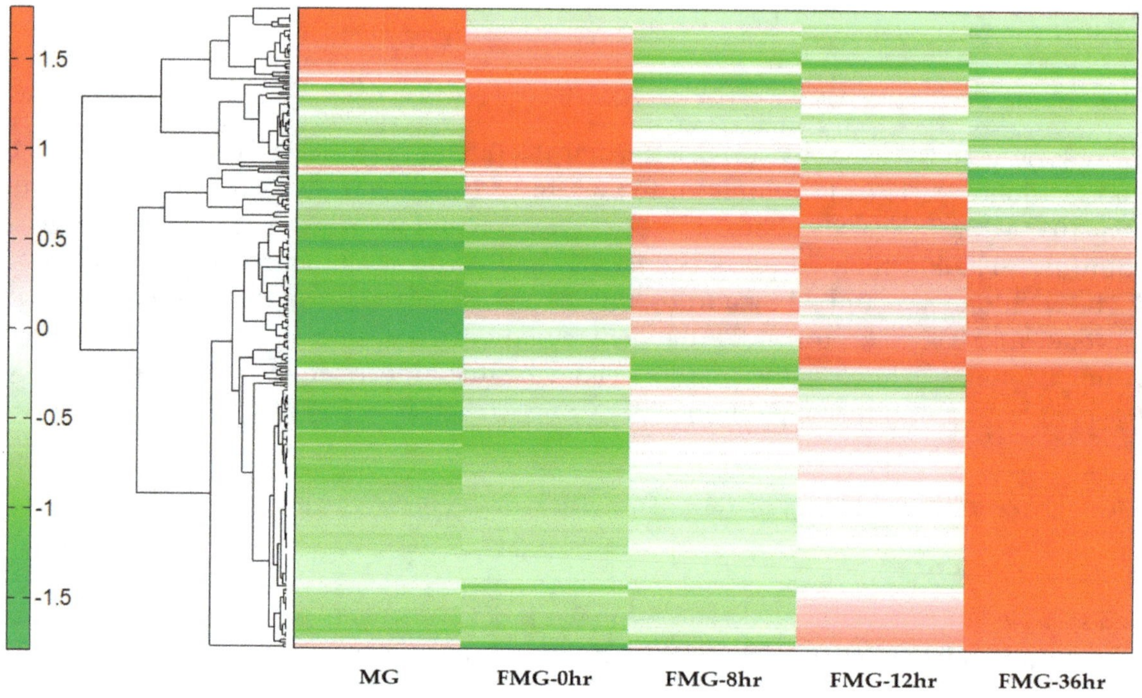

Figure 1. An hierarchical cluster analysis (HCA) heatmap comparing the metabolites from the mixed grains (MG) during fermentation. The x-axis shows MG (a grain mixture before steaming), fermented mixed grains (FMG)-0hr (a mixture of grain steamed for 30 min at 100 °C), FMG-8hr (a mixture of grain fermented for 8 h), FMG-12hr (a mixture of grain fermented for 12 h), and FMG-36hr (a mixture of grain fermented for 36 h) for each metabolite. The green and red colors indicate lower and higher contents of the metabolites, respectively.

The CE-TOF-MS-based metabolite profiling of the biological samples revealed noticeable changes in the components involved in amino acid pathways during fermentation (Figure 2). All the essential amino acids were increased with fermentation time. In non-essential amino acids, the contents of glutamic acid, cysteine, proline, and tyrosine were also gradually elevated during fermentation. Interestingly, the expression of alanine, aspartic acid, glycine, and serine was decreased at the middle phase of fermentation but elevated in the late phase.

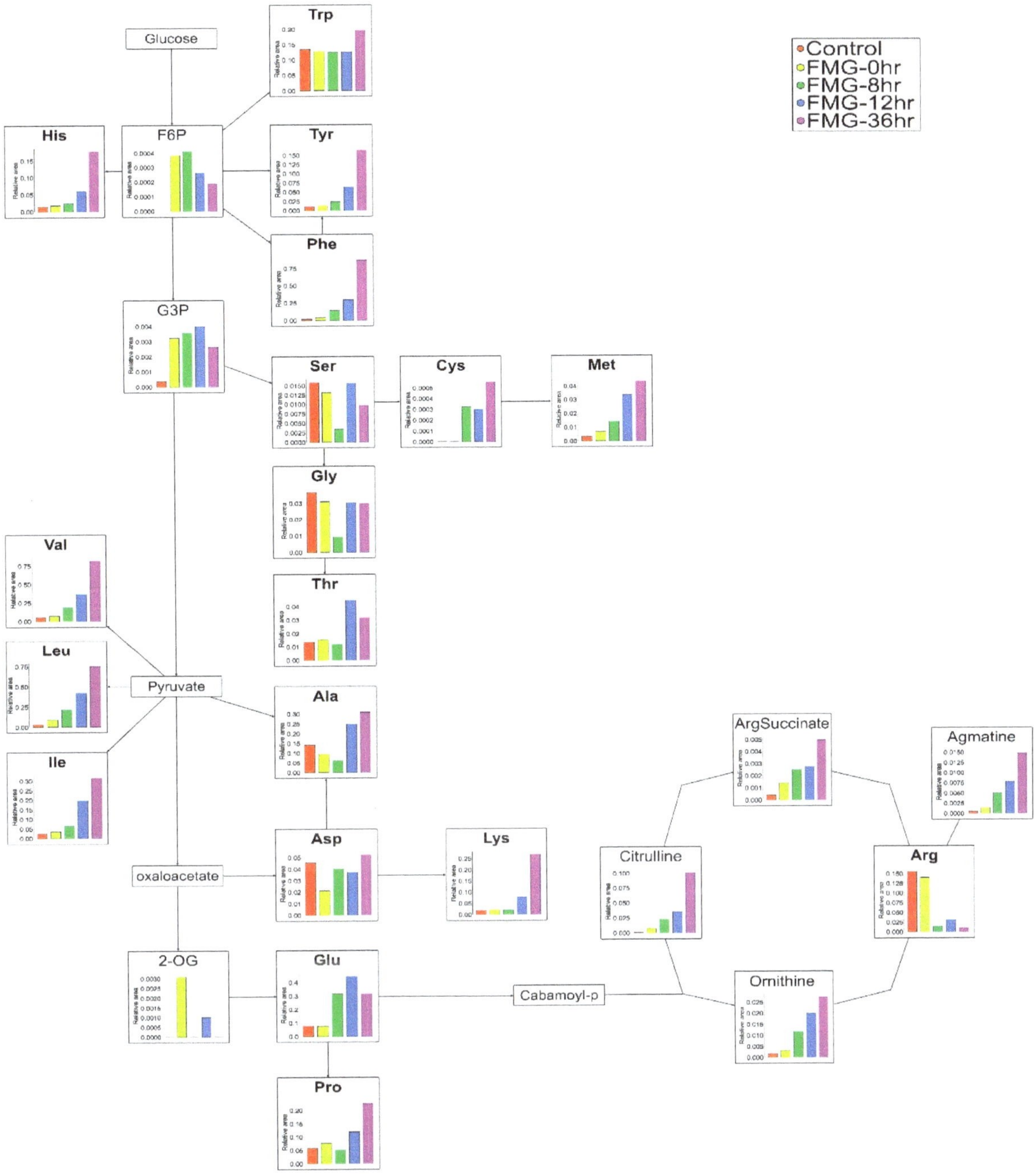

Figure 2. Scheme of the amino acid and the urea and polyamine pathways. The metabolic pathway was adopted from Kyoto Encyclopedia of Genes and Genomes (KEGG database. Changes in the levels of MG metabolites produced by *Bacillus amyloliquefaciens* 245 during fermentation were detected by capillary electrophoresis time-of-flight mass spectrometry (CE-TOF-MS). Each bar represents the relative metabolite abundance. Red, yellow, green, blue, and purple squares indicate MG (a grain mixture before steaming), FMG-0hr (a mixture of grain steamed for 30 min at 100 °C), FMG-8hr (a mixture of grain fermented for 8 h), FMG-12hr (a mixture of grain fermented for 12 h), and FMG-36hr (a mixture of grain fermented for 36 h), respectively.

The changes in the metabolites of the urea and polyamine pathway were shown to decrease the amount of arginine during fermentation (Figure 2). Meanwhile, the amount of citrulline, a precursor for the biosynthesis of arginine in the urea cycle, was increased. A similar ascending pattern was observed for the production of ornithine from arginine by arginase. The amount of agmatine transformed from arginine by arginine decarboxylase was also augmented with increasing fermentation time.

3.2. The Contents of Free Amino Acids during the Fermentation of MG

To validate the data for the amino acid metabolites during MG fermentation (File S1 and Figure 2), we quantitatively analyzed 18 amino acids at different fermentation stages.

Specifically, the total contents of amino acids were 368.76 mg/100 g in MG, 287.35 mg/100 g in FMG-0hr, 457.59 mg/100 g in FMG-8hr, 925.26 mg/100 g in FMG-12hr, and 1610.19 mg/100 g in FMG-36hr (Table 1). The contents of the essential amino acids such as histidine, isoleucine, leucine, lysine, methionine, phenylalanine, threonine, valine, and tryptophan in FMG-36hr increased about 4.5-, 9.0-, 7.1-, 9.5-, 1.5-, 18.9-, 2.2-, 12.8-, and 3.2-fold, respectively, compared to in MG. In the non-essential amino acids alanine, aspartic acid, glutamic acid, proline, serine, and tyrosine in FMG-36hr were 0.5-, 3.1-, 4.7-, 9.6-, 1.8-, and 10.1-fold, respectively, higher in quantity than in MG. However, the contents of arginine decreased from 76.9 mg/g in MG to 35 mg/g in FMG-36hr. The amount of glycine also decreased from 23.6 mg/g in MG to 14.3 mg/g in FMG-36hr. Additionally, no cysteine was detected during fermentation.

Table 1. The contents of free amino acids during the fermentation of MG.

Amino Acids	MG	FMG-0hr	FMG-8hr	FMG-12hr	FMG-36hr
			(mg/100 g)		
			Essential Amino Acids		
Histidine	13.27 ± 0.31 c	ND	13.88 ± 0.46 c	26.47 ± 1.03 b	60.37 ± 1.83 a
Isoleucine	7.43 ± 0.21 d	6.40 ± 0.72 d	9.86 ± 1.51 c	31.30 ± 1.01 b	66.52 ± 1.8 a
Leucine	19.74 ± 0.65 d	14.17 ± 0.23 e	33.44 ± 0.88 c	70.39 ± 2.12 b	139.21 ± 1.25 a
Lysine	19.46 ± 1.05 d	19.46 ± 0.11 d	23.7 ± 0.89 c	61.64 ± 1.74 b	184.25 ± 1.12 a
Methionine	16.19 ± 0.17 b	ND	ND	13.45 ± 0.52 c	24.21 ± 2.33 a
Phenylalanine	12.65 ± 0.67 d	9.34 ± 0.20 e	39.86 ± 1.41 c	81.46 ± 2.61 b	239.46 ± 1.5 a
Threonine	10.71 ± 0.73 b	8.51 ± 0.15 b	9.35 ± 1.65 b	22.50 ± 1.18 a	23.38 ± 2.25 a
Tryptophan	13.92 ± 0.56 d	11.40 ± 0.20 e	34.61 ± 1.04 c	78.95 ± 1.89 b	178.23 ± 1.68 a
Valine	29.00 ± 0.50 d	32.00 ± 2.65 cd	33.83 ± 0.76 c	43.00 ± 2.00 b	91.67 ± 1.53 a
			Non-Essential Amino Acids		
Alanine	36.49 ± 0.38 c	26.47 ± 0.42 d	23.36 ± 0.75 e	91.32 ± 1.63 b	113.88 ± 1.84 a
Arginine	76.90 ± 1.30 a	69.46 ± 0.29 b	29.78 ± 1.88 d	34.16 ± 2.32 c	35.29 ± 1.69 c
Aspartic acid	13.48 ± 0.80 d	11.14 ± 0.09 e	20.48 ± 1.04 c	22.81 ± 1.30 b	41.28 ± 2.13 a
Glutamic acid	37.07 ± 1.37 d	32.38 ± 0.77 e	149.96 ± 1.89 c	227.08 ± 2.52 a	175.07 ± 0.9 b
Glycine	23.61 ± 0.29 a	15.29 ± 0.68 b	6.78 ± 0.2 d	15.26 ± 0.20 b	14.30 ± 0.33 c
Cysteine	ND	ND	ND	ND	ND
Proline	8.23 ± 0.21 e	12.33 ± 1.53 d	18.33 ± 1.53 c	46.33 ± 3.21 b	79.00 ± 1.00 a
Serine	11.22 ± 0.86 b	7.96 ± 0.55 c	ND	10.73 ± 0.45 b	20.21 ± 2.56 a
Tyrosine	12.02 ± 0.53 d	ND	18.56 ± 0.76 c	44.69 ± 1.55 b	121.38 ± 1.10 a
Total	368.76	287.35	457.59	925.26	1615.07

Data from one representative experiment of three independent experiments were presented as the mean with standard deviation of three technical replicates. Different letters indicate significant differences at the $p < 0.05$ according to Duncan's multiple-comparison test. MG, a grain mixture before steaming; FMG-0hr, a mixture of grain steamed for 30 min at 100 °C; FMG-8hr, a mixture of grain fermented for 8 h; FMG-12hr, a mixture of grain fermented for 12 h; and FMG-36hr, a mixture of grain fermented for 36 h. ND: not detected.

Consistent with these results, the fermentation of maize and other grains improved protein quality and increased the contents of lysine, methionine, and tryptophan [23]. Kang et al. [24] also found that fermented soybeans contained 11- and 28-fold greater contents of peptides and amino acid groups, respectively, than unfermented soybeans. In particular, the health benefits of the essential amino acids produced during fermentation have been extensively investigated. For example, phenylalanine, a precursor to tyrosine, is used for the biosynthesis of catecholamines that are known to be effective in depression, pain, and skin disorders [25]. Jansen et al. [26] also demonstrated that lysine was required for healthy tissue function, growth, calcium uptake, and healing as well as the immune system. In addition, leucine, isoleucine, and valine are branched-chain amino acids (BCAAs) that exhibit effective anti-fatigue and ergogenic activities in an animal model of power exercise training [27].

The contents of each essential amino acid continued to increase, showing a similar pattern to the data for the metabolites during fermentation. FMG with larger amounts of essential amino acids could be dietary supplements with health benefits, especially in the areas of muscle growth and the brain.

3.3. Content of Arginine Metabolites during Fermentation

To confirm the differential patterns of metabolites in the urea cycle and polyamine pathways, we quantitatively analyzed arginine and its metabolites such as citrulline, ornithine, and agmatine during fermentation (Figure 3). As expected, the arginine contents of MG, FMG-0hr, FMG-8hr, FMG-12hr, and FMG-36hr gradually decreased to 76.9, 69.5, 29.8, 34.2, and 35.3 mg/100 g, respectively. The citrulline contents were 8.3 mg/100 g in MG, 29.1 mg/100 g in FMG-0hr, 21.1 mg/100 g in FMG-8hr, 58.8 mg/100 g in FMG-12hr, and 87.8 mg/100 g in FMG-36hr. The ornithine contents were 2.6 mg/100 g in FMG-8hr, 6.8 mg/100 g in FMG-12hr, and 8.7 mg/100 g in FMG-36hr, but no ornithine was detected in MG and FMG-0hr. The agmatine contents of MG, FMG-0hr, FMG-8hr, FMG-12hr, and FMG-36hr were 20.7, 20.8, 26.2, 48.6, and 125.0 mg/100 g, respectively.

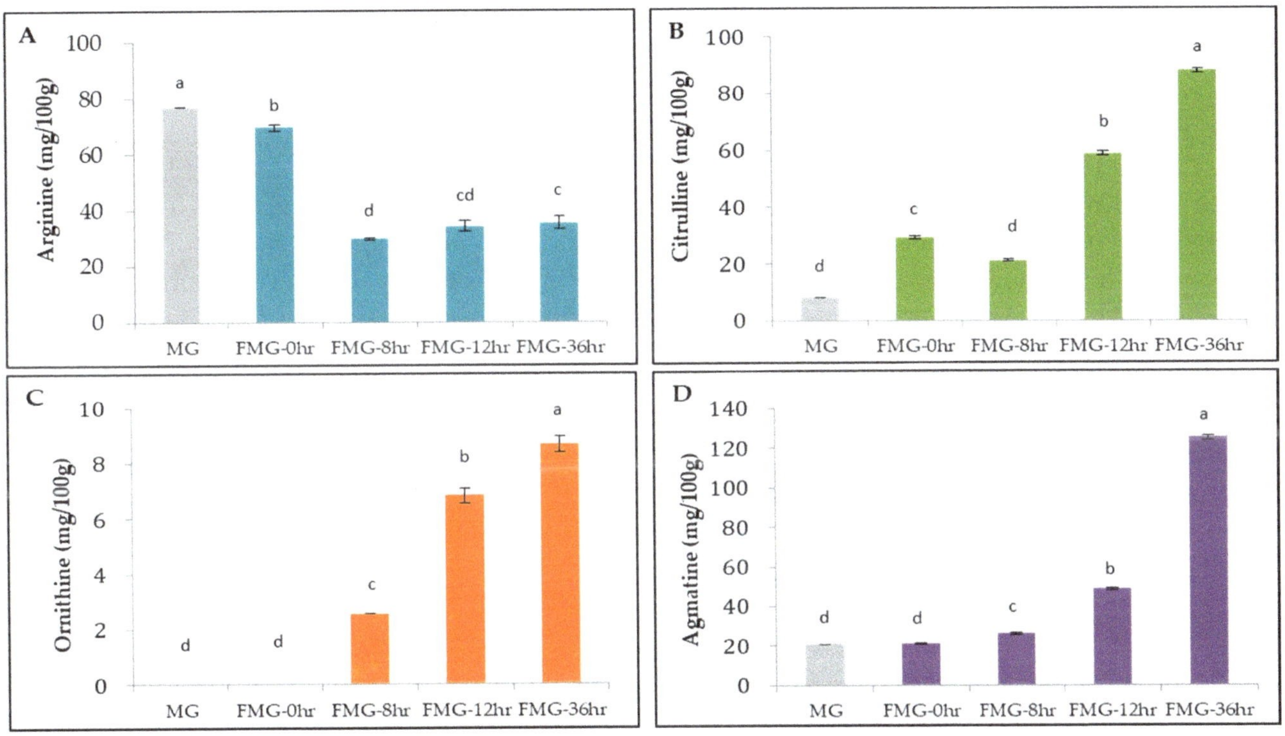

Figure 3. Arginine metabolites during fermentation. Content changes of (**A**) arginine, (**B**) citrulline, (**C**) ornithine, and (**D**) agmatine were measured using HPLC. MG, a grain mixture before steaming; FMG-0hr, a mixture of grain steamed for 30 min at 100 °C; FMG-8hr, a mixture of grain fermented for 8 h; FMG-12hr, a mixture of grain fermented for 12 h; and FMG-36hr, a mixture of grain fermented for 36 h. Data from one representative experiment of three independent experiments were presented as the mean with standard deviation of three technical replicates. Values with different letters are significantly different with $p < 0.05$ according to Duncan's multiple-comparison test.

The data imply that *Bacillus amyloliquefaciens* 245 modulated the arginine–deiminase system for arginine decomposition. Our speculation was supported by other investigators demonstrating that *Bacillus amyloliquefaciens* utilized arginine deiminase to effectively produce citrulline from arginine in fermented grains [28]. In addition to *Bacillus amyloliquefaciens*, *Lactobacillus brevis* and *Weissella confusa* showed arginine catabolism as well as citrulline and ornithine anabolism [29]. A comparable situation was also found in *Aspergillus oryzae*, widely used in the production of various Asian fermented foods [30].

There is growing evidence for the superior biological health benefits of arginine metabolites over arginine itself. A dietary supplement of citrulline malate increased endothelial-dependent vasodilation in healthy, normotensive, and physically active young adults [31]. Furthermore, L-citrulline supplementation increased nitric oxide (NO) availability, resulting in better protection of the aorta from senescence in diabetic rats than L-arginine supplementation [32]. Citrulline supplementation appeared to more efficiently increase arginine bioavailability than the supplementation of arginine itself in an animal study [33]. Ornithine, another arginine metabolite with therapeutic potential, has been demonstrated to modulate lipid metabolism and the urea cycle, leading to less fatigue in healthy subjects under physical load [34]. Agmatine has also been reported to improve the cardiovascular system by suppressing the inducible nitric oxide synthase (NOS)-mediated induction of NO synthesis [35].

Bacillus amyloliquefaciens 245 may therefore be a suitable microorganism for transforming arginine to citrulline, ornithine, and agmatine. The nutritional value of FMG consisting of a large number of arginine metabolites could make them attractive functional ingredients for maintaining cardiovascular health in a broad manner.

3.4. Enzymatic Activities in FMG

Amylase, protease, and fibrinolytic enzymes are traditionally produced by certain microorganisms in the fermentation process [2,10,36–39]. We examined whether the activity of amylase, protease, and fibrinolysis was affected by *Bacillus amyloliquefaciens* 245 in MG during fermentation.

We found that amylase activity was 0, 0, 594.0, 1525.8, and 3210.0 U/g in MG, FMG-0hr, FMG-8hr, FMG-12hr, and FMG-36hr, respectively (Figure 4A). Kunamnei et al. [37] demonstrated that the SSF of wheat bran by a thermophilic fungus at 50 °C for 120 h with an initial moisture content of 90% resulted in the highest amylase activity, at 534 U/g. We observed the maximum level of amylase activity (3210.0 U/g) in our mixture inoculated with a 10% ratio of *Bacillus amyloliquefaciens* 245 at 37 °C and 95% humidity for 36 h. Thus, further investigation is needed to determine whether bacterial microbiota rather than fungal communities are cost-effective for elevating amylase activity during fermentation with the same substances.

Under the same fermentation conditions, the protease activity of MG, FMG-0hr, FMG-8hr, FMG-12hr, and FMG-36hr was 0, 0, 1409.2, 2401.1, and 2818.6.0 U/g, respectively (Figure 4B). We confirmed that enzymatic activity was maximized at FMG-36hr. These data suggest that high proteolysis by *Bacillus amyloliquefaciens* 245 led to increased and balanced amounts of essential amino acids (Table 1). Consistent with our findings, *Bacillus amyloliquefaciens* U304 produced a highly active protease, increasing the degree to which large-molecular-weight proteins broke down into small-molecular-weight peptides and amino acids in fermented soybean meal [2,10].

A fibrinolytic enzyme that converts plasminogen to plasmin directly prevents intravascular coagulation without the risk of hemorrhage [40]. According to our results, the fibrinolytic activities induced by *Bacillus amyloliquefaciens* 245 in MG, FMG-0hr, FMG-8hr, FMG-12hr, and FMG-36hr were 0, 53.9, 133.3, 198.6, and 181.6 FU/g, respectively (Figure 4C). FMG-36hr displayed about 3-fold higher fibrinolysis than FMG-0hr ($p < 0.05$). Yao et al. [41] also demonstrated that *Bacillus amyloliquefaciens* RSB34 produced the strongest activity among nine Bacillus strains used as starters for traditional Korean fermented soy foods such as doenjang. Various microorganisms besides *Bacillus amyloliquefaciens* and substances have been used to produce fibrinolytic properties. For example, the fibrinolytic activity of roasted soybean flour and mixed grains (barley and brown rice) fermented by *Bacillus* spp. was higher than that of fermented roasted soybean flour [38]. In particular, Vijayaraghavan et al. [39] demonstrated that the highest fibrinolysis by *Bacillus cereus* IND1 was in wheat bran compared to different agroresidues including banana peel, tapioca peel, rice bran, and green gram husk.

Our results showed that MG with wheat bran, wheat germ, oats, brown rice, barley, and lentils inoculated with *Bacillus amyloliquefaciens* 245 displayed effective enzymatic activities for amylase, protease, and fibrinolysis.

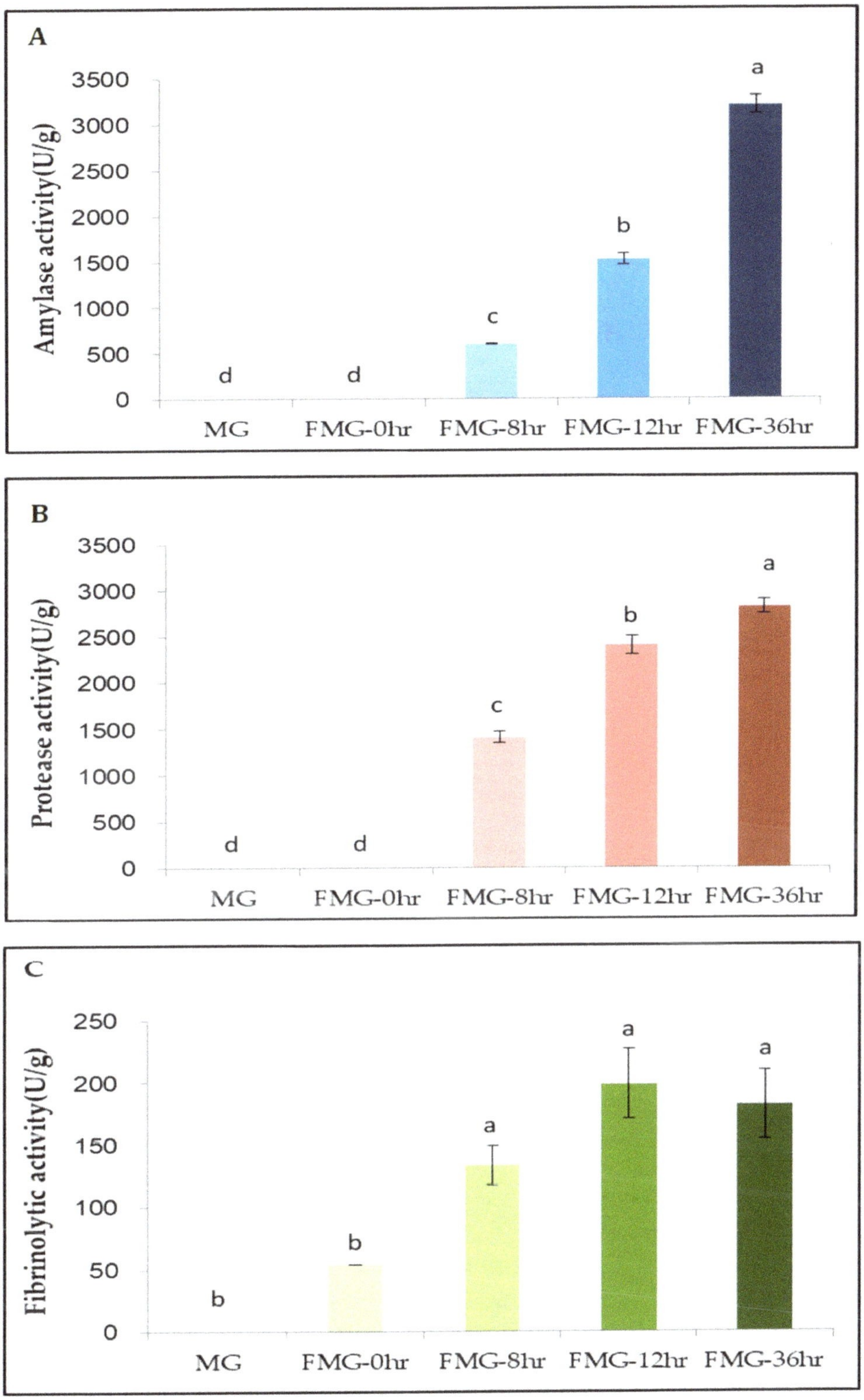

Figure 4. Enzymatic activity during MG fermentation. (**A**) Amylase, (**B**) protease, and (**C**) fibrinolytic activities were measured in each extracted sample. MG, a grain mixture before steaming; FMG-0hr, a mixture of grain steamed for 30 min at 100 °C; FMG-8hr, a mixture of grain fermented for 8 h; FMG-12hr, a mixture of grain fermented for 12 h; and FMG-36hr, a mixture of grain fermented for 36 h. Data from one representative experiment of three independent experiments were presented as the mean with standard deviation of three technical replicates. Values with different letters are significantly different with $p < 0.05$ according to Duncan's multiple-comparison test.

3.5. Total Phenolic Content (TPC) and ABTS+ Radical Scavenging Capacity in MG during Fermentation

It is extensively established that the increased contents of polyphenols following grain fermentation are strongly correlated with their antioxidant activity [42]. We also measured the TPC and antioxidant activities in the MG during fermentation.

As shown in Figure 5A, the TPCs in MG, FMG-0hr, FMG-8hr, FMG-12hr, and FMG-36hr were found to be 44.2, 92.5, 110.7, 167.5, and 373.5 mg GAE/100 g, respectively. FMG-36hr displayed about 8.4-fold higher TPC than MG, a statistically significant difference. The increase in TPC with the time of fermentation is due to the elevation of phenolic compounds including homovanillic acid, 2.5-dihydroxybenzoic acid, and α-hydroxybenzoic acid, which we observed by metabolomic analysis using CE-TOF-MS (File S1). These data indicate that during fermentation, bacterial enzymes are able to modify the grain constituents affecting the TPC.

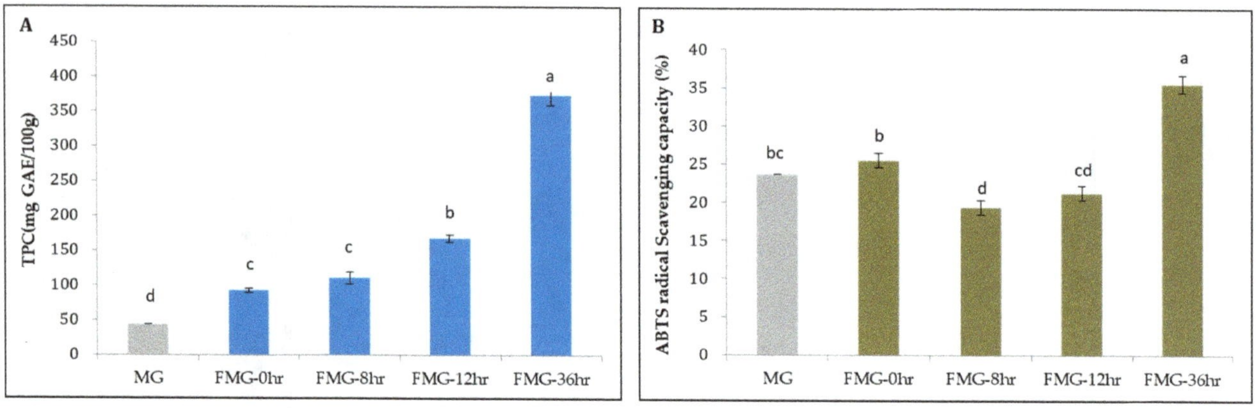

Figure 5. The contents and activities of antioxidant during MG fermentation. (**A**) Total Phenolic Content (TPC) and (**B**) ABTS+ radical scavenging capacity during fermentation. MG, a grain mixture before steaming; FMG-0hr, a mixture of grain steamed for 30 min at 100 °C; FMG-8hr, a mixture of grain fermented for 8 h; FMG-12hr, a mixture of grain fermented for 12 h; and FMG-36hr, a mixture of grain fermented for 36 h. Data from one representative experiment of three independent experiments were presented as the mean with standard deviation of three technical replicates. Values with different letters are significantly different with $p < 0.05$ according to Duncan's multiple-comparison test. GAE: gallic acid equivalent.

In parallel with the TPC, the antioxidant activity during fermentation was measured via the ABTS+ assay. The ABTS+ radical scavenging capacity of MG, FMG-0hr, FMG-8hr, FMG-12hr, and FMG-36hr was found to be 23.6, 25.5, 19.4, 21.3, and 35.6%, respectively (Figure 5B). FMG-36hr had the highest radical scavenging activity, in association with the largest TPC. However, unlike for the TPC, we did not observe an incremental increase in ABTS+ activity with fermentation time. Cao et al. [43] demonstrated that while phenolic compounds with double hydroxyls on the flavonoid B-ring displayed strong antioxidant activity, those with a single hydroxyl group on the B-ring showed minimal free radical scavenging ability. This indicates that antioxidant activity can vary depending on the composition of the total phenol compounds. Furthermore, it has been reported that the essential amino acids of protein hydrolysates from Cucurbitaceae seeds can be a potent source of antioxidants [44]. Thus, the ABTS+ radical savaging capacity of MG and FMG may be determined by the number of amino acid metabolites in addition to the composition of phenolic compounds.

4. Conclusions

In this study, we established the conditions for the SSF of MG containing wheat germ, wheat bran, oats, brown rice, barley, quinoa, and lentils using our patented microorganism, Bacillus amyloliquefaciens 245. Under these conditions, we demonstrated that the number of essential amino acids and arginine metabolites incremented with fermentation time. Amylase, protease, and fibrinolysis were also gradually activated according to the fermentation stage. Furthermore, 36-hr cultured FMG exhibited significant increases in antioxidant capability and total polyphenol content compared to MG. Thus, we provide compelling evidence that the nutritional value and functional capacity of FMG produced by SSF in the presence of Bacillus amyloliquefaciens 245 could render them potential sources of dietary supplements.

Author Contributions: Conceptualization, D.Y.S.; formal analysis, S.J.H., A.-J.K., and M.-J.P.; investigation, S.J.H., A.-J.K., and M.-J.P.; methodology, S.J.H., A.-J.K., and M.-J.P.; project administration, S.J.H., A.-J.K., and M.-J.P.; software, S.J.H., A.-J.K., and M.-J.P.; supervision, K.K. and D.Y.S.; validation, K.K. and D.Y.S.; visualization, S.J.H. and A.-J.K.; writing—original draft, S.J.H. and A.-J.K.; writing—review and editing, K.K. and D.Y.S. All authors have read and agreed to the published version of the manuscript.

References

1. Aguilar Gorodecki, A. *USDA: World Agricultural Supply and Demand Estimates*; USDAGOV: Washington, DC, USA, 2012.
2. Sefatie, R.S.; Fatoumata, T.; Eric, K.; Shi, Y.H.; Guo-Wei, L. In Vitro Antioxidant Activities of Protein Hydrolysate from Germinated Black Soybean (*Glycine Max* L.). *Adv. J. Food Sci. Technol.* **2013**, *5*, 453–459. [CrossRef]
3. Brandolini, A.; Hidalgo, A. Wheat Germ: Not Only a by-Product. *Int. J. Food Sci. Nutr.* **2012**, *63*, 71–74. [CrossRef] [PubMed]
4. Coda, R.; Kärki, I.; Nordlund, E.; Heiniö, R.-L.; Poutanen, K.; Katina, K. Influence of Particle Size on Bioprocess Induced Changes on Technological Functionality of Wheat Bran. *Food Microbiol.* **2014**, *37*, 69–77. [CrossRef] [PubMed]
5. Rizzello, C.G.; Nionelli, L.; Coda, R.; Di Cagno, R.; Gobbetti, M. Use of Sourdough Fermented Wheat Germ for Enhancing the Nutritional, Texture and Sensory Characteristics of the White Bread. *Eur. Food Res. Technol.* **2010**, *230*, 645–654. [CrossRef]
6. Castro-Alba, V.; Lazarte, C.E.; Perez-Rea, D.; Sandberg, A.-S.; Carlsson, N.-G.; Almgren, A.; Bergenståhl, B.; Granfeldt, Y. Effect of Fermentation and Dry Roasting on the Nutritional Quality and Sensory Attributes of Quinoa. *Food Sci. Nutr.* **2019**, *7*, 3902–3911. [CrossRef] [PubMed]
7. Pepper, T.; Olinger, P.M. Xylitol in Sugar-Free Confections. *Food Technol. Chic.* **1988**, *42*, 98–106.
8. Webber, D.M.; Hettiarachchy, N.S.; Li, R.; Horax, R.; Theivendran, S. Phenolic Profile and Antioxidant Activity of Extracts Prepared from Fermented Heat-Stabilized Defatted Rice Bran. *J. Food Sci.* **2014**, *79*, H2383–H2391. [CrossRef]
9. Manan, M.A.; Webb, C. Design Aspects of Solid State Fermentation as Applied to Microbial Bioprocessing. *J. Appl. Biotechnol. Bioeng.* **2017**, *4*, 91.
10. Chi, C.-H.; Cho, S.-J. Improvement of Bioactivity of Soybean Meal by Solid-State Fermentation with Bacillus amyloliquefaciens Versus Lactobacillus Spp. and Saccharomyces Cerevisiae. *LWT-Food Sci. Technol.* **2016**, *68*, 619–625. [CrossRef]
11. Shahzad, R.; Shehzad, A.; Bilal, S.; Lee, I.-J. Bacillus amyloliquefaciens RWL-1 as a New Potential Strain for Augmenting Biochemical and Nutritional Composition of Fermented Soybean. *Molecules* **2020**, *25*, 2346. [CrossRef]
12. Bacillus amyloliquefaciens Strain BA245 16S Ribosomal RNA Gene, Partial Sequence. Available online: https://www.ncbi.nlm.nih.gov/nuccore/kr535604 (accessed on 18 July 2015).
13. Park, M.-J.; Kim, A.-J.; Han, S.W.; Heo, S.J.; Yang, T.J.; Park, S.W.; Lee, S.B.; Jang, J.H.; Cho, S.J.; Hong, Y.H.; et al. Novel Strain Derived from Traditional Fermented Food and Having Excellent Enzyme Productivity, and Method for Preparing Fermented Cereal Enzyme Food by Using Same. U.S. Patent WO2017074037A1, 4 May 2017.
14. Soga, T.; Ueno, Y.; Naraoka, H.; Ohashi, Y.; Tomita, M.; Nishioka, T. Simultaneous Determination of Anionic Intermediates for *Bacillus subtilis* Metabolic Pathways by Capillary Electrophoresis Electrospray Ionization Mass Spectrometry. *Anal. Chem.* **2002**, *74*, 2233–2239. [CrossRef] [PubMed]

15. Soga, T.; Ohashi, Y.; Ueno, Y.; Naraoka, H.; Tomita, M.; Nishioka, T. Quantitative Metabolome Analysis Using Capillary Electrophoresis Mass Spectrometry. *J. Proteome Res.* **2003**, *2*, 488–494. [CrossRef] [PubMed]
16. Henderson, J.W.; Brooks, A. *Improved Amino Acid Methods Using Agilent ZORBAX Eclipse Plus C18 Columns for a Variety of Agilent LC Instrumentation and Separation Goals*; Agilent Technologies: Santa Clara, CA, USA, 2010.
17. Caro, G.M.; Meierhenrich, U.J.; Schutte, W.A.; Barbier, B.; Segovia, A.A.; Rosenbauer, H.; Thiemann, W.-P.; Brack, A.; Greenberg, J.M. Amino Acids from Ultraviolet Irradiation of Interstellar Ice Analogues. *Nature* **2002**, *416*, 403–406. [CrossRef] [PubMed]
18. Pfueller, S.L.; Elliott, W.H. The Extracellular α-Amylase of Bacillus Stearothermophilus. *J. Biol. Chem.* **1969**, *244*, 48–54.
19. Kum, S.-J.; Yang, S.-O.; Lee, S.M.; Chang, P.-S.; Choi, Y.H.; Lee, J.J.; Hurh, B.S.; Kim, Y.-S. Effects of Aspergillus Species Inoculation and Their Enzymatic Activities on the Formation of Volatile Components in Fermented Soybean Paste (Doenjang). *J. Agric. Food Chem.* **2015**, *63*, 1401–1418. [CrossRef]
20. Chang, C.-T.; Fan, M.-H.; Kuo, F.-C.; Sung, H.-Y. Potent Fibrinolytic Enzyme from a Mutant of Bacillus s Ubtilis IMR-NK1. *J. Agric. Food Chem.* **2000**, *48*, 3210–3216. [CrossRef]
21. Singleton, V.L.; Orthofer, R.; Lamuela-Raventós, R.M. [14] Analysis of Total Phenols and Other Oxidation Substrates and Antioxidants by Means of Folin-Ciocalteu Reagent. In *Methods in Enzymology*; Elsevier: Amsterdam, The Netherlands, 1999; Volume 299, pp. 152–178.
22. Puchalska, P.; Marina, M.L.; García, M.C. Isolation and Identification of Antioxidant Peptides from Commercial Soybean-Based Infant Formulas. *Food Chem.* **2014**, *148*, 147–154. [CrossRef]
23. Hamad, A.M.; Fields, M.L. Evaluation of the Protein Quality and Available Lysine of Germinated and Fermented Cereals. *J. Food Sci.* **1979**, *44*, 456–459. [CrossRef]
24. Kang, H.J.; Yang, H.J.; Kim, M.J.; Han, E.-S.; Kim, H.-J.; Kwon, D.Y. Metabolomic Analysis of Meju during Fermentation by Ultra Performance Liquid Chromatography-Quadrupole-Time of Flight Mass Spectrometry (UPLC-Q-TOF MS). *Food Chem.* **2011**, *127*, 1056–1064. [CrossRef]
25. Akram, M.; Daniyal, M.; Ali, A.; Zainab, R.; Shah, S.M.A.; Munir, N.; Tahir, I.M. Role of Phenylalanine and Its Metabolites in Health and Neurological Disorders. In *Synucleins-Biochemistry and Role in Diseases*; IntechOpen: London, UK, 2020.
26. Jansen, G.R. Lysine in Human Nutrition. *J. Nutr.* **1962**, *76*, 1–35. [CrossRef]
27. Chen, Y.-M.; Lin, C.-L.; Wei, L.; Hsu, Y.-J.; Chen, K.-N.; Huang, C.-C.; Kao, C.-H. Sake Protein Supplementation Affects Exercise Performance and Biochemical Profiles in Power-Exercise-Trained Mice. *Nutrients* **2016**, *8*, 106. [CrossRef] [PubMed]
28. Qiu, Y.; Fang, F.; Zhou, X.; Chen, X.; Zhang, L.; Du, G.; Chen, J. Characterization of Arginine Utilization Strains from Fermented Grains and Evaluation of Their Contribution to Citrulline Accumulation in Chinese Luzhou-Flavor Spirits. *Acta Microbiol. Sin.* **2016**, *56*, 1638–1646.
29. Hwang, H.; Lee, J.-H. Characterization of Arginine Catabolism by Lactic Acid Bacteria Isolated from Kimchi. *Molecules* **2018**, *23*, 3049. [CrossRef] [PubMed]
30. Akasaka, N.; Fujiwara, S. The Therapeutic and Nutraceutical Potential of Agmatine, and Its Enhanced Production Using Aspergillus oryzae. *Amino Acids* **2020**, *52*, 181–197. [CrossRef] [PubMed]
31. Rogers, J.M.; Gills, J.; Gray, M. Acute Effects of Nitrosigine®and Citrulline Maleate on Vasodilation. *J. Int. Soc. Sports Nutr.* **2020**, *17*, 1–8. [CrossRef] [PubMed]
32. Tsuboi, T.; Maeda, M.; Hayashi, T. Administration of L-Arginine plus L-Citrulline or L-Citrulline Alone Successfully Retarded Endothelial Senescence. *PLoS ONE* **2018**, *13*, e0192252. [CrossRef] [PubMed]
33. Agarwal, U.; Didelija, I.C.; Yuan, Y.; Wang, X.; Marini, J.C. Supplemental Citrulline Is More Efficient than Arginine in Increasing Systemic Arginine Availability in Mice. *J. Nutr.* **2017**, *147*, 596–602. [CrossRef] [PubMed]
34. Sugino, T.; Shirai, T.; Kajimoto, Y.; Kajimoto, O. L-Ornithine Supplementation Attenuates Physical Fatigue in Healthy Volunteers by Modulating Lipid and Amino Acid Metabolism. *Nutr. Res.* **2008**, *28*, 738–743. [CrossRef]
35. Raghavan, S.A.; Dikshit, M. Vascular Regulation by the L-Arginine Metabolites, Nitric Oxide and Agmatine. *Pharmacol. Res.* **2004**, *49*, 397–414. [CrossRef]
36. Li, P.; Liang, H.; Lin, W.-T.; Feng, F.; Luo, L. Microbiota Dynamics Associated with Environmental Conditions and Potential Roles of Cellulolytic Communities in Traditional Chinese Cereal Starter Solid-State Fermentation. *Appl. Environ. Microbiol.* **2015**, *81*, 5144–5156. [CrossRef]

37. Kunamneni, A.; Permaul, K.; Singh, S. Amylase Production in Solid State Fermentation by the Thermophilic Fungus Thermomyces Lanuginosus. *J. Biosci. Bioeng.* **2005**, *100*, 168–171. [CrossRef] [PubMed]
38. Son, S.-J.; Lee, S.-P. Evaluation of Rheological and Functional Properties of Roasted Soybean Flour and Mixed Cereals Fermented by Bacillus Sp. *J. Korean Soc. Food Sci. Nutr.* **2011**, *40*, 450–457. [CrossRef]
39. Vijayaraghavan, P.; Prakash Vincent, S.G. Statistical Optimization of Fibrinolytic Enzyme Production Using Agroresidues by Bacillus Cereus IND1 and Its Thrombolytic Activity in Vitro. *BioMed Res. Int.* **2014**, *2014*, 725064. [CrossRef] [PubMed]
40. Hsia, C.-H.; Shen, M.-C.; Lin, J.-S.; Wen, Y.-K.; Hwang, K.-L.; Cham, T.-M.; Yang, N.-C. Nattokinase Decreases Plasma Levels of Fibrinogen, Factor VII, and Factor VIII in Human Subjects. *Nutr. Res.* **2009**, *29*, 190–196. [CrossRef]
41. Choi, H.-K.; Yoon, J.-H.; Kim, Y.-S.; Kwon, D.Y. Metabolomic Profiling of Cheonggukjang during Fermentation by 1H NMR Spectrometry and Principal Components Analysis. *Process Biochem.* **2007**, *42*, 263–266. [CrossRef]
42. Velioglu, Y.S.; Mazza, G.; Gao, L.; Oomah, B.D. Antioxidant Activity and Total Phenolics in Selected Fruits, Vegetables, and Grain Products. *J. Agric. Food Chem.* **1998**, *46*, 4113–4117. [CrossRef]
43. Cao, X.; Yang, L.; Xue, Q.; Yao, F.; Sun, J.; Yang, F.; Liu, Y. Antioxidant Evaluation-Guided Chemical Profiling and Structure-Activity Analysis of Leaf Extracts from Five Trees in *Broussonetia* and *Morus* (Moraceae). *Sci. Rep.* **2020**, *10*, 4808. [CrossRef]
44. Dash, P.; Ghosh, G. Amino Acid Composition, Antioxidant and Functional Properties of Protein Hydrolysates from Cucurbitaceae Seeds. *J. Food Sci. Technol.* **2017**, *54*, 4162–4172. [CrossRef]

3

Application of Hydroxytyrosol in the Functional Foods Field: From Ingredient to Dietary Supplements

Andreia F. R. Silva, Daniela Resende, Mariana Monteiro, Manuel A. Coimbra, Artur M. S. Silva and Susana M. Cardoso *

LAQV-REQUIMTE, Department of Chemistry, University of Aveiro, 3810-193 Aveiro, Portugal; afrs@ua.pt (A.F.R.S.); danielaresende@outlook.com (D.R.); marianaicnamonteiro@gmail.com (M.M.); mac@ua.pt (M.A.C.); artur.silva@ua.pt (A.M.S.S.)

* Correspondence: susanacardoso@ua.pt.

Abstract: Hydroxytyrosol (HT) is an amphipathic functional phenol found in the olive tree, both in its leaves and fruits, in free or bound forms, as well as in olive oil and by-products of olive oil manufacture. The European Food Safety Authority recommends regular consumption of HT due to its several beneficial effects on human health, which are closely associated to its antioxidant activity. These reasons make HT an excellent candidate for application as a functional ingredient in the design of novel food products. Patents already exist for methodologies of extraction, purification, and application of HT in supplements and food products. The present review discusses the impact of HT incorporation on food properties and its effects on consumers, based on relevant data related to the use of HT as a functional ingredient, both as a pure compound or in the form of HT-rich extracts, in various food products, namely in edible oils, beverages, bakery products, as well animal-based foods such as meat, fishery and dairy products.

Keywords: phenol; olive oil; by-products; table olives; antioxidant; functional ingredient; novel foods

1. Introduction

The assumption that "diet is the best medicine" embraces the valorization of food ingredients and, in particular, of health-promoting bioactive compounds. Hydroxytyrosol (HT) is a dietary constituent that has received much attention in the last decade due to the many benefits of the ingestion of virgin olive oil, relative to antioxidant capacity and properties against cardiovascular diseases. This phenolic is recognized as safe by the European Food Safety Authority (EFSA) and Food and Drug Administration (FDA). Based on the opinion of the EFSA, in 2017, the European Commission (EC) authorized the placing on the market of HT as a novel food ingredient under Regulation (EC) No 258/97 [1,2], which assumes its use for the general population, excluding children under the age of three years, pregnant women, and lactating women [3]. To promote its widespread consumption, HT has been integrated into the concept of functional foods, i.e., a natural-based food product provider of health benefits beyond the primary nutrition value, which has exponentially increased over the last few years.

HT, i.e., 3,4-dihydroxyphenylethanol, is an amphipathic phenol with the potential to be used as an ingredient in functional foods. In fact, it is stated by EFSA opinion of 2011 and EC regulation 432/2012 that HT is the only "food" officially accepted to have an obvious health effect when consumed regularly with the prerequisite to contain at least 5 mg/20 g oil of HT and related compounds [4]. The main dietary sources of HT include olive oil and table olives, in free and/or bound forms, although this is also present in olive leaves [5] and in lower amounts in grapes [6] and wine [7]. Its formation occurs during the ripening process of olives, as well as during the preparation of table oils and oil storage, by hydrolysis of oleuropein [8]. In olives, this may be a consequence of the acidic conditions (resulting from the brining of fruits), the activity of endogenous olive enzymes [9] or from the fermentation of lactic acid bacteria [10], whereas in wine, HT results from the conversion of tyrosol through alcoholic fermentation, or enzymatic oxidation by polyphenol oxidase present in the fruits [6,11]. Note that oleuropein is composed of a glycosylated ester of elenolic acid with HT, which makes it suitable to be hydrolyzed by β-glucosidase enzymes. However, oleuropein and HT share catecholic structures, conferring them similar antioxidant activity [9].

According to the EFSA, the average HT content, in mg/kg of product, ranges from 3.5–7.7 in olive oils and it is approximately 556 and 660 in green and black olives, respectively [1]. Thus, considering the dietary data from the European Union, it is estimated that the mean values of HT consumption in adults vary between 0.15–4.0 and 19–185 μg of HT/kg body weight (bw) per day, as a result of olive oil and table olives intake, respectively [1], far from the daily recommended intake. In addition, table olives and olive oil are not consumed by everyone, which relays the importance of the incorporation of HT in other types of products.

The health-promoting abilities of dietary HT are dependent on metabolism, bioaccessibility and bioavailability issues. Similar to most phenolic compounds, no salivary digestion was reported for HT, possibly due to its inhibitory effect on α-amylase [12]. In the gastric phase, most of HT is released from the food matrix and remains stable [13] while metabolization is triggered in the intestinal phase, due to the basic pH conditions and the presence of enzymes in enterocytes. The compound is absorbed by the enterocytes of the epithelium and reaches the liver through the hepatic portal vein, where metabolism continues. Afterward, HT and its metabolites are further excreted into systemic circulation or can be reabsorbed by the intestine through bile [14]. During this process, it is gradually converted into other metabolites such as 3,4-dihydroxyphenylacetaldehyde, 3,4-dihydroxyphenylacetic acid (DOPAC) and 4-hydroxy-3-methoxyphenylacetic acid (or homovanillic acid), which can be detected in human plasma [15]. Hydroxytyrosol acetate is another metabolite often detected in human plasma, resulting from the alkaline hydrolysis and acetylation of HT in the lumen [16,17]. For the study of the health benefits of HT consumption, it is of utmost relevance to know which metabolites are generated once, similar to HT, some of them exert antioxidant activity, due to the hydroxy group in the 3,4-ortho position [18], such as DOPAC [19] and homovanillic acid [20]. Hydroxytyrosol acetate exhibits less antioxidant activity than HT due to the acetate group of the ester that may hide the scavenging effect of the hydroxyl groups by intra- or intermolecular hydrogen bonding [21]. Still, it inhibits platelet aggregation in rats [22], an important cardiovascular comorbidity. Otherwise, 3,4-dihydroxyphenylacetaldehyde is a reactive and toxic metabolite [23], which may interfere in the bioactivity of the remaining compounds.

As HT is well absorbed and rapidly metabolized [24], its concentrations in plasma can be very low, although other factors such as the vehicle of ingestion may also interfere. For example, after ingesting 25 mL of extra olive oil with 61.4 μg HT/g olive oil [25] or 50 mL of olive oil extract that contains 6.0 μg HT/mL extract, along with bread [14], the maximum HT concentration detected in human plasma was 0.004 μg/L after 15 min of intake and 25.8 μg/L after 32 min, respectively. Additionally, the input of a single dose of 2.5 mg of HT/kg bw in aqueous solution reached 169 μg HT/L 13 min upon ingestion but quickly decreased to undetectable levels after 1 h [26]. Differences between the amount ingested and the levels detected in plasma support the hypothesis that the main part of HT has undergone the first-pass metabolism in great extension and was converted into other metabolites [14]. Moreover, in the study of Tuck and coworkers [27], the authors demonstrated that the estimated HT plasma concentration was significantly reduced if HT was administered to rats as an aqueous solution (solution of radiolabelled HT, 12 mCi/mmol H^3-HT) when compared to a close amount administered as an olive oil solution (17 mCi/mmol). In addition, López de las Hazas and collaborators [24] noticed that the absorption of HT could be improved after dietary supplementation with oleuropein. Overall, it is crucial to further understand the extension of HT metabolization and mechanisms of action in order to establish HT dose effects. In addition, the possible contribution of other phenols such as tyrosol (which may be converted in the human body into HT and vice-versa) to the levels of bioavailable HT and its claimed bioactivities should be clarified [28].

2. Antioxidant Properties of HT

HT is claimed to exert many bioactive properties, including antioxidant, anti-inflammatory, anticancerogenic, neuroprotector, immunomodulatory, cardioprotective, antidiabetic, cytoprotective, antimicrobial, antiviral, endothelial and vascular regulatory, and skin protective properties [15,29–31]. Among these, antioxidant abilities are undoubtedly one of the most relevant properties for application of HT in the food industry, not only because they can impact on the quality of the fortified food products, but also in parameters related to consumers' health. Regarding prevention of cardiovascular diseases, in addition to its antioxidant capacity, HT was also claimed to inhibit platelet aggregation, chronic cardiac toxicity, the expression of proteins related to ageing, as well as attenuation of the metabolic alterations of glucose, triglyceride and total cholesterol [29].

The mechanisms of action of the antioxidant activity of HT include the breakdown of peroxidation chain reactions, such as lipid peroxidation, the scavenging of free radicals, e.g., radical superoxide ($O_2^{\bullet-}$), hydrogen peroxide (H_2O_2) and hypochlorous acid (HOCl), and the prevention of metal ions catalyzing the production of reactive oxygen species (ROS) [15,29]. These properties are due to its catechol group [18] and its ability to act as a chelate of the intracellular iron [32].

The antiradical potential of HT or of HT-rich extracts was confirmed by distinct authors through in vitro assays [33–35], albeit contradictory observations were reported in some cases. Visioli et al. [33] reported the intense radical-scavenging activity of HT and oleuropein towards 2,2-diphenyl-1-picrylhydrazyl radical ($DPPH^{\bullet}$), which was superior to those of 2,6-di-*t*-butyl-4-methylphenol (BHT) and vitamin E, and the ability to eliminate $O_2^{\bullet-}$ and HOCl, in equivalent or higher extension as the reference vitamins E and C. However, in another study, despite both oleuropein and HT being potent hydroxy radical ($OH^{\bullet}$), $O_2^{\bullet-}$, and peroxynitrous acid (ONOOH) scavengers, none of these compounds showed potential to sequester HOCl or H_2O_2 [35]. Moreover, O'Dowd et al. [34] reported that HT had no potential to scavenge $O_2^{\bullet-}$ whereas it was effective towards H_2O_2.

Despite the inconsistency described for the HT scavenging ability in chemical models, cellular studies support its high antioxidant capacity. As shown by Peng and coworkers [36], in rat adrenal pheochromocytoma cells, the pre-treatment of the cells with this phenolic compound at non-toxic concentrations (1–50 μM) remarkably reduced toxic effects induced by H_2O_2 and 6-hydroxydopamine, including amelioration of cellular viability to values above 80%, decreasing of ROS production and prevention of the loss of cellular thiols, which are essential in the intracellular redox balance. Another study performed with kidney cell lines of distinct animals (Madin–Darby canine MDCK, a pig kidney LLC-PK1, and a rabbit kidney RK 13) revealed that 10 μM HT effectively prevented cytotoxicity and the increment of ROS levels induced by ochratoxin-A (a toxic able to cause kidney disorders) [37]. Similarly, in human hepatocarcinoma HepG2 cells oxidized by *t*-butyl hydroperoxide, the pre-treatment with 10–40 μM of HT completely prevented the cell damage and maintained glutathione (GSH; a thiol antioxidant) levels [38]. In addition, cell damage prevention in apoptosis-responsive-cellular models (human monocytoid U937 and murine proliferating muscle C2C12 myoblasts) exposed to H_2O_2 was also noticed with pretreatments of 20 μM of HT or its ester HT laurate [39], and with 0.05 mM and 0.1 mM of HT in Jurkat cells (clone E6-1, peripheral human blood), 30 min before H_2O_2 exposure [32]. Notably, in the work of Rietjens et al. [35], the authors demonstrated that the exposure of low-density lipoproteins (LDL) of healthy human volunteers' blood to 5 μM HT prevented copper (II) sulphate-induced oxidation increased the lag time of conjugated dienes formation (products of oxidation) from 30 to 240 min. The ability to hamper lipid oxidation is extended to HT-rich extracts, as previously demonstrated, e.g., for a purified extract from the solid olive residue (the base of the supplement Oleaselect™ (Milan, Italy)). This extract, containing HT and other phenols, effectively restored the cells and reduced the lipid oxidation in haemolysis-induced cellular rat erythrocytes and endothelial cells [40].

The antioxidant effect of HT also occurs through its ability to stimulate the expression and the activity of antioxidant enzymes. In fact, HT has been claimed to modulate the gene expression of antioxidant enzymes such as catalase (CAT), superoxide dismutase (SOD) and glutathione peroxidase (GPx), which are key regulators of oxidative stress, and the expression of inflammation transcription factors [30,41,42]. According to Zhu et al. [42], at a concentration of 100 μmol/L, HT effectively regulated the transcription of the nuclear factor erythroid 2 (Nfr2) in acrolein-stimulated human retinal pigment epithelial cells (ARPE-19 cells), activating phase II detoxifying enzymes, such as γ-glutamyl cysteine ligase (produces reduced GSH), GPx, nicotinamide adenine dinucleotide phosphate (NADPH)-quinone-oxidoreductase, heme-oxygenase, SOD, peroxiredoxin and thioredoxin. HT also activated peroxisome proliferator-activated receptor coactivator 1α (PPARGC1α), which enhanced mitochondria biogenesis. As a result, it blocked the oxidative damage induced by acrolein and, therefore, the degeneration of these cells. Additionally, Giordano and Visioli [43] reported that HT modulated GSH-driven antioxidant enzymatic machinery of mice pre-adipocyte cells (murine 3T3-L1), thus mitigating the H_2O_2-induced alterations regarding the reduced/oxidized GSH ratio, an oxidative stress indicator.

Antioxidant-related health effects of HT are supported by animal studies. Granados-Principal et al. [44] demonstrated that the administration of 0.5 mg HT/kg, five days/week for six weeks in Sprague-Dawley rats with breast cancer, mitigated the cardiotoxicity caused by doxorubicin (a chemotherapy drug), reduced ROS production and restored the redox chain in mitochondria. In another work, González-Santiago and coworkers [45] reported that the supply of 4 mg of HT/kg bw to hyperlipidemic male New Zealand rabbits for one month led to an improvement in the antioxidant status and the blood lipid profile of the animals, as well as to a decrease in the levels of total cholesterol and total triglycerides. Additionally, the same study noticed a reduction in the size of arteriosclerosis lesions in a histological cross-section of the aortic arch, a consequence of the hyperlipidemic rabbits. Furthermore, the supply of 40–80 mg HT/kg bw to lipopolysaccharide (LPS)-induced inflammation Balb/c mice subjected to different time points of administration caused an overall increment of the plasma antioxidant power, prevented the LPS-induced DNA damage and decreased the levels of several pro-inflammatory markers such as cyclooxygenase-2 and tumor necrosis factor-α (TNFα) [46]. Pan and coworkers [47] also highlighted a decrease in the levels of TNFα and other inflammatory proteins (interleukin-6 and macrophage inflammatory protein 2) in the liver tissues of male mice Balb/c and an increase in CAT and SOD activity after HT treatment (1 or 10 mg HT/kg), overall preventing ischemia/reperfusion injury of the liver. In addition, Feng et al. [48] reported that HT was able to regulate dynamic mitochondrial remodeling and enhance antioxidant enzyme activity of the respiratory chain in the muscle of rats subjected to strenuous physical exercise.

In vivo studies performed with HT-rich extracts also support HT antioxidant-related capacities. In a study conducted by Jemai et al. [49], the authors used olive leaf extract (OLE) and its corresponding acid and enzymatic hydrolysate extracts (1.4 g HT/100 g and 3.82 g HT/100 g dry weight, respectively) to supplement the cholesterol-rich diet of rats over sixteen weeks, having shown that these promote the activity of hepatic antioxidant enzymes and a simultaneous decrease in the levels of total cholesterol, triglycerides and LDL, compared to rats fed with a non-supplemented cholesterol diets. Additionally, the feeding of diabetic rats with a pellet diet fortified with a purified-HT extract from olive milled waste origin (20 mg HT/kg bw) was shown to increase the activity of SOD, CAT and GPx in the liver and kidney, as well as other enzymes that catalyze the phosphorylation of glucose. As a result, the glucose level in plasma decreased by 55% [50]. Moreover, in an European clinical trial (EUROLIVE study, Effects of Olive Oil Consumption on Oxidative Damage in European Populations), the daily intake of virgin olive oil (VOO), with 366 mg of phenolic content/kg, over three weeks was demonstrated to increase high-density lipoprotein (HDL) content while also reducing lipid oxidation in human volunteers [51]. This is consistent with other pre-clinical studies that remarked the ability of HT in reducing thrombogenic, platelet aggregation factors and markers of inflammation at a cellular level [15,29], thus inhibiting arteriosclerosis, among other comorbidities [29,31].

3. Applicability of Hydroxytyrosol in Food Products

3.1. Consumption Recommendations

The minimum recommended HT amount (including its derivatives) for manutention of cardiovascular health by the EFSA and FDA panel [1,2] reinforces the necessity to incorporate HT in other food products. As an integrated part of a food product, the EFSA has established HT concentrations for fishery products and vegetable oils, as well as for margarine, of 215 mg/kg and 175 mg/kg, respectively. For other types of food, the amount of HT is suggested to be adjusted, taking into account the HT content in the background diet [1]. Moreover, according to the FDA, final concentrations should comprise between 8 and 21 mg/kg for energy drinks and vegetables/fruits beverages, respectively; 167 to 250 mg/kg for snacks and baked goods; 44 to 333 mg/kg for sauces, condiments, fat and oil products and, finally, about 1.1 g/kg for meat, poultry and fish coating mixes [2].

So far, the HT toxicological data are mainly based on cell and animal studies. Among them, the study of D'Angelo and coworkers [52] represented a hallmark, with no adverse effects (NOAEL) being registered upon the induction of acute toxicity in rats by injection of a single dose of 2 g of HT/kg bw. Afterward, subchronic toxicity studies with oral gavage administration through a daily dose of aqueous olive pulp extract at levels of 500, 1000 or 2000 mg/kg [53], as well as 5, 50 or 500 mg HT/kg bw per day [54], did not cause any adverse effects. Auñon-Calles and his collaborator [54] assumed the lowest observed adverse effect level at 500 mg of HT/kg bw per day and a NOAEL of 250 mg/kg bw per day. The only difference noted was salivation before and after administration in all animals, which the authors attributed to the bitter taste of HT and the oily and dense formulation. Considering these studies, the EFSA panel recommended a maximum daily HT intake of 100 mg/kg body weight per day for children and 200 mg/kg body weight per day for adolescents, adults and elderly [1].

3.2. Application of HT in the Functional Food Market

As for other natural bioactive compounds, obtaining pure HT and its use in food products is hardly considered economically viable. Therefore, a variety of approaches to meet market requirements for a lower cost HT, including its exploitation from natural sources or the use of biocatalysis, have been proposed [55]. Part of this solution involves the use of by-products. In fact, the cheapest sources of HT comprise olive pomace, olive mill wastewaters (OMWW), and olive leaves, from which the obtention of HT-rich extracts or pure HT requires the combination of solvent extraction, membrane filtration technology and stabilization by lyophilization or spray-drying [56]. Thus, it is possible to find many patented adaptations of the olive pressing systems, extraction procedures [57–59] and purification methods [60], aiming at the full use of these resources [61], and at the promotion of circular economy processes, through the usage of olive oil by-products for the development of the extracts.

Supplements and Patented HT-Rich Extracts

HT-rich extracts are widely marketed as food supplements or healthy ingredients. Among them, Hidrox (CreAgri, Hayward, CA, USA) is a formulation of olive polyphenols rich in HT obtained from vegetative waters, certified as Generally Recognized as Safe (GRAS) and patented (patent EP06025262A). It is used to formulate other supplements such as the OLIVACTIV™ (20–35 weight % of HT), the OLEASELECT™ (total content of HT of ≥1.5 weight %), the OLIVE(OLEA)DRY, i.e., a powder containing from 22 to 24 g of HT per kg, and Prolivols (20 mg of HT per g) [62]. Hytolive (Genosa, Spain) is a patented olive extract [63], which was previously shown to be effective in reducing inflammation among early-stage breast cancer patients [64]. Phenolea® (Phenofarm, Scandriglia, Italy) is an active complex also derived from a natural standardized olive pulp extract through a patented mechanical process, in which HT accounts for 30% of all phenols. Evidence has shown that its administration to mice modulates the level of cytokines, having a role in the process of inflammation [65]. Moreover, Aponte et al. [66] used Phenolea® as a source of HT to produce oral granules for co-delivery of *L. plantarum* and a standardized OLE. Through in vivo data, they noticed that co-administration of live *L. plantarum* bacteria with the olive phenol-containing extract provided higher amounts of bioavailable HT compared to the extract alone. Another example is the Oleaselect® (Indena, Milan, Italy), obtained by a patented process (patent US 6358542B2) from olive-based starting materials, including olives, olive pulps, olive oil, and wastewater from olive oil manufacturing, and claimed to achieve an extract with antioxidant activity four to five times higher than the hydroalcoholic extract of solid olive residue [40]. Mediteanox® (Euromed S.A., Barcelona, Spain) is another registered supplement. Notably, oral administration of three capsules of supplement that contains a combined 3.3 mg of HT from Mediteanox® and 65 mg of punicalagin from Pomanox® (a pomegranate natural extract, Euromed S.A., Barcelona, Spain), per day for eight weeks, significantly improved the endothelial function and blood pressure, and reduced LDL oxidation in middle-aged subjects [67]. In the case of Mediteanox®, the studied dosage gets closer to the minimum daily recommendation (5 mg HT per day).

3.3. HT as a Food Ingredient

3.3.1. Plant-Based Products

HT has also been proposed as a functional ingredient in various food matrices, including edible oils [68], beverages, bakery products, as reported in Table 1 [69–95].

Table 1. Applicability of free or extract-based hydroxytyrosol (HT) on edible oils, beverages, and vegetable-based and bakery food products.

Formulation	Dosage Applied to Food Products	Main Findings	Ref
	Edible oils		
HT Rosemary EXT	200 mg/kg HT in *Echium* oil	↑ oil antioxidant status (1.4-fold) HT > rosemary EXT	[69]
Olive cake/dried *Thymus zygis EXT*	VOO supplementation Three oils doses tested (25 mL): 0.01 [a], 0.12 [b] and 0.21 [c] mg of HT	Thirty-three hypercholesterolemic individuals ingested VOO [a], olive EXT supplemented VOO [b] and olive/thyme EXT supplemented VOO [c] (25 mL of olive oil/day, 3 weeks): ↑ HDL antioxidant compounds; ↑ blood plasma antioxidant activity; No consequences on levels of fat intake	[70]
OMWW EXTHT	200 mg/kg of HT and EXT in husk and olive oils (EXT with 1225.6 mg HT/L)	↓ oxidation rate; ↓ peroxide values HT antioxidant effect > BHT	[71]
Olivefen® DHPG, HT, and α-tocopherol mixes	8, 20, 40 and 80 mg Olivefen® to 50 g vegetable oil; Olivefen (37.75% HT) Mixes (0.125–3 mmol/kg vegetable oil)	↑ oxidative stability of oils (DHPG/HT combination > Olivefen®); Antioxidant synergic effect in HT/DHPG mixtures	[72]
OMWW EXT	350 to 531 mg HT/kg refined olive oil for French fries	↓ α-tocopherol oxidation; ↓ formation acrolein and hexanal Preservation of French fries sensory and nutritional values; ↑ color, texture score and taste	[73]
Olive cake EXT	Olive oil supplementation Olive cake EXT = 6.64 mg HT/kg olive oil cake	Single-dose of 30 mL enriched olive oil administered to thirteen pre- and stage-1 hypertensive patients: ↓ oxidation of LDL; more benefits on endothelial function than a standard VOO - ↑ ischemic reactive hyperemia	[74]
PO + gallic acid, caffeic acid and HT	PO/EVO: 20:80, 40:60 and 80:20 (100 mg each phenol /kg PO)	No PO oxidation stability by HT (gallic acid > caffeic acid > HT); PO stabilize mixtures < 20% EVO	[75]
HT	Patented application of HT to supplements and edibles oils 30–300 mg HT/kg edible oils 300–30,000 mg HT/kg dietary supplements	Prevention/treatment of cardiovascular diseases, plaque build-up, arterial hypertension, metabolic syndrome	[76]
	Beverages		
Olive by-products HT EXT	80 mg HT or EXT/L white wine (Sauvignon blanc)	↑ yellowness; ↑ visual appearance score (first six months of bottling); preservation of VC; ↓ Sauvignon blanc wines character (≠ aromas)	[80]

Table 1. *Cont.*

Formulation	Dosage Applied to Food Products	Main Findings	Ref
Olive by-products HT EXT	50 mg HT or EXT/L red wine (Syrah)	better red wine chromatic parameters (at bottling); ↓ fruit aroma scents and oxidation odors; ↓ Syrah characteristics after six months	[82]
Olive leaf EXT (OLE)	30 and 60 mg OLE/100 mL fruit smoothies "strawberry-banana"	↑ bitterness perception; recommended < 20 mg OLE/100 g (to prevent bitterness)	[83]
HT	0.02, 0.2 and 1 mg HT/mL tomato juice	0.2 and 1 mg/mL of HT ↑ antioxidant activity (3 and 8-fold, respectively); 1 mg/mL of HT ↓ lipid peroxidation (> BHA); No changes in sensory quality and color. Favorable olive oil taste.	[84]
Olive leaves (dry, infusion, atomized extract)	0.34,1.01, 1.74 and 3 g atomized/L; 0.34, 1.01 and 132 mL infusion/L, 9.9 g leaves/L dry leaves (1.27 mg HT/g), infusion (3.43 mg HT/g), and atomized extract (5.58 mg HT/g)	↑ PC, antioxidant, HT content; Sour/astringent taste, herbal aroma; colloidal instability of beer	[85]
	Vegetable-based products		
OLE	Table olives fermentation (0.7 kg of olives and 0.7 L of brine solution with 200 mg OLE/L)	↑ antioxidant, anti-inflammatory, and antimicrobial substances; ↓ bitter taste; No adverse effect on their sensorial qualities	[88]
OLE	30 kg table olives for 30 L OLE with 8% NaCl brine solution and starter culture	↑ PC, mostly HT (1700 mg/kg flesh olives vs. 900 mg/kg control olives)	[89]
HT/OLEUR EXT	Table olives submerged in EXT (200 mg HT/kg EXT)	↑ HT content in table olive (↑ 109%); ↑ bitterness; good overall acceptability	[87]
OMWW EXT	0.44, 1.00, 2.25 or 5.06 g EXT/kg vegetable meals: bean purée, potato purée, tomato juice	↑ PC (from 3.7 to 13%); ↑ bitterness, sourness, astringency and pungency	[90]
	Bakery products		
HT	5.25 mg HT/30 g Biscuit (20% of HT is lost during baking)	↓ oxidized LDL levels; No changes in antioxidant activity of human serum (pharmacokinetic assay)	[91]
Olive pomace EXT*	Biscuit enriched in olive pomace extract (PreBiÒ®) (8.11 μg HT/g biscuit),	Human intake study (90 g biscuit/day, 8 weeks): subtle change on bacteria abundance of gut microbiota ↑ homovanillic acid and DOPAC; ↓ oxidative LDL cholesterol	[92]

Table 1. *Cont.*

Formulation	Dosage Applied to Food Products	Main Findings	Ref
HT/OLE	2.55, 5.11 and 10.22 mg of HT/g dough; 0.127 and 0.537 mg of OLE/g dough OLE (0.15 mg HT/mL)	↑ slight the darkens the biscuits; ↑ antiglycative effect	[93]
OLE	17% OLE (weight/weight) OLE (24.08 mg gallic acid equivalent/g dry weight)	↑ antioxidant activity, total flavonoids and PC ↑ dark color	[94]
OMWW EXT Ascorbic acid α-Tocopherol (powder and emulsion)	50, 200, 500, 1000, 2000, 3000 mg olive PC/kg bread 100, 200, 400 mg olive PC/kg Rusk	200 mg PC/kg was the most efficient as antimicrobial; ↑ antimicrobial emulsification effect and shelf life of both bread (from 10 to 15 days) and rusk samples (up to 12 weeks)	[95]

Abbreviations: BHA—3-*t*-butyl-4-hydroxyanisole; BHT—2,6-di-*t*-butyl-4-methylphenol; DHPG—3,4-dihydroxyphenylglycol; DOPAC—3,4-dihydroxyphenylacetic acid; EVO—extra virgin oil; EXT—extract; HDL—high-density lipoprotein; HT—hydroxytyrosol; LDL—low-density lipoproteins; OLE—olive leaf extract; OMWW—olive mill wastewater; PC—phenolic compounds; PO—palm oil; VC—volatile compounds; VOO—virgin olive oil. ([a]—dose of VOO containing 0.01 mg of HT; [b]—dose of olive EXT supplemented with VOO with 0.12 mg of HT; [c]— dose of olive/thyme EXT supplemented with VOO with 0.21 mg of HT; ↑—increase; ↓—decrease).

Edible Oils

Edible oils, particularly refined ones, are prone to oxidation [68], but fortification with HT can delay this phenomenon [69–74]. The fortification of edible oils has been obtained by the addition of the pure compound or through extracts. OMWW extract (containing 1225.6 mg/L of HT, among other phenols), added to refined olive oils at a concentration of 200 mg/kg, reduced the peroxide values and delayed the oxidation rate, even better than BHT [71]. In addition to HT, this OMWW extract also contained DOPAC, an HT derivative, which could contribute to these effects [71]. Additionally, with OMWW extract, the supplementation of oils for French fries significantly hampered the oxidation of α-tocopherol and the formation of unwanted compounds (e.g. acrolein and hexanal) during the frying process. Curiously, this supplementation increased the number of available sugars and, consequently, the extension of Maillard reactions, resulting in French fries with a more positive taste and better color [73]. In echium oil, which is more susceptible to oxidation than other vegetable oils, 200 mg of HT/kg substantially protected the oil from the oxidation process [69]; however, this was only verified under non-thermal conditions [75].

In addition to HT, other compounds that exist in HT-rich extracts may exhibit a synergic effect. This observation was made by Lama-Muñoz and coworkers [72], who reported that a mixture of HT with 3,4-dihydroxyphenylglycol (DHPG) (proportion 2:1) was more efficient in delaying the oxidation of the vegetable oil than the commercial Olivefen®. This reinforces the idea that natural antioxidants' activity is affected by multicomponent foods and varies according to the extract composition.

Nevertheless, regarding the health effects of HT in oils, the main studies focus on olive oil, which is the best natural source of HT through diet. For example, Valls et al. [74] tested a single dose of 30 mL of olive oil supplemented with a phenolic-rich extract from olive cake (with 6.64 mg HT/kg olive oil cake) in hypertensive patients (in pre- and stage 1). They found that the olive oil supplement caused more positive effects on the patient's endothelial function than the ingestion of a standard virgin olive oil, especially in terms of the decrease in oxidized LDL and blood stimulation flow (reactive hyperemia). Similarly, Farràs et al. [70] evaluated the regular intake of 25 mL per day of distinct olive oil that provided 0.01, 0.12 and 0.21 mg of HT, for three weeks in hypercholesterolemic patients, and they noticed benefits, namely in the improvement of HDL levels and blood plasma antioxidant activity, without increasing the individual's fat intake. Thus, in addition to the ability of HT to stabilize oily matrices, edible oils fortified with HT may also be suitable to act as a functional food to prevent cardiovascular comorbidities.

At present, there are also several patented applications of HT in edible oils, Más et al. [76] patented fortified edible oils, fortified edible oil-containing products and dietary supplements in the form of soft gel capsules containing fortified edible oils, with increased antioxidant capacity to be used as a source of HT for prevention or treatment of cardiovascular diseases, plaque build-up in the arteries, arterial hypertension and metabolic syndrome [76]. In the same line, Bulbarello and collaborators [77] patented capsules for oral consumption of an edible oil fortified with HT (more than 250 mg HT/kg fortified oil). Moreover, the addition of an extract of bisphenol with more than 60% of HT and a terpene extract with more than 80% of maslinic acid to an extra VOO or olive oil was also patented [78].

Beverages

In beverages, wine is valorized as a functional food towards cardiovascular diseases due to its polyphenol content, especially resveratrol and HT, the latter resulting from tyrosol through alcoholic fermentation [7]. However, the use of sulfur additives, such as a sulfur oxide (SO_2), to prevent the degradation of wine, including oxidation, may induce a range of adverse health effects in sensitive individuals [79]. Thus, efforts have been made to reduce or replace its usage, betting on the use of HT as a promising natural antioxidant alternative [80,81], although the characteristic aroma of HT-rich extracts may hinder its application [82]. In fact, Raposo et al. [80] demonstrated that the use of 80 mg of HT/L in white wine (Sauvignon Blanc) intensified its color when compared to control samples, even after six months of storage in a bottle, but its score was injured with regard to the olfactometric profile. In red wines (Syrah), Raposo and coworkers [82] reported that its fortification with 50 mg of HT/L improved color parameters (namely the red chromatid) and the scent and tasting at bottling. However, after six months of storage, the bottle HT wines were more oxidized than SO_2 wines, showing new odorant zones from the added product and oxidation. Hence, the authors recommended the combined use of HT with sulfur dioxide, reducing the sulfur content without compromising the wine oxidation.

The application of HT was also demonstrated in fruit juices [83,84] to improve their nutritional properties. In fruit smoothies, the addition of OLE (HT-rich extract) increased their bitterness, but this could be masked if lower concentrations were used (below 20 mg/100 g), or by adding ingredients with known bitterness-masking properties [83]. However, the lower concentrations proposed had lower phenolic content compared to coffee or tea [83]. In an attempt to formulate a functional juice, Larrosa et al. [84] added enzymatically-synthesized HT at a concentration of 1 mg/mL to tomato juice and claimed that 200 mL of this juice would provide 4 mg of HT, which is close to the minimum recommended by the ESFA. In this matrix, the HT was more efficient than a commercial antioxidant (3-t-butyl-4-hydroxyanisole, BHA) in improving antioxidant activity and deaccelerating lipid oxidation (over eight- and three-fold, respectively). Additionally, HT remained stable in the tomato juice matrix at room temperature and light exposure storage conditions for 48 days without affecting the sensory properties (flavor and color) in great extension [84].

More recently, Guglielmotti and coworkers [85] incorporated HT as part of brewing to fortify a beer. They used olive leaves as an ingredient of beer, in the form of dry crumbled leaves (1.27 mg of HT/g), infusion (3.43 mg of HT/g), and an atomized extract (5.58 mg of HT/g), that were added near to the boiling phase of brewing, thus promoting the hydrolysis of oleuropein of the leaves to HT. The addition of 10 g/L of olive leaves conferred to the beers a sour/astringent taste and herbal aroma, whereas 5 g/L olive left a more soft and pleasant sensory profile. Both results could be interesting to formulate distinct beers, especially with increased antioxidant capacity and polyphenol content.

Regarding HT's sensorial impact, efforts have been made to overcome HT's bitter taste in the products. An example of this is a patented beverage with HT (in the amount of 0.5–50 mg/100 mL) that claims to be easily drinkable due to the presence of ethanol, propylene glycol, and caffeine at a specific rate that disguises the characteristics of the flavor of HT [86].

Vegetable-Based Products

Although table olives are a source of HT, their fermentation process often changes and/or reduces their phenolic fraction. Some authors proposed the supplementation with HT or HT-rich extracts to balance this loss (Table 1). In fact, even supplemented with OLE, there was a decrease in the concentration of total phenolics during the fermentation of table olives, but, in the case of HT, it increased upon 120 days in brine and olive flesh samples, achieving in the final of fermentation the levels of 2489 mg/L of HT and 187 mg HT/kg, respectively, with no or only slight changes in their sensory acceptability [88]. These observations were consistent with the work of Schaide et al. [89], who reported that the addition of OLE to table olives increased the levels of HT (1700 mg/kg in olive flesh and 3500 mg/L in brined olive flesh) as compared to control conditions (900 and 2500 mg/L respectively), and provided olives without bitterness after 121 days of fermentation. In line with the previous studies, the sensory acceptability was unchanged in Lalas et al.'s study [87], after the addition of OLE (200 mg HT/kg extract) to table olives fermented for a week, while the HT content increased from 408 to 855 mg/kg in flesh table olives.

In addition to table olives, the fortification of bean purée, potato purée, and tomato juice with an OMWW extract (0.44, 1.00, 2.25, or 5.06 g extract/kg food product) increased bitterness and intensified the sourness and astringency. Pungency was suppressed in bean purée and perceived at a weak-moderate intensity in potato purée and tomato juice samples at the highest phenol concentration [90]. As table olives are already a natural source of HT, their application should be more explored in other vegetable-based products.

Bakery Products

Bakery products are attractive food products for HT supplementation since they are largely consumed by different populational groups of all ages. Among bakery products, a major part of the studies investigated biscuits. For instance, Mateos et al. [91] reported that the human intake of HT-fortified biscuits (30 g biscuits that provide 5.25 mg of HT, after an overnight fast) was able to reduce the levels of oxidized LDL in blood, even though there was no increase in the antioxidant activity in blood serum. In the same line but with a different source of HT, Conterno et al. [92] found that the 90 g daily doses of biscuits supplemented with an olive pomace extract (8.11 μg of HT/g biscuit, provides 729.9 μg of HT), consumed daily for eight weeks, increased homovanillic acid and DOPAC levels, which were suggested by the authors to be involved in the reduction in oxidative LDL cholesterol. Note, however, that sensory changes may occur, as noticed by Navarro and Morales [93] in HT and OLE-fortified biscuits (at different concentrations of HT, 2.55, 5.11 and 10.22 mg of HT/g dough, and OLE, 0.127 and 0.537 mg of OLE/g dough), which became darker than the plain products. Yet, in some conditions, a synergy between components of the extract can contribute to the antiglycative effect; hence, suppressing these changes. A similar pattern of results was obtained in the work of Cedola et al. [94]. In the Italian biscuit "taralli", the replacement of the ingredient white wine by OLE (17% weight/weight, 24.08 mg gallic acid equivalent/g dry weight) turned the biscuit color darker without changing the overall quality score. Moreover, the addition of OLE improved the nutritional quality of "taralli", increasing antioxidant activity, total phenols and, especially, flavonoid content from 0.09 mg quercetin/g dry weight in plain samples to 0.39 and 0.36 mg quercetin/g dry weight of uncooked and cooked, respectively [94].

Apart from this, one must also remark the promising application of HT as a functional ingredient in bakery products, aiming to improve their quality. In this regard, the fortification of bread and rusk with olive polyphenols by emulsion was reported to extend their shelf-life from 10 to 15 days. Among the tested concentrations (50–3000 mg olive phenols/kg bread, 100–400 mg olive phenols/kg rusk), that of 200 mg of polyphenols/kg was the most efficient in terms of antimicrobial activity, particularly in rusk [95]. Furthermore, related to this topic, a bread containing Hytolive 2 developed from Genosa (Spain), and the Puratos' Nostrum brand bread is possible to find on the market [96]. However, in vivo tests are needed to support the potential of these breads as a functional food.

3.3.2. Animal-Based Food Products

Animal-based products such as meat, fish and dairy products [97–119], using HT as an ingredient, are summarized in Table 2.

Table 2. Applicability of free or extract-based HT on animal-based products and its effect on product quality.

Formulation	Dosage Applied to Food Products	Main Findings	Ref
		Meat products	
Olive EXT	100 mg HT/kg low-fat frankfurters sausages	↓ lipid oxidation; HT antioxidant potential > BHA/BHT	[102]
OMWW EXT/OLE/Olive oil, walnut	50 mg of HT/kg chicken sausages	↓ lipid and protein oxidation; ↓ sausage acceptability with olive oil. ↓ stale odor of sausages with OMWW EXT and walnuts (7 and 14 days); ↑ cooking loss, change the color, texture, and taste	[103]
OMWW EXT	150 mg OMWW (66.8% of HT)/kg lard	↓ peroxidation	[104]
Olive vegetative water EXT	0.075 and 0.15 g EXT/100 g pork sausage	↓ pH, diacylglycerols, peroxide value and cholesterol oxidation; no unpleasant sensory properties	[105]
Olive waste EXT (Hytolive®)	Hytolive®: 10.5% HT in EXT 100, 200 or 400 mg GAE/kg lamb meat patties	↓ lipid oxidation and protein carbonylation; ↑ loss of thiol groups during 6 days of storage; ↓ meat discoloration; change in odor and flavor; texture stable	[106]
Olive pomace HT with grape seed or chestnut EXT	10 g EXT/kg sausages (EXT with11.65 g of HT/L)	↓ lipid oxidation; ↓ microbial growth, comparable to nitrites Changes in profile, color, and texture; good acceptability	[107]
OMWW EXT	100.23 ± 5.25 mg HT/g EXT Fermented sausages dipped 2.5% of OMWW	↓ undesired fungal species growth; ↓ VC (from fatty acids oxidative degradation)	[108]
Olive oil EXT	Olive oil, 1 and 3% to ground beef	↓ E. coli cell count; ↓ amine formation	[110]
HT	3.6 g HT/kg fresh pork	Aged rats fed with high cholesterol/high saturated fat diets: ↓ body weight; ↓ cholesterol content in very-low-density lipoprotein (VLDL) (74% less); ↓ VLDL total mass (63% less)	[109]
OLE	1, and 5% of OLE with 7.32% of HT	↑ antioxidant activity; ↓ microbial growth no impact on overall acceptability	[111]
HT and OMWW extract	200 mg/kg lamb burgers patties HT 99.2% purity; OMWW extract: 7.3% HT	Both induced ↓ lipid oxidation and ↓ the microbiological growth; good color maintenance and general acceptability; ↑ loss of thiol maintenance and general acceptability. HT more efficient	[112]

Table 2. *Cont.*

Formulation	Dosage Applied to Food Products	Main Findings	Ref
		Fishery products	
HT	50 and 100 mg HT/kg fresh horse mackerel (*Trachurus trachurus*), cod (*Gadus morhua*) liver oil	↓ lipid oxidation in bulk oil and minced horse mackerel during frozen storage; ↓ generation of oxidation products; preservation of PUFAs content	[113]
OLE	Anchovy fillets: marinade (1:1) marinade = 10 mg/mL of OLE	in vitro antimicrobial activity, inclusive psychrophilic bacteria ↓ oxidation; preservation of texture, appearance, and organoleptic characteristics	[114]
OLE Fruit EXT	200 mg OLE/kg fish patties	↑ antioxidant activity; ↓ VC (oxidation indicators); ↓ viable count patties, after 11 days (*S. Aureus* > *E. coli* and *L. monocytogenes*)	[115]
		Dairy products	
OMWW EXT	100 or 200 mg PC/mL functional milk beverage (yogurt-like)	No interference with the fermentation/lactic acid bacteria; No impact on the VC	[116]
Medoliva© (Polyhealth S.A. Larissa, Greece)	olive PC encapsulated in maltodextrin (0.5 mg HT/g powder) Greek yogurt 2% fat	Human intake of 50 mg olive PC + 400 g yogurt/day, 2 weeks: ↓ body weight, body mass index, hip circumference and systolic blood pressure; ↓ LDL cholesterol levels In yogurt: ↑ lactic acid bacteria during fermentation, ↓ spoilage	[117]
Olive oil extract	0.625 mg EXT/mL milk	↓ vegetative cells to undetectable levels	[118]
VOO EXT Vinegar Wine	VOO (52.8 mg HT/kg); olive oil (14.1 mg HT/kg) VOO EXT (36.9 mg HT/kg); olive oil EXT (13.5 mg HT/kg to milk and egg mayonnaises	↑ bactericidal effect (vinegar > aqueous VOO EXT > wines > olive oil EXT); ↓ *Salmonella Enteritidis and Listeria monocytogenes* (VOO mayonnaise ~ 3 log CFU/g > olive oil mayonnaise)	[119]

Abbreviations: BHA—3-*t*-butyl-4-hydroxyanisole; BHT—2,6-di-*t*-butyl-4-methylphenol; CFU—colony-forming unit; EXT—extract; GAE—gallic acids equivalent; HT—hydroxytyrosol; LDL—low-density lipoproteins; OLE—olive leaf extract; OMWW—olive mill wastewater; PC—phenolic compounds; PUFAs—polyunsaturated fatty acids; VC—volatile compounds; VLDL—very-low-density lipoprotein; VOO—virgin olive oil. (↑—increase; ↓—decrease).

Meat-Based Products

Meat products with high-fat content, such as lard or sausages, are prone to lipid oxidation either during manufacturing, storage or cooking, and this may lead to a decline in nutritional quality, color changes, texture deterioration, off-odors and off-flavors, and generation of toxic compounds [97]. Concerns about the negative health impacts of the industrial use of nitrites and synthetic antioxidants, such as BHT or BHA [98–100], have increased over the last few years and they have clearly prompted the search for natural antioxidant alternatives, such as HT. The fortification of HT in meat-based products has been reported by several authors (Table 2), most of them already considered in the review of Martínez et al. [101].

In this context, Cofrades et al. [102] studied the antioxidant activity of HT-fortified sausage frankfurters with 100 mg of HT/kg meat batter, highlighting that HT effectively inhibited oxidation to the same extent of BHA and BHT. A smaller amount was applied by Nieto et al. [103], 50 mg of HT/kg sausages, which still prevented the lipid oxidation and the loss of thiol groups, in comparison with control samples. The authors suggested that the replacement of animal fat by olive oil and walnuts could be an alternative to produce healthier meat products. Similar antioxidant potential was noticed with the application of 150 mg OMWW extract/kg of lard (HT representing 66.8%) [104], as well through the use of a purified phenolic-rich extract obtained from olive vegetation water in fresh pork sausages [105]. In the same line, in lamb meat patties enriched with omega-3 (n-3) fatty acids, the addition of the olive waste extract Hytolive® (containing 10.5% of HT), at concentrations of 100, 200 or 400 mg gallic acid equivalent/kg muscle, was demonstrated to delay meat discoloration, lipid oxidation, and protein carbonylation, and increased the loss of thiol groups relative to controls, during six days of storage [106].

Nevertheless, Nieto et al. [103] reported changes in the general acceptability of the sausages supplemented with olive oil and HT-rich extract (50 mg/kg), mostly in flavor and odor, especially when supplemented with olive oil, which lowered the sensorial acceptability score. Yet, the opposite trend was observed by Aquilani et al. [107] and Chaves-López et al. [108] in HT-fortified fermented sausages under different concentrations (higher, around 11.65 mg HT/kg) or even using a distinct supplementation method (submersion in 2.5% of OMWW extract), for which the authors only noticed a color change. Additionally, it was also pointed out that the HT supplementation resulted in a more compact meat emulsion, less porous structure, and more reddish color as a consequence of the possible interaction of HT with fat and protein particles with myoglobin [103].

In the context of in vivo experiments supporting the health-promoting effects caused by HT-fortified meat products, Santos-López et al. [109] studied the impact on pork meat supplemented with 3.6 g HT/kg of fresh batter on the lipoprotein profile of aged rats fed high cholesterol/high saturated fat diets. The results show a decrease in adverse effects associated with the diet, mainly by reducing the amount of total cholesterol.

In addition to preventing lipid oxidation, HT-rich extracts have also been claimed to be able to inhibit the growth of major foodborne pathogens, such as *Escherichia coli*, *Listeria monocytogenes*, *Staphylococcus* spp., *Clostridium* spp. and *Salmonella* spp. This effect was comparable to sodium nitrite, i.e., a commercial preservative usually used in meat products [107]. In the study of Chaves-López et al. [108], fermented sausages dipped in 2.5% of OMWW extract (100.23 mg HT/g of extract) resisted the development of fungal species and volatile compound characteristics of fatty acid oxidation. In the work of Rounds and colleagues [110], the authors demonstrated that the addition of an olive oil extract to ground beef (1 and 3%) reduced the *E. coli* population to levels below detectable limits, as well as the amine formation (i.e., carcinogenic compounds that resulted from the heating process) to about half of their initial values. Moreover, the application of olive leaf extracts from *Olea europaea* var. sylvestris (rich in oleuropein and HT) to raw halal minced beef at 1 and 5% was shown to improve the levels of antioxidants in the food products, and simultaneously reduce psychrotrophic counts and pathogens, without any influence on the overall acceptability [111].

More recently, the effect of a HT-rich extract from vegetative waters on the shelf-life of lamb meat burger patties was tested [112], allowing the conclusion that the fortification of this product in 200 mg/kg patties prevented lipid oxidation and microbiological growth, although with less efficiency when compared to pure HT.

Fishery-Based Products

In addition to meat products, fishery products are a great source of lipids, particularly of long-chain polyunsaturated fatty acids ω-3 (PUFAs), which makes them well recommended by the World Health Organization for preventing cardiovascular diseases. Within this scope, their preservation becomes essential and many antioxidant compounds have been tested to prevent oxidative deterioration of PUFAs during processing and storage. Curiously, the fortification of horse mackerel, bulk cod liver oil and cod liver oil-in-water emulsions with HT (50 mg of HT/kg) showed comparable results with the propyl gallate (a synthetic phenol) (Table 2) regarding the prevention of lipid oxidation, while in cod liver bulk oil and cod liver oil-in-water emulsions, the best oxidative stability was obtained at 100 mg of HT/kg. In horse mackerel muscle, the peroxide values stayed below 20 milliequivalent (meq) oxygen/kg fat even after four weeks of frozen storage (control showed 100 meq oxygen/kg fat). Furthermore, HT allowed good preservation of the original content of docosahexaenoic acid (DHA, 22:6ω-3), as well as of α-tocopherol (decrements are often used as a reflection of oxidative stress of fish) [113]. Moreover, the application of an OLE was effective to hinder the microbial growth of psychrophilic bacteria in anchovy fillets [114], as well to preserve fish patties against *Staphilococcus aureus*, *E. coli*, and *L. monocytogenes* [115], simultaneously contributing favorable sensory and preventive oxidation properties.

Dairy Products

Consumers of a wide range of ages consume dairy products, which make them promising functional foods. A functional milk beverage (yogurt-like) was developed by mixing an OMWW extract in pasteurized cow's milk concentrated to a final concentration of 100–200 mg/L (expressed in HT equivalent) (Table 2). The added phenols did not interfere either with the fermentation nor with functional lactic acid bacteria, and the HT content increased during the storage. In fact, the authors claimed that, in terms of phenolic content, the consumption of 100 mL of this beverage is almost equivalent to 20 g of VOO (containing 500 mg/kg phenols), and hence extends the health benefits of olive phenols to a milk beverage [116]. Curiously, a HT-rich product obtained from olive fruits (Medoliva©, 0.5 g HT/g powder) added to yogurt was shown to improve the growth of lactic acid bacteria and to contribute to preventing spoilage during fermentation, as well as to promote benefits towards the lipid metabolism of consumers. In non-declared pathology individuals, the daily consumption of two yogurts (200 g each) for two weeks did not change blood redox status but reduced LDL cholesterol [117]. Thus, this yogurt may be integrated into the concept of functional food. In fact, another HT-fortified yogurt (HT concentration ranges of 0.1 and 0.01%) was developed and patented by Villanova and her collaborators [120], which suggests some competition regarding this type of food.

In addition to yogurt, the application of HT in regular milk has also been reported before. In this regard, Fei et al. [118] described that the addition of an olive oil extract (at concentrations of 0.625 mg/mL, containing ≥ 6% HT) exhibited antimicrobial activity, decreasing the vegetative cells to undetectable levels. In milk or egg-based mayonnaise, the addition of VOO also showed bactericidal activity for *Salmonella enteritidis* and *L. monocytogenes* [119], which may be relevant considering mayonnaise's application in raw products, such as salads.

4. Conclusions

The vastness of information regarding bioactivity, metabolism, and absorption of HT makes it an exciting compound to be considered as a potential functional ingredient. The valorization of HT towards diet improvement is an excellent opportunity to use it as a source of natural antioxidants to replace (or reduce) synthetic additives. Among bioactive properties, HT has been claimed to activate endogenous defense systems, such as the antioxidant enzymes that control and regulate the detoxifying mechanism of mitochondrial biogenesis. So far, clinical studies have been focused on HT ingestion together with olive oil, hindering possible conclusions on the real potential of HT. Additionally, information related to the metabolization process and absorption of the compound is still scarce. Although the bioactivity of some HT metabolites is known, further studies are required to investigate their potential applications.

A great diversity of food products supplemented with HT have been reported. However, the impact of the food matrix on the delivery of HT requires further studies. As HT may provide a bitter taste to food, a sensorial analysis should be considered more often to predict the acceptability of consumers to HT supplementation. The costs of the process of HT recovery, pure or in extracts, and the overall impact of HT-fortification on the price of new HT-enriched food products are also important factors to be considered, in order to obtain a fair balance between the valorization of the product and the acquisition price.

Author Contributions: A.F.R.S. contributed to conceptualization and writing the original draft. D.R. contributed to writing the original draft. M.M. contributed to writing the original draft. M.A.C. contributed to supervision, writing—review. A.M.S.S. contributed to project coordination, resources, supervision, writing—review. S.M.C. contributed to conceptualization, supervision, and writing—review. All authors have read and agreed to the published version of the manuscript.

Funding: Project NETDIAMOND (POCI-01-0145-FEDER-016385)-New targets in diastolic heart failure: from comorbidities to personalized medicine, for financial support of experimental work and of the fellowship grants of Andreia Silva, Mariana Monteiro and Daniela Resende. University of Aveiro and to Fundação para a Ciência e a Tecnologia/Ministério da Ciência, Tecnologia e Ensino Superior (FCT/MCTES) for financial support to the associated laboratory LAQV-REQUIMTE (project reference UIDB/50006/2020), through national funds and co-financed by Fundo Europeu de Desenvolvimento Regional (FEDER), within the PT2020 Partnership Agreement. FCT for the Ph.D. grant of Andreia Silva (SFRH/BD/142100/2018). Project AgroForWealth (CENTRO-01-0145-FEDER-000001), funded by Centro2020, through FEDER and PT2020, for the research contract of Susana M. Cardoso.

References

1. Turck, D.; Bresson, J.; Burlingame, B.; Dean, T.; Fairweather-Tait, S.; Heinonen, M.; Hirsch-Ernst, K.I.; Mangelsdorf, I.; McArdle, H.J.; Naska, A.; et al. Safety of hydroxytyrosol as a novel food pursuant to Regulation (EC) No 258/97. *EFSA J.* **2017**, *15*. [CrossRef]
2. Nova Mentis GRAS Notice (GRN) No. 876. Office of Food Additive Safety. 2019. Available online: https://www.fda.gov/media/134474/download (accessed on 17 July 2020).
3. Europeo COMMISSION IMPLEMENTING DECISION (EU) 2017/2373 of 14 December 2017 authorising the placing on the market of hydroxytyrosol as a novel food ingredient under Regulation (EC) No 258/97 of the European Parliament and of the Council. *Off. J. Eur. Union* **2017**, *2017*, 56–59.
4. Parliament, E.; States, M. COMMISSION REGULATION (EU) No 432/2012 of 16 May 2012 establishing a list of permitted health claims made on foods, other than those referring to the reduction of disease risk and to children's development and health. *Off. J. Eur. Union* **2012**, *13*, 22.
5. Boskou, D. Phenolic Compounds in Olives and Olive Oil. In *Olive oil:Minor Constituents and Health*; Boskou, D., Ed.; CRC Press: Boca Raton, FL, USA, 2008; pp. 12–36. ISBN 9780429136900.
6. García-García, M.I.; Hernández-García, S.; Sánchez-Ferrer, Á.; García-Carmona, F. Kinetic Study of Hydroxytyrosol Oxidation and Its Related Compounds by Red Globe Grape Polyphenol Oxidase. *J. Agric. Food Chem.* **2013**, *61*, 6050–6055. [CrossRef]
7. Fernández-Mar, M.I.; Mateos, R.; García-Parrilla, M.C.; Puertas, B.; Cantos-Villar, E. Bioactive compounds in wine: Resveratrol, hydroxytyrosol and melatonin: A review. *Food Chem.* **2012**, *130*, 797–813. [CrossRef]
8. Cardoso, S.M.; Guyot, S.; Marnet, N.; Lopes-da-Silva, J.A.; Renard, C.M.G.C.; Coimbra, M.A. Characterisation of phenolic extracts from olive pulp and olive pomace by electrospray mass spectrometry. *J. Sci. Food Agric.* **2005**, *85*, 21–32. [CrossRef]
9. Ramírez, E.; Brenes, M.; García, P.; Medina, E.; Romero, C. Oleuropein hydrolysis in natural green olives: Importance of the endogenous enzymes. *Food Chem.* **2016**, *206*, 204–209. [CrossRef]

10. Santos, M.M.; Piccirillo, C.; Castro, P.M.L.; Kalogerakis, N.; Pintado, M.E. Bioconversion of oleuropein to hydroxytyrosol by lactic acid bacteria. *World J. Microbiol. Biotechnol.* **2012**, *28*, 2435–2440. [CrossRef]
11. Di Tommaso, D.; Calabrese, R.; Rotilio, D. Identification and Quantitation of Hydroxytyrosol in Italian Wines. *J. High. Resolut. Chromatogr.* **1998**, *21*, 549–553. [CrossRef]
12. Domínguez-Avila, J.A.; Wall-Medrano, A.; Velderrain-Rodríguez, G.R.; Chen, C.-Y.O.; Salazar-López, N.J.; Robles-Sánchez, M.; González-Aguilar, G.A. Gastrointestinal interactions, absorption, splanchnic metabolism and pharmacokinetics of orally ingested phenolic compounds. *Food Funct.* **2017**, *8*, 15–38. [CrossRef]
13. Pereira-Caro, G.; Sarriá, B.; Madrona, A.; Espartero, J.L.; Escuderos, M.E.; Bravo, L.; Mateos, R. Digestive stability of hydroxytyrosol, hydroxytyrosyl acetate and alkyl hydroxytyrosyl ethers. *Int. J. Food Sci. Nutr.* **2012**, *63*, 703–707. [CrossRef] [PubMed]
14. Miro-Casas, E. Hydroxytyrosol Disposition in Humans. *Clin. Chem.* **2003**, *49*, 945–952. [CrossRef] [PubMed]
15. Robles-Almazan, M.; Pulido-Moran, M.; Moreno-Fernandez, J.; Ramirez-Tortosa, C.; Rodriguez-Garcia, C.; Quiles, J.L.; Ramirez-Tortosa, M.C. Hydroxytyrosol: Bioavailability, toxicity, and clinical applications. *Food Res. Int.* **2018**, *105*, 654–667. [CrossRef] [PubMed]
16. Mateos, R.; Pereira-Caro, G.; Saha, S.; Cert, R.; Redondo-Horcajo, M.; Bravo, L.; Kroon, P.A. Acetylation of hydroxytyrosol enhances its transport across differentiated Caco-2 cell monolayers. *Food Chem.* **2011**, *125*, 865–872. [CrossRef]
17. Rubió, L.; Macià, A.; Valls, R.M.; Pedret, A.; Romero, M.-P.; Solà, R.; Motilva, M.-J. A new hydroxytyrosol metabolite identified in human plasma: Hydroxytyrosol acetate sulphate. *Food Chem.* **2012**, *134*, 1132–1136. [CrossRef]
18. De La Cruz, J.P.; Ruiz-Moreno, M.I.; Guerrero, A.; López-Villodres, J.A.; Reyes, J.J.; Espartero, J.L.; Labajos, M.T.; González-Correa, J.A. Role of the catechol group in the antioxidant and neuroprotective effects of virgin olive oil components in rat brain. *J. Nutr. Biochem.* **2015**, *26*, 549–555. [CrossRef]
19. Raneva, V.; Shimasaki, H.; Ishida, Y.; Ueta, N.; Niki, E. Antioxidative activity of 3,4-dihydroxyphenylacetic acid and caffeic acid in rat plasma. *Lipids* **2001**, *36*, 1111–1116. [CrossRef]
20. Deiana, M.; Incani, A.; Rosa, A.; Corona, G.; Atzeri, A.; Loru, D.; Paola Melis, M.; Assunta Dessì, M. Protective effect of hydroxytyrosol and its metabolite homovanillic alcohol on H2O2 induced lipid peroxidation in renal tubular epithelial cells. *Food Chem. Toxicol.* **2008**, *46*, 2984–2990. [CrossRef]
21. Gordon, M.H.; Paiva-Martins, F.; Almeida, M. Antioxidant Activity of Hydroxytyrosol Acetate Compared with That of Other Olive Oil Polyphenols. *J. Agric. Food Chem.* **2001**, *49*, 2480–2485. [CrossRef]
22. González-Molina, E.; Moreno, D.A.; García-Viguera, C. Aronia-Enriched Lemon Juice: A New Highly Antioxidant Beverage. *J. Agric. Food Chem.* **2008**, *56*, 11327–11333. [CrossRef]
23. Burke, W.J.; Li, S.W.; Williams, E.A.; Nonneman, R.; Zahm, D.S. 3,4-Dihydroxyphenylacetaldehyde is the toxic dopamine metabolite in vivo: Implications for Parkinson's disease pathogenesis. *Brain Res.* **2003**, *989*, 205–213. [CrossRef]
24. López de las Hazas, M.C.; Piñol, C.; Macià, A.; Romero, M.P.; Pedret, A.; Solà, R.; Rubió, L.; Motilva, M.J. Differential absorption and metabolism of hydroxytyrosol and its precursors oleuropein and secoiridoids. *J. Funct. Foods* **2016**, *22*, 52–63. [CrossRef]
25. Pastor, A.; Rodríguez-Morató, J.; Olesti, E.; Pujadas, M.; Pérez-Mañá, C.; Khymenets, O.; Fitó, M.; Covas, M.-I.; Solá, R.; Motilva, M.-J.; et al. Analysis of free hydroxytyrosol in human plasma following the administration of olive oil. *J. Chromatogr. A* **2016**, *1437*, 183–190. [CrossRef] [PubMed]
26. González-Santiago, M.; Fonollá, J.; Lopez-Huertas, E. Human absorption of a supplement containing purified hydroxytyrosol, a natural antioxidant from olive oil, and evidence for its transient association with low-density lipoproteins. *Pharmacol. Res.* **2010**, *61*, 364–370. [CrossRef] [PubMed]
27. Tuck, K.L.; Freeman, M.P.; Hayball, P.J.; Stretch, G.L.; Stupans, I. The In Vivo Fate of Hydroxytyrosol and Tyrosol, Antioxidant Phenolic Constituents of Olive Oil, after Intravenous and Oral Dosing of Labeled Compounds to Rats. *J. Nutr.* **2001**, *131*, 1993–1996. [CrossRef]
28. Tsimidou, M.Z.; Nenadis, N.; Servili, M.; García-González, D.L.; Gallina Toschi, T. Why Tyrosol Derivatives Have to Be Quantified in the Calculation of "Olive Oil Polyphenols" Content to Support the Health Claim Provisioned in the EC Reg. 432/2012. *Eur. J. Lipid Sci. Technol.* **2018**, *120*, 1800098. [CrossRef]
29. Bulotta, S.; Celano, M.; Lepore, S.M.; Montalcini, T.; Pujia, A.; Russo, D. Beneficial effects of the olive oil phenolic components oleuropein and hydroxytyrosol: Focus on protection against cardiovascular and metabolic diseases. *J. Transl. Med.* **2014**, *12*, 219. [CrossRef]

30. Echeverría, F.; Ortiz, M.; Valenzuela, R.; Videla, L. Hydroxytyrosol and Cytoprotection: A Projection for Clinical Interventions. *Int. J. Mol. Sci.* **2017**, *18*, 930. [CrossRef]
31. Bertelli, M.; Kiani, A.K.; Paolacci, S.; Manara, E.; Kurti, D.; Dhuli, K.; Bushati, V.; Miertus, J.; Pangallo, D.; Baglivo, M.; et al. Hydroxytyrosol: A natural compound with promising pharmacological activities. *J. Biotechnol.* **2020**, *309*, 29–33. [CrossRef]
32. Kitsati, N.; Mantzaris, M.D.; Galaris, D. Hydroxytyrosol inhibits hydrogen peroxide-induced apoptotic signaling via labile iron chelation. *Redox Biol.* **2016**, *10*, 233–242. [CrossRef]
33. Visioli, F.; Bellomo, G.; Galli, C. Free Radical-Scavenging Properties of Olive Oil Polyphenols. *Biochem. Biophys. Res. Commun.* **1998**, *247*, 60–64. [CrossRef] [PubMed]
34. O'Dowd, Y.; Driss, F.; Dang, P.M.-C.; Elbim, C.; Gougerot-Pocidalo, M.-A.; Pasquier, C.; El-Benna, J. Antioxidant effect of hydroxytyrosol, a polyphenol from olive oil: Scavenging of hydrogen peroxide but not superoxide anion produced by human neutrophils. *Biochem. Pharmacol.* **2004**, *68*, 2003–2008. [CrossRef] [PubMed]
35. Rietjens, S.J.; Bast, A.; Haenen, G.R.M.M. New Insights into Controversies on the Antioxidant Potential of the Olive Oil Antioxidant Hydroxytyrosol. *J. Agric. Food Chem.* **2007**, *55*, 7609–7614. [CrossRef] [PubMed]
36. Peng, S.; Zhang, B.; Yao, J.; Duan, D.; Fang, J. Dual protection of hydroxytyrosol, an olive oil polyphenol, against oxidative damage in PC12 cells. *Food Funct.* **2015**, *6*, 2091–2100. [CrossRef]
37. Crupi, R.; Palma, E.; Siracusa, R.; Fusco, R.; Gugliandolo, E.; Cordaro, M.; Impellizzeri, D.; De Caro, C.; Calzetta, L.; Cuzzocrea, S.; et al. Protective Effect of Hydroxytyrosol Against Oxidative Stress Induced by the Ochratoxin in Kidney Cells: In vitro and in vivo Study. *Front. Vet. Sci.* **2020**, *7*, 136. [CrossRef]
38. Goya, L.; Mateos, R.; Bravo, L. Effect of the olive oil phenol hydroxytyrosol on human hepatoma HepG2 cells. *Eur. J. Nutr.* **2007**, *46*, 70–78. [CrossRef]
39. Burattini, S.; Salucci, S.; Baldassarri, V.; Accorsi, A.; Piatti, E.; Madrona, A.; Espartero, J.L.; Candiracci, M.; Zappia, G.; Falcieri, E. Anti-apoptotic activity of hydroxytyrosol and hydroxytyrosyl laurate. *Food Chem. Toxicol.* **2013**, *55*, 248–256. [CrossRef]
40. Aldini, G.; Piccoli, A.; Beretta, G.; Morazzoni, P.; Riva, A.; Marinello, C.; Maffei Facino, R. Antioxidant activity of polyphenols from solid olive residues of c.v. Coratina. *Fitoterapia* **2006**, *77*, 121–128. [CrossRef]
41. Vlavcheski, F.; Young, M.; Tsiani, E. Antidiabetic Effects of Hydroxytyrosol: In Vitro and In Vivo Evidence. *Antioxidants* **2019**, *8*, 188. [CrossRef]
42. Zhu, L.; Liu, Z.; Feng, Z.; Hao, J.; Shen, W.; Li, X.; Sun, L.; Sharman, E.; Wang, Y.; Wertz, K.; et al. Hydroxytyrosol protects against oxidative damage by simultaneous activation of mitochondrial biogenesis and phase II detoxifying enzyme systems in retinal pigment epithelial cells. *J. Nutr. Biochem.* **2010**, *21*, 1089–1098. [CrossRef]
43. Giordano, E.; Dávalos, A.; Visioli, F. Chronic hydroxytyrosol feeding modulates glutathione-mediated oxido-reduction pathways in adipose tissue: A nutrigenomic study. *Nutr. Metab. Cardiovasc. Dis.* **2014**, *24*, 1144–1150. [CrossRef] [PubMed]
44. Granados-Principal, S.; El-azem, N.; Pamplona, R.; Ramirez-Tortosa, C.; Pulido-Moran, M.; Vera-Ramirez, L.; Quiles, J.L.; Sanchez-Rovira, P.; Naudí, A.; Portero-Otin, M.; et al. Hydroxytyrosol ameliorates oxidative stress and mitochondrial dysfunction in doxorubicin-induced cardiotoxicity in rats with breast cancer. *Biochem. Pharmacol.* **2014**, *90*, 25–33. [CrossRef] [PubMed]
45. González-Santiago, M.; Martín-Bautista, E.; Carrero, J.J.; Fonollá, J.; Baró, L.; Bartolomé, M.V.; Gil-Loyzaga, P.; López-Huertas, E. One-month administration of hydroxytyrosol, a phenolic antioxidant present in olive oil, to hyperlipemic rabbits improves blood lipid profile, antioxidant status and reduces atherosclerosis development. *Atherosclerosis* **2006**, *188*, 35–42. [CrossRef]
46. Fuccelli, R.; Fabiani, R.; Rosignoli, P. Hydroxytyrosol Exerts Anti-Inflammatory and Anti-Oxidant Activities in a Mouse Model of Systemic Inflammation. *Molecules* **2018**, *23*, 3212. [CrossRef] [PubMed]
47. Pan, S.; Liu, L.; Pan, H.; Ma, Y.; Wang, D.; Kang, K.; Wang, J.; Sun, B.; Sun, X.; Jiang, H. Protective effects of hydroxytyrosol on liver ischemia/reperfusion injury in mice. *Mol. Nutr. Food Res.* **2013**, *57*, 1218–1227. [CrossRef]
48. Feng, Z.; Bai, L.; Yan, J.; Li, Y.; Shen, W.; Wang, Y.; Wertz, K.; Weber, P.; Zhang, Y.; Chen, Y.; et al. Mitochondrial dynamic remodeling in strenuous exercise-induced muscle and mitochondrial dysfunction: Regulatory effects of hydroxytyrosol. *Free Radic. Biol. Med.* **2011**, *50*, 1437–1446. [CrossRef]

49. Jemai, H.; Bouaziz, M.; Fki, I.; El Feki, A.; Sayadi, S. Hypolipidimic and antioxidant activities of oleuropein and its hydrolysis derivative-rich extracts from Chemlali olive leaves. *Chem. Biol. Interact.* **2008**, *176*, 88–98. [CrossRef]
50. Hamden, K.; Allouche, N.; Damak, M.; Elfeki, A. Hypoglycemic and antioxidant effects of phenolic extracts and purified hydroxytyrosol from olive mill waste in vitro and in rats. *Chem. Biol. Interact.* **2009**, *180*, 421–432. [CrossRef]
51. Covas, M.-I.; Nyyssönen, K.; Poulsen, H.E.; Kaikkonen, J.; Zunft, H.-J.F.; Kiesewetter, H.; Gaddi, A.; de la Torre, R.; Mursu, J.; Bäumler, H.; et al. The Effect of Polyphenols in Olive Oil on Heart Disease Risk Factors. *Ann. Intern. Med.* **2006**, *145*, 333. [CrossRef]
52. D'Angelo, S.; Manna, C.; Migliardi, V.; Mazzoni, O.; Morrica, P.; Capasso, G.; Pontoni, G.; Galletti, P.; Zappia, V. Pharmacokinetics and metabolism of hydroxytyrosol, a natural antioxidant from olive oil. *Drug Metab. Dispos.* **2001**, *29*, 1492–1498.
53. Christian, M.S.; Sharper, V.A.; Hoberman, A.M.; Seng, J.E.; Fu, L.; Covell, D.; Diener, R.M.; Bitler, C.M.; Crea, R. The Toxicity Profile of Hydrolyzed Aqueous Olive Pulp Extract. *Drug Chem. Toxicol.* **2004**, *27*, 309–330. [CrossRef]
54. Auñon-Calles, D.; Canut, L.; Visioli, F. Toxicological evaluation of pure hydroxytyrosol. *Food Chem. Toxicol.* **2013**, *55*, 498–504. [CrossRef]
55. Achmon, Y.; Fishman, A. The antioxidant hydroxytyrosol: Biotechnological production challenges and opportunities. *Appl. Microbiol. Biotechnol.* **2015**, *99*, 1119–1130. [CrossRef] [PubMed]
56. Veneziani, G.; Novelli, E.; Esposto, S.; Taticchi, A.; Servili, M. Applications of recovered bioactive compounds in food products. In *Olive Mill Waste*; Elsevier: Amsterdam, The Netherlands, 2017; pp. 231–263, ISBN 9780128053140.
57. Changping, L.; Zhuo, L. A Kind of Extracting Process of Hydroxytyrosol. Patent CN107382675 A, 24 November 2017.
58. Más, J.A.L.; Mellado, M.P.; Ortiz, P.M.; Streitenberger, S.A. Process and Apparatus for the Production of Hydroxytyrosol Containing Extract from Olives and Solids Containing Residues of Olive Oil Extraction. Patent EP2049458 A1, 24 June 2010.
59. Weiping, H. The Method that Hydroxytyrosol Is Extracted from Processing Olive Oil Waste Water. Patent CN106946662A, 14 July 2017.
60. Lingxiao; Shende, J.; Xinyan, G.; Chao, X. Method for Preparing High-Purity Hydroxytyrosol. Patent CN103420804 A, 4 December 2013.
61. Milczarek, R.; Larson, D.; Li, Y.O.; Sedej, I.; Wang, S. Olive. In *Integrated Processing Technologies for Food and Agricultural By-Products*; Elsevier: Amsterdam, The Netherlands, 2019; ISBN 9780128141380.
62. Ulm, J.; Leuenberger, B.H. Novel Powders Based on Vegetation Water from Olive Oil Production. Patent EP2106218 A1, 7 October 2009.
63. Raederstorff, D.; Richard, N.; Schwager, J.; Wertz, K. Compositions. U.S. Patent US8841264 B2, 23 September 2010.
64. Martínez, N.; Herrera, M.; Frías, L.; Provencio, M.; Pérez-Carrión, R.; Díaz, V.; Morse, M.; Crespo, M.C. A combination of hydroxytyrosol, omega-3 fatty acids and curcumin improves pain and inflammation among early stage breast cancer patients receiving adjuvant hormonal therapy: Results of a pilot study. *Clin. Transl. Oncol.* **2019**, *21*, 489–498. [CrossRef] [PubMed]
65. Carito, V.; Ciafrè, S.; Tarani, L.; Ceccanti, M.; Natella, F.; Iannitelli, A.; Tirassa, P.; Chaldakov, N.G.; Ceccanti, M.; Boccardo, C.; et al. TNF-α and IL-10 modulation induced by polyphenols extracted by olive pomace in a mouse model of paw inflammation. *Ann. Ist Super Sanità* **2015**, *5*, 382–386. [CrossRef]
66. Aponte, M.; Ungaro, F.; D'Angelo, I.; De Caro, C.; Russo, R.; Blaiotta, G.; Dal Piaz, F.; Calignano, A.; Miro, A. Improving in vivo conversion of oleuropein into hydroxytyrosol by oral granules containing probiotic Lactobacillus plantarum 299v and an *Olea europaea* standardized extract. *Int. J. Pharm.* **2018**, *543*, 73–82. [CrossRef] [PubMed]
67. Quirós-Fernández, R.; López-Plaza, B.; Bermejo, L.; Palma-Milla, S.; Gómez-Candela, C. Supplementation with Hydroxytyrosol and Punicalagin Improves Early Atherosclerosis Markers Involved in the Asymptomatic Phase of Atherosclerosis in the Adult Population: A Randomized, Placebo-Controlled, Crossover Trial. *Nutrients* **2019**, *11*, 640. [CrossRef]

68. Kehili, M.; Choura, S.; Zammel, A.; Allouche, N.; Sayadi, S. Oxidative stability of refined olive and sunflower oils supplemented with lycopene-rich oleoresin from tomato peels industrial by-product, during accelerated shelf-life storage. *Food Chem.* **2018**, *246*, 295–304. [CrossRef]
69. Bañares, C.; Martin, D.; Reglero, G.; Torres, C.F. Protective effect of hydroxytyrosol and rosemary extract in a comparative study of the oxidative stability of Echium oil. *Food Chem.* **2019**, *290*, 316–323. [CrossRef]
70. Farràs, M.; Fernández-Castillejo, S.; Rubió, L.; Arranz, S.; Catalán, Ú.; Subirana, I.; Romero, M.-P.; Castañer, O.; Pedret, A.; Blanchart, G.; et al. Phenol-enriched olive oils improve HDL antioxidant content in hypercholesterolemic subjects. A randomized, double-blind, cross-over, controlled trial. *J. Nutr. Biochem.* **2018**, *51*, 99–104. [CrossRef]
71. Fki, I.; Allouche, N.; Sayadi, S. The use of polyphenolic extract, purified hydroxytyrosol and 3,4-dihydroxyphenyl acetic acid from olive mill wastewater for the stabilization of refined oils: A potential alternative to synthetic antioxidants. *Food Chem.* **2005**, *93*, 197–204. [CrossRef]
72. Lama-Muñoz, A.; Rubio-Senent, F.; Bermúdez-Oria, A.; Fernández-Prior, Á.; Fernández-Bolaños, J.; Rodríguez-Gutiérrez, G. Synergistic effect of 3,4-dihydroxyphenylglycol with hydroxytyrosol and α-tocopherol on the Rancimat oxidative stability of vegetable oils. *Innov. Food Sci. Emerg. Technol.* **2019**, *51*, 100–106. [CrossRef]
73. Sordini, B.; Veneziani, G.; Servili, M.; Esposto, S.; Selvaggini, R.; Lorefice, A.; Taticchi, A. A quanti-qualitative study of a phenolic extract as a natural antioxidant in the frying processes. *Food Chem.* **2019**, *279*, 426–434. [CrossRef]
74. Valls, R.-M.; Farràs, M.; Suárez, M.; Fernández-Castillejo, S.; Fitó, M.; Konstantinidou, V.; Fuentes, F.; López-Miranda, J.; Giralt, M.; Covas, M.-I.; et al. Effects of functional olive oil enriched with its own phenolic compounds on endothelial function in hypertensive patients. A randomised controlled trial. *Food Chem.* **2015**, *167*, 30–35. [CrossRef] [PubMed]
75. De Leonardis, A.; Macciola, V. Heat-oxidation stability of palm oil blended with extra virgin olive oil. *Food Chem.* **2012**, *135*, 1769–1776. [CrossRef] [PubMed]
76. Más, J.A.L.; Streitenberger, S.A.; Mellado, M.P.; Ortiz, P.M. Fortification of Nutritional Products with Olive Extracts Containing Hydroxytyrosol and Hydroxytyrosol Fortified Nutritional Products. Patent WO2009013596 A2, 29 January 2009.
77. Bulbarello, A.; Leuthardt, B. Fortification of Edible Oils with Hyrdoxytyrosol. Patent WO2016087428 A1, 9 June 2016.
78. De Hierro, A.G.-G.L.; Sánchez, A.P. Olive Oil Composition and Use Thereof as Functional Food. Patent WO2008102047 A1, 28 August 2008.
79. Vally, H.; Misso, N.L.A.; Madan, V. Clinical effects of sulphite additives. *Clin. Exp. Allergy* **2009**, *39*, 1643–1651. [CrossRef] [PubMed]
80. Raposo, R.; Ruiz-Moreno, M.J.; Garde-Cerdán, T.; Puertas, B.; Moreno-Rojas, J.M.; Zafrilla, P.; Gonzalo-Diago, A.; Guerrero, R.F.; Cantos-Villar, E. Replacement of sulfur dioxide by hydroxytyrosol in white wine: Influence on both quality parameters and sensory. *LWT Food Sci. Technol.* **2016**, *65*, 214–221. [CrossRef]
81. Ruiz-Moreno, M.J.; Raposo, R.; Moreno-Rojas, J.M.; Zafrilla, P.; Cayuela, J.M.; Mulero, J.; Puertas, B.; Guerrero, R.F.; Piñeiro, Z.; Giron, F.; et al. Efficacy of olive oil mill extract in replacing sulfur dioxide in wine model. *LWT Food Sci. Technol.* **2015**, *61*, 117–123. [CrossRef]
82. Raposo, R.; Ruiz-Moreno, M.J.; Garde-Cerdán, T.; Puertas, B.; Moreno-Rojas, J.M.; Gonzalo-Diago, A.; Guerrero, R.F.; Ortiz, V.; Cantos-Villar, E. Effect of hydroxytyrosol on quality of sulfur dioxide-free red wine. *Food Chem.* **2016**, *192*, 25–33. [CrossRef]
83. Kranz, P.; Braun, N.; Schulze, N.; Kunz, B. Sensory quality of functional beverages: Bitterness perception and bitter masking of olive leaf extract fortified fruit smoothies. *J. Food Sci.* **2010**, *75*. [CrossRef]
84. Larrosa, M.; Espín, J.C.; Tomás-Barberán, F.A. Antioxidant capacity of tomato juice functionalised with enzymatically synthesised hydroxytyrosol. *J. Sci. Food Agric.* **2003**, *83*, 658–666. [CrossRef]
85. Guglielmotti, M.; Passaghe, P.; Buiatti, S. Use of olive (*Olea europaea* L.) leaves as beer ingredient, and their influence on beer chemical composition and antioxidant activity. *J. Food Sci.* **2020**, *85*, 2278–2285. [CrossRef] [PubMed]
86. Takashi, F.; Yuki, N.; Hideki, M. Beverage Containing Hydroxytyrosol. Patent WO2017094654 A1, 8 June 2017.

87. Lalas, S.; Athanasiadis, V.; Gortzi, O.; Bounitsi, M.; Giovanoudis, I.; Tsaknis, J.; Bogiatzis, F. Enrichment of table olives with polyphenols extracted from olive leaves. *Food Chem.* **2011**, *127*, 1521–1525. [CrossRef]
88. Caponio, F.; Difonzo, G.; Calasso, M.; Cosmai, L.; De Angelis, M. Effects of olive leaf extract addition on fermentative and oxidative processes of table olives and their nutritional properties. *Food Res. Int.* **2019**, *116*, 1306–1317. [CrossRef] [PubMed]
89. Schaide, T.; Cabrera-Bañegil, M.; Pérez-Nevado, F.; Esperilla, A.; Martín-Vertedor, D. Effect of olive leaf extract combined with Saccharomyces cerevisiae in the fermentation process of table olives. *J. Food Sci. Technol.* **2019**, *56*, 3001–3013. [CrossRef] [PubMed]
90. De Toffoli, A.; Monteleone, E.; Bucalossi, G.; Veneziani, G.; Fia, G.; Servili, M.; Zanoni, B.; Pagliarini, E.; Gallina Toschi, T.; Dinnella, C. Sensory and chemical profile of a phenolic extract from olive mill waste waters in plant-base food with varied macro-composition. *Food Res. Int.* **2019**, *119*, 236–243. [CrossRef]
91. Mateos, R.; Martínez-López, S.; Baeza Arévalo, G.; Amigo-Benavent, M.; Sarriá, B.; Bravo-Clemente, L. Hydroxytyrosol in functional hydroxytyrosol-enriched biscuits is highly bioavailable and decreases oxidised low density lipoprotein levels in humans. *Food Chem.* **2016**, *205*, 248–256. [CrossRef]
92. Conterno, L.; Martinelli, F.; Tamburini, M.; Fava, F.; Mancini, A.; Sordo, M.; Pindo, M.; Martens, S.; Masuero, D.; Vrhovsek, U.; et al. Measuring the impact of olive pomace enriched biscuits on the gut microbiota and its metabolic activity in mildly hypercholesterolaemic subjects. *Eur. J. Nutr.* **2019**, *58*, 63–81. [CrossRef]
93. Navarro, M.; Morales, F.J. Effect of hydroxytyrosol and olive leaf extract on 1,2-dicarbonyl compounds, hydroxymethylfurfural and advanced glycation endproducts in a biscuit model. *Food Chem.* **2017**, *217*, 602–609. [CrossRef]
94. Cedola, A.; Palermo, C.; Centonze, D.; Del Nobile, M.A.; Conte, A. Characterization and Bio-Accessibility Evaluation of Olive Leaf Extract-Enriched "Taralli". *Foods* **2020**, *9*, 1268. [CrossRef]
95. Galanakis, C.M.; Tsatalas, P.; Charalambous, Z.; Galanakis, I.M. Control of microbial growth in bakery products fortified with polyphenols recovered from olive mill wastewater. *Environ. Technol. Innov.* **2018**, *10*, 1–15. [CrossRef]
96. Hayata, M.; özuğur, G. Phytochemical fortification of flour and bread. In *Flour and Breads and Their Fortification in Health and Disease Prevention*; Academic Press: Cambridge, MA, USA, 2011; pp. 293–298, ISBN 978-0-12-380886-8.
97. Pateiro, M.; Barba, F.J.; Domínguez, R.; Sant'Ana, A.S.; Mousavi Khaneghah, A.; Gavahian, M.; Gómez, B.; Lorenzo, J.M. Essential oils as natural additives to prevent oxidation reactions in meat and meat products: A review. *Food Res. Int.* **2018**, *113*, 156–166. [CrossRef] [PubMed]
98. De Mey, E.; De Maere, H.; Paelinck, H.; Fraeye, I. Volatile N -nitrosamines in meat products: Potential precursors, influence of processing, and mitigation strategies. *Crit. Rev. Food Sci. Nutr.* **2017**, *57*, 2909–2923. [CrossRef] [PubMed]
99. Kawano, S.; Nakao, T.; Hiraga, K. Species and Strain Differences in the Butylated Hydroxytoluene (BHT)-Producing Induction of Hepatic Drug Oxidation Enzymes. *Jpn. J. Pharmacol.* **1980**, *30*, 861–870. [CrossRef] [PubMed]
100. Park, S.; Lee, J.-Y.; Lim, W.; You, S.; Song, G. Butylated Hydroxyanisole Exerts Neurotoxic Effects by Promoting Cytosolic Calcium Accumulation and Endoplasmic Reticulum Stress in Astrocytes. *J. Agric. Food Chem.* **2019**, *67*, 9618–9629. [CrossRef] [PubMed]
101. Martínez, L.; Ros, G.; Nieto, G. Hydroxytyrosol: Health Benefits and Use as Functional Ingredient in Meat. *Medicines* **2018**, *5*, 13. [CrossRef]
102. Cofrades, S.; Salcedo Sandoval, L.; Delgado-Pando, G.; López-López, I.; Ruiz-Capillas, C.; Jiménez-Colmenero, F. Antioxidant activity of hydroxytyrosol in frankfurters enriched with n-3 polyunsaturated fatty acids. *Food Chem.* **2011**, *129*, 429–436. [CrossRef]
103. Nieto, G.; Martínez, L.; Castillo, J.; Ros, G. Hydroxytyrosol extracts, olive oil and walnuts as functional components in chicken sausages. *J. Sci. Food Agric.* **2017**, *97*, 3761–3771. [CrossRef]
104. De Leonardis, A.; Macciola, V.; Lembo, G.; Aretini, A.; Nag, A. Studies on oxidative stabilisation of lard by natural antioxidants recovered from olive-oil mill wastewater. *Food Chem.* **2007**, *100*, 998–1004. [CrossRef]
105. Balzan, S.; Taticchi, A.; Cardazzo, B.; Urbani, S.; Servili, M.; Di Lecce, G.; Zabalza, I.B.; Rodriguez-Estrada, M.T.; Novelli, E.; Fasolato, L. Effect of phenols extracted from a by-product of the oil mill on the shelf-life of raw and cooked fresh pork sausages in the absence of chemical additives. *LWT Food Sci. Technol.* **2017**, *85*, 89–95. [CrossRef]

106. Muíño, I.; Díaz, M.T.; Apeleo, E.; Pérez-Santaescolástica, C.; Rivas-Cañedo, A.; Pérez, C.; Cañeque, V.; Lauzurica, S.; Fuente, J. de la Valorisation of an extract from olive oil waste as a natural antioxidant for reducing meat waste resulting from oxidative processes. *J. Clean. Prod.* **2017**, *140*, 924–932. [CrossRef]
107. Aquilani, C.; Sirtori, F.; Flores, M.; Bozzi, R.; Lebret, B.; Pugliese, C. Effect of natural antioxidants from grape seed and chestnut in combination with hydroxytyrosol, as sodium nitrite substitutes in Cinta Senese dry-fermented sausages. *Meat Sci.* **2018**, *145*, 389–398. [CrossRef] [PubMed]
108. Chaves-López, C.; Serio, A.; Mazzarrino, G.; Martuscelli, M.; Scarpone, E.; Paparella, A. Control of household mycoflora in fermented sausages using phenolic fractions from olive mill wastewaters. *Int. J. Food Microbiol.* **2015**, *207*, 49–56. [CrossRef] [PubMed]
109. Santos-López, J.A.; Garcimartín, A.; Bastida, S.; Bautista-Ávila, M.; González-Muñoz, M.J.; Benedí, J.; Sánchez-Muniz, F.J. Lipoprotein Profile in Aged Rats Fed Chia Oil- or Hydroxytyrosol-Enriched Pork in High Cholesterol/High Saturated Fat Diets. *Nutrients* **2018**, *10*, 1830. [CrossRef]
110. Rounds, L.; Havens, C.M.; Feinstein, Y.; Friedman, M.; Ravishankar, S. Concentration-dependent inhibition of Escherichia coli O157:H7 and heterocyclic amines in heated ground beef patties by apple and olive extracts, onion powder and clove bud oil. *Meat Sci.* **2013**, *94*, 461–467. [CrossRef]
111. Djenane, D.; Gómez, D.; Yangüela, J.; Roncalés, P.; Ariño, A. Olive Leaves Extract from Algerian Oleaster (*Olea europaea* var. sylvestris) on Microbiological Safety and Shelf-life Stability of Raw Halal Minced Beef during Display. *Foods* **2018**, *8*, 10. [CrossRef]
112. Martínez-Zamora, L.; Ros, G.; Nieto, G. Synthetic vs. Natural Hydroxytyrosol for Clean Label Lamb Burgers. *Antioxidants* **2020**, *9*, 851. [CrossRef]
113. Pazos, M.; Alonso, A.; Sánchez, I.; Medina, I. Hydroxytyrosol Prevents Oxidative Deterioration in Foodstuffs Rich in Fish Lipids. *J. Agric. Food Chem.* **2008**, *56*, 3334–3340. [CrossRef]
114. Testa, B.; Lombardi, S.J.; Macciola, E.; Succi, M.; Tremonte, P.; Iorizzo, M. Efficacy of olive leaf extract (*Olea europaea* L. cv Gentile di Larino) in marinated anchovies (*Engraulis encrasicolus*, L.) process. *Heliyon* **2019**, *5*, e01727. [CrossRef]
115. Martínez, L.; Castillo, J.; Ros, G.; Nieto, G. Antioxidant and Antimicrobial Activity of Rosemary, Pomegranate and Olive Extracts in Fish Patties. *Antioxidants* **2019**, *8*, 86. [CrossRef]
116. Servili, M.; Rizzello, C.G.; Taticchi, A.; Esposto, S.; Urbani, S.; Mazzacane, F.; Di Maio, I.; Selvaggini, R.; Gobbetti, M.; Di Cagno, R. Functional milk beverage fortified with phenolic compounds extracted from olive vegetation water, and fermented with functional lactic acid bacteria. *Int. J. Food Microbiol.* **2011**, *147*, 45–52. [CrossRef]
117. Georgakouli, K.; Mpesios, A.; Kouretas, D.; Petrotos, K.; Mitsagga, C.; Giavasis, I.; Jamurtas, A. The Effects of an Olive Fruit Polyphenol-Enriched Yogurt on Body Composition, Blood Redox Status, Physiological and Metabolic Parameters and Yogurt Microflora. *Nutrients* **2016**, *8*, 344. [CrossRef] [PubMed]
118. Fei, P.; Xu, Y.; Zhao, S.; Gong, S.; Guo, L. Olive oil polyphenol extract inhibits vegetative cells of Bacillus cereus isolated from raw milk. *J. Dairy Sci.* **2019**, *102*, 3894–3902. [CrossRef] [PubMed]
119. Medina, E.; Romero, C.; Brenes, M.; de Castro, A. Antimicrobial Activity of Olive Oil, Vinegar, and Various Beverages against Foodborne Pathogens. *J. Food Prot.* **2007**, *70*, 1194–1199. [CrossRef] [PubMed]
120. Villanova, A.; Villanova, L.; Merendino, A.; Fasiello, G. Yoghurt Containing Hydroxytyrosol and Other Biophenols with a Preventive Nutritional Activity Beneficial to Human Beings. Patent EP2170089 A2, 7 April 2010.

4

Food (Matrix) Effects on Bioaccessibility and Intestinal Permeability of Major Olive Antioxidants

Dubravka Vitali Čepo, Kristina Radić *, Petra Turčić, Dora Anić, Barbara Komar and Mirela Šalov

Faculty of Pharmacy and Biochemistry, University of Zagreb, Ante Kovačića 1, 10000 Zagreb, Croatia; dvitali@pharma.hr (D.V.Č.); pturcic@pharma.hr (P.T.); danic@student.pharma.hr (D.A.); bkomar@student.pharma.hr (B.K.); msalov@pharma.hr (M.Š.)

* Correspondence: kradic@pharma.hr.

Abstract: Background: olive pomace extract (OPE) is a rich source of health promoting polyphenols (hydroxytyrosol (HTS) and tyrosol (TS)) and can be used as a nutraceutical ingredient of dietary supplements and functional foods. Its adequate bioavailability is a prerequisite for excreting biological activity and can be significantly and specifically affected by different food matrices. Methods: in order to investigate food effects on polyphenol bioaccessibility, OPE was co-digested with different foods according to internationally harmonized in vitro digestibility method. Impact of particular nutrients on HTS and TS permeability was assessed on Caco-2 cell monolayer. Results: HTS and TS bioaccessibility and transepithelial permeability can be significantly affected by foods (nutrients), especially by casein and certain types of dietary fiber. Those effects are polyphenol-and nutrient-specific and are achieved either through complexation in gastrointestinal lumen and/or through direct effects of nutrients on intestinal monolayer. Conclusions: obtained results emphasize the significance and complexity of polyphenol interactions within the food matrix and the necessity of individual investigational approaches with respect to particular food/nutrient and interacting phenolic compounds.

Keywords: olive pomace; hydroxytyrosol; tyrosol; polyphenol-food interaction; Caco-2 monolayer; in vitro digestion

---

1. Introduction

The well-established health effects of olive oil can be attributed to its high monounsaturated fatty acid content; it is principally made of oleic acid (56% to 84% of the total fraction of fatty acids) and its phenolic compounds are effective at decreasing the risk of cardiovascular disease, mostly due to its ability to reduce the peroxidation of blood lipids [1,2]. The main antioxidants in olive oil are two groups of phenolic compounds: lipophilic and hydrophilic. While lipophilic phenols, including tocopherols and tocotrienols, can be found in other types of vegetable oils, hydrophilic phenols (hydroxytyrosol, tyrosol, and oleuropein) are characteristic of olive oil, and are not found in other oils and fats. They demonstrate unusual sensory properties, exert antioxidant, immunomodulatory, antimicrobial, and anticancer activity, and may decrease the risk of numerous, chronic, non-infectious diseases, such as atherosclerosis, different types of cancer (colorectal, prostate, breast, etc.), chronic inflammation, strokes (e.g., ischemic stroke), and other degenerative diseases (primarily neurodegenerative diseases, such as Alzheimer's disease) [2]. Olive pomace and olive pomace wastewater, the residues left after the production of olive oil, are secondary raw materials that contain significantly higher amounts of olive polyphenols compared to olive oil, particularly hydroxytyrosol (HTS) and tyrosol (TS). Numerous green extraction methods for efficient extraction of polyphenols from olive mill waste were recently developed [3–6], and significant steps forward have been taken in developing functional formulations of olive pomace extracts (OPEs) that will ensure satisfactory composition, stability, bioavailability, and biological activity of major active compounds, primarily HTS and TS [7,8].

Bioavailability of polyphenols is essential for their biological activity. Since it differs greatly among various phenolic compounds and depends on the characteristics of the food source, polyphenols that are the most abundant in food are not necessarily the ones with the most important health-related impacts. Since the current knowledge on health-effects of polyphenols arise mainly from epidemiological studies, it is necessary to gain better insight into their bioavailability in order to establish conclusive evidence for their effectiveness in disease prevention [9].

Bioavailability can be defined as the fraction of aa particular compound available for physiological functions in the body. In the case of polyphenols, it depends on release of polyphenols from the food matrix and/or interactions with meal (1); structural changes that occur during gastro-intestinal digestion (2); cellular uptake of glycoside forms of polyphenols and respective aglycons by enterocytes (3); fermentation of nonabsorbed polyphenols by gut microbiota and formation and absorption of metabolites (4); and metabolism of all absorbed compounds (5) [10].

Impact of food matrix (food components) on bioavailability of nutraceutical is particularly important in cases when it is necessary to compare different food matrices as the sources of the same bioactive compounds (for example olive oil vs. OPE as sources of HTS and TS). Assessing polyphenol-food interactions is also of great importance because nutraceuticals may be isolated from their natural environment, purified, and then used as nutraceutical ingredients in processed (functional) food [11]. Additionally, sufficient knowledge on the significance and the type of polyphenol-food (nutrient) interactions enables targeted use of absorption, promoting interactions and subsequent formulation of excipient foods that would improve bioavailability of particular polyphenols [12].

Mechanisms of polyphenol–food interactions are numerous. Presence of food in the gastrointestinal system changes the physiological conditions in the human gastrointestinal tract (fluid volumes, gastric, and intestinal motility, gastric emptying, luminal pH values, enzyme capacity, osmolality, bile salt content) and, consequently, affects stability and solubility of particular phenolic compounds. Moreover, polyphenols can form complexes with nutrients (components of the meal) such as dietary fiber, carbohydrates, lipids, and proteins, which can significantly affect their bioaccessibility. Additionally, nutrients can also interact with the process of absorption of polyphenols through interactions with influx and efflux intestinal transporters, interactions with intestinal monolayer permeability, or interactions with intestinal metabolizing enzymes bioaccessibility [13–15].

Bioavailability of HTS and TS from olive oil has been investigated in more in vivo studies and it was found to be satisfactory, with plasma HTS and TS concentrations rising early after virgin olive oil ingestion and reaching a peak at around 1 h in plasma and 0–2 h in urine [16]. It is important to emphasize that complex secoiridoids from olive oil are biotransformed by gut microflora, giving additional rise to postprandial HTS and TS [17,18]. OPEs are generally richer sources of HTS and TS in comparison to extra-virgin olive oil, but they have rarely been investigated in terms of bioavailability. Recent data obtained by Radić and co-authors [8] show that OPE polyphenols are stable during gastrointestinal digestion (88–187%; due to degradation of secoiridoids and formation of HTS and TS during digestion). Investigation of permeability showed that HTS and TS are primarily absorbed by passive diffusion and that absorbed oleuropein is extensively metabolized in Caco-2 cells. OPE matrix negatively influenced the permeability of HTS and TS, but the negative effect could be partially neutralized by absorption-promotive effects of particular cyclodextrins [8].

This research builds up on the work of Radić and co-authors [8], and its main focus is to investigate the impact of particular foods on gastrointestinal bioaccessibility and permeability of HTS and TS from OPE. As mentioned before, functional extracts, rich in bioactive health promoting compounds, such as OPE, are nowadays being extensively used as nutraceutical ingredients of dietary supplements and functional foods. It is therefore of great importance to understand the nature and significance of polyphenol–food interactions in order to provide efficient and accurate dosing instructions and enable targeted formulation of dietary supplements or excipient foods that will result in optimized bioavailability of those health-promoting compounds.

2. Materials and Methods

2.1. Chemical and Reagents

Petrol ether, dimethyl sulfoxide (DMSO) ethanol, methanol (≥99.9%), sodium acetate, Folin-Ciocalteu reagent, Dulbecco's Phosphate Buffered Saline (PBS liquid, sterile-filtered, without calcium, without magnesium, suitable for cell culture), tert-butyl hydroperoxide (tBOOH), 3-hydroxytyrosol (HTS) and tyrosol (TS) (≥98%), bile salts, thermostable α-amylase (A3306), pancreatin from porcine pancreas (4 × USP), Dulbecco's Modified Eagle's Medium, D-glucose, ethylenediaminetetraacetic acid (EDTA), and sodium caseinate were from Sigma–Aldrich (St. Louis, MO, USA). Acetonitrile (≥99.9%) was from Honeywell (Charlotte, NC, USA). Acetic acid and Na_2CO_3 were from Kemika (Zagreb, Croatia). Pepsin (from porcine gastric mucosa) 0.7 FIP-U/mg was from Merck (Darmstadt, Germany). Heat inactivated fetal bovine serum (FBS), nonessential amino acids (NEAA), penicillin/streptomycin/amphotericin B (A/A), and trypsin were from Capricorn Scientific (Ebsdorfergrund, Germany). The 3-(4,5-dimethylthiazole-2-yl)-2,5-diphenyltetrazolium bromide (MTT) was from Panreac AppliChem (Darmstadt, Germany). Caco-2 cells were from American Type Culture Collection (ATCC, Manassas, VA, SAD). Hydroxypropyl β cyclodextrin (HPB) was purchased from Wacker–Chemie GmbH (Burghausen, Germany), Cellulose Alba Fiber®C200 from Mikro-Technik (Bürgstadt, Germany), and Inulin Orafti®HSI from Beneo (Mannheim, Germany). Pectin was from Foodchem (Zhangjiang, China). Ultrapure water (18 MΩ) was obtained from SG Reinstwassersystem Ultra Clear UV Plus coupled with SG Wasservollentsalzer-Patrone SG 2800 (Günzburg, Germany). Sunflower oil and full-fat milk and food matrices were obtained from local suppliers, unless noted otherwise. All other chemicals were from Kemika (Zagreb, Croatia).

The exact composition of simulated salivary fluid (SSF), simulated gastric fluid (SGF), and simulated intestinal fluid (SIF) is presented in Table S1. Fed state simulated gastric fluid (FeSSGF) contained sodium chloride (237 mM), acetic acid (17.1 mM), and sodium acetate (29.8 mM) and was mixed with full fat milk in 1:1 ratio. The pH was adjusted to 3 by using hydrochloric acid. Fed state simulated intestinal fluid (FeSSIF) contained $CaCl_2$ (1.67 mM), $MgSO_4$ (0.81 mM), KCl (5.37 mM), KH_2PO_4 (0.44 mM), $NaHCO_3$ (0.42 mM), NaCl (137 mM), Na_2HPO_4 (0.34 mM), D-glucose (5.55 mM), L-glutamine (2 mM), lecithin (7.5 mM), sodium taurocholate (1 mM) and MES (1 M) to adjust pH to 6. Standardized food model (SFM) was prepared according to the procedure of Zhang and co-workers [19] with slight modifications (Table S2). Briefly, sodium caseinate (1%, *w/w*) was dissolved in phosphate buffer solution (10 mM, pH 7) and then filtered to remove any residual insoluble matter. Sunflower oil was gradually added (7.6%, *w/w*) and vortexed for 5 min. Powdered sodium caseinate was gradually added into the emulsion to reach a final concentration of 7.7% *w/w* protein and continuously stirred for 30 min. An aqueous pectin (1.6% *w/v*) solution was obtained by dispersing pectin powder into distilled water and then mixing at 50 °C for 60 min. The mixture was then cooled to room temperature and stirred continuously to fully dissolve the pectin. Then 44.8 g of the prepared pectin solution was mixed with 44.8 g of emulsion (1:1, *w/w*). At the end, 5.15 g of corn starch was slowly poured into the previous mixture with continuous stirring until it was fully dissolved (around 30 min). Pepsin solution was prepared by dissolving 50 mg of pepsin in 1 ml of SGF (25 000 U/mL). Pancreatin solution was prepared by dissolving 8 mg of pancreatin in 1 mL of SIF (800 U/mL). Bile salt solution was prepared by dispersing 65.37 mg of bile salt in 1 mL of water. The α-amylase solution was prepared by dissolving thermostable α-amylase in SSF (1500 U/mL). Hank's balanced salt solution (HBSS) pH 6.0 was prepared by dissolving KCl (0.4 mg/mL), $NaHCO_3$ (0.35 mg/mL), NaCl (8.0 mg/mL), D-glucose monohydrate (1.1 mg/mL), KH_2PO_4 (0.06 mg/mL), $Na_2HPO_4 \times 2H_2O$ (0.06 mg/mL), $CaCl_2 \times 2H_2O$ (0.185 mg/mL), $MgCl_2 \times 6H_2O$ (0.1 mg/mL), $MgSO_4 \times 7H_2O$ (0.1 mg/mL), and HEPES (7.15 mg/mL) in ultrapure water. All of the solvents needed for chromatographic separation were degassed with Branson 1210 Ultrasonic

Cleaner (Danbury, CT, USA) before analysis. Acetate buffer was prepared by mixing sodium acetate 0.1 M:acetic acid 0.1 M (2:1 *v/v*) and adjusting the pH to 5 with pH meter (702 SM Titrino, Metrohm, Herisau, Switzerland).

2.2. Preparation of Samples

Olive pomace extract (OPE) was prepared according to previously published procedure [8] with some modifications. Briefly, olive pomace was dried at 60 °C for 24 h in an incubator (INKO, Zagreb, Croatia), sieved through Φ 0.8 mm sieve (Prüfsieb DIN 4188, Kassel, Germany), and defatted with petrol ether using the Soxhlet apparatus (INKO SK6ESS, Zagreb, Croatia). Pre-treated olive pomace was mixed with 20% ethanol (20 g/L) and the extraction was performed by 2 h maceration in a shaking water bath at 70 °C and 100 rpm (Thermostat, Inko, Zagreb, Croatia). The mixture was filtered to remove the crude parts, ethanol was removed from the filtrate under reduced pressure (Rotavapor R-220 EX, BÜCHI Labortechnik AG, Flawil, Switzerland) and obtained water extracts were dried for 48 h in a lyophilizator (Alpha 1-4 LOC-1, Martin Christ Gefriertrocknungsanlagen GmbH, Osterode am Harz, Germany). Dry OPE was used for the simulation of gastrointestinal digestion. Chemical composition of OPE is presented in Table S3. Olive oil (OO) was obtained from the local supplier. Prior to simulation of gastrointestinal digestion OO was diluted with water in 1:10 ratio and vortexed thoroughly (VTY-3000L, Mixer UZUSIO, Tokyo, Japan). For the investigation of polyphenol-food interactions the following materials were used: dietary fiber (cellulose, pectin, inulin), tuna (canned), sour cream (12% milk fat), milk (fresh, 3.2% milk fat), yogurt (2.8% milk fat), milk formula, banana (raw minced), breakfast cereals, soy flakes, fresh cheese, meat sauce, apple (grated, skinless), silver beat (blanched, minced), bread, potato (boiled), honey, and corn starch. Basic nutritive composition was obtained from producers' nutrition data labels or from nutrition data tables [20] and are presented in supplementary materials (Table S4).

2.3. Determination of Total Phenols

Total polyphenols (total reductive capacity) of analyzed samples was assessed by Folin–Ciocalteu method that relies on the transfer of electrons in alkaline medium from phenolic (or other reductive) compounds to phosphomolybdic/phosphotungstic acid complexes, which are determined spectroscopically at 765 nm. Experiments were conducted according to the protocol described by Ainsworth and co-workers [21]. Moreover, 20 μL of adequately diluted sample/standard/solvent (blank) were added in triplicate to 96-well plate (Thermo Fisher Scientific 130188, Rochester, NY, USA) and incubated at 37 °C with 50 μL of Folin Ciocalteu reagent (10% (*v/v*)) for 5 min. The 160 μL of Na_2CO_3 (700 mM) was added into each well, shaken, and incubated at 37 °C for 30 min. Absorbance was read at 765 nm and results were expressed as gallic acid equivalents (GAE).

2.4. HPLC-FLD Determination of Hydroxytyrosol and Tyrosol

HTS and TS were identified and quantified by HPLC system (Waters Alliance 2695, Milford, MA, USA) coupled with a 2475 Multi λ detector (FLD) with Xenon lamp, according to slightly modified method of Tsarbopoulos and co-workers [22]. Samples were prepared by filtration through 0.45 μm polyethersulfone (PES) syringe filters (Macherey–Nagel, Düren, Germany). Chromatographic separation was conducted by injecting 20 μL of sample on a reversed phase column (250 × 4.6 mm, 5 μm) (Agilent Zorbax Eclipse Plus C18, Santa Clara, CA, USA). Mobile phases were 0.05 M sodium acetate buffer pH 5 and acetonitrile with the flow rate of 1 mL/min. Elution was conducted over 25 min at 25 °C. Identification was performed with FLD set at the excitation wavelength of 280 nm, and emission wavelength of 316 nm. Polyphenols were identified by comparing the retention times of the eluting peaks with those of the standards. Peaks were quantified by using the Empower2 software (Waters, Milford, MA, USA) and compared to external standard calibration. Standard stock solutions were prepared by dissolving reference compounds in DMSO.

2.5. Simulation of Gastrointestinal Digestion

In vitro simulation of gastrointestinal digestion and the assessment of bioaccessibility of hydroxytyrosol and tyrosol from OPE was conducted by standardized static in vitro digestion method suitable for food [23]. Three-phase digestion process was applied consisting of short salivary phase, simulation of gastric digestion and simulation of duodenal digestion. Briefly, 200 mg of OPE was used alone or mixed with 600 mg of food matrix (Table S4) in 50 mL Falcon tube. The 875 µL of SSF, 125 µL of salivary α amylase solution, 6.25 µL of $CaCl_2$ (0.3 mol/L), and 243.8 µL of water was added, and the mixture incubated at 37 °C for 2 min with constant shaking. The 2.5 mL of reaction mixture were transferred to another Falcon tube and mixed with 1.875 mL of SGF, 1.25 µL of $CaCl_2$ (0.3 mol/L), and 50 µL of HCl (1 mol/L). The pH of the mixture was adjusted to 3, and total volume was adjusted to 5 mL with water. The content of the Falcon tube was vortexed and incubated for 2 h at 37 °C with constant shaking. Every 15 min pH of the mixture was checked and adjusted to 3 if necessary. At the end of simulation of the gastric digestion step, 5 mL of aliquot were transferred to another 50 mL Falcon tube for the simulation of intestinal digestion. The 2.75 mL of SIF, 1.25 mL of pancreatin solution, 0.625 mL of bile salt (160 mmol/L), 10 µL of $CaCl_2$ (0.3 mol/L), and 37.5 µL of NaOH (1 mol/L) were added. The pH was checked and adjusted to 7. Total volume of reaction mixture was adjusted to 10 with water, mixtures were vortexed and incubated for 2 h at 37 °C with constant shaking. Every 15 min, pH of the mixture was checked and adjusted to 7 if necessary. After digestion, simulation samples were cooled at −20 °C for 10 min and centrifuged (Heraeus Biofuge Stratos, Hanau, Germany) for 20 min at 4 °C and 4100 rpm. For HPLC analysis of hydroxytyrosol and tyrosol, obtained supernatants were additionally filtered through 0.45 µm polyether sulfone (PES) syringe filters. Supernatants were collected and used for the assessment of bioaccessible HTS and TS fractions. Aliquots of samples to be used on cell monolayers were kept at 100 °C for 5 min in Thermomixer R (Eppendorf, Hamburg, Germany) for enzyme inactivation. For each sample blank was prepared, by omitting the addition of OPE to reaction mixture. Simulations of gastrointestinal digestion were conducted in duplicates. For fed state simulation using biorelevant media FeSSGF and FeSSIF were used instead of SGF and SIF and gastrointestinal digestion of OPE was simulated according to the procedure described above. For simulation of food effects on bioaccessibility of polyphenols using SFM, SFM was mixed with SSF in 1:1 ratio in the beginning of the experiment and gastrointestinal digestion of OPE was simulated according to the procedure described above. Total amount of polyphenols/HTS/TS in OPE was determined by dissolving dry OPE in distilled water. Bioaccessibility of polyphenols was calculated according to Equation (1):

$$\text{Bioaccessibility (\%)} = \frac{\text{bioaccessible amount}}{\text{total amount}} \times 100 \quad (1)$$

Impact of food on bioaccessibility of investigated compounds was expressed as relative bioaccessibility, that compares the bioaccessibility after digestion with food with bioaccessibility from OPE digested without the presence of food using SSF/SGF/SIF, and it was calculated according to Equation (2):

$$\text{Relative bioaccessibility (\%)} = \frac{\text{bioaccessibility with food (\%)}}{\text{bioacessibility without food (\%)}} \times 100 \quad (2)$$

2.6. Transepithelial Transport of HTS and TS in Caco-2 Monolayers

For investigation of transepithelial transport human epithelial colorectal adenocarcinoma cell line (Caco-2) was used. Caco-2 cells (ATCC) were cultured in DMEM supplemented with 10% heat-inactivated FBS, 1% NEAA, and 1% A/A. Cell cultures were maintained at 37 °C, in a humidity saturated atmosphere consisted of 5% CO_2 (Sanyo MCO 20AIC CO_2 Incubator, Osaka, Japan). Medium was changed every 2 days. Cells were passaged at 80–90% confluence. The study of transepithelial transport was conducted by using 40 µg/mL of TS and HTS diluted in HBSS (MIX) in the presence of one of the following substances: 10 mM glucose (GLU); 0.25% nonessential amino acids (NEAA); 0.125% nonessential amino acids (NEAA2x); 2.4 mg/mL hydroxypropyl β cyclodextrin (HPB); 1% cellulose (alba fiber); 1% inulin (inulin). The highest non-toxic concentration of samples was determined by MTT assay [24]. The 3×10^5 cells/well were seeded in 96-well plates (Thermo Fisher Scientific 130188, Rochester, NY, USA) and grown until reaching confluence (approximately 48 h). The medium was aspirated, and the cells washed with 100 μL PBS/well. Cells were incubated for 4 h with either 100 μL of samples or Hank's balanced salt solution (HBSS) for positive control or 350 μM tBOOH for negative control. Samples were then removed, and cells were washed with 100 μL PBS/well. Cell viability was assessed by the addition of 40 μL of MTT 0.5 mg/mL (diluted in PBS) and incubation for 3 h at 37 °C, followed by dissolution of the formazan crystals in 170 μL of DMSO. Absorbance (A) was measured at 490 nm and cell viability was expressed as percentage (%) relative to the positive control according to Equation (3). Blank absorbance was measured in wells containing MTT without cells.

$$\%\ \text{viability} = \frac{\text{Asample} - \text{Ablank}}{\text{Acontrol} - \text{Ablank}} \times 100 \quad (3)$$

Transepithelial transport was investigated in 12-well plate with Transwell® permeable supports (Costar 3401, Corning Incorporated, Kennebunk, ME, USA) [25]. The 3×10^5 cells were seeded per well and maintained at 37 °C, in a humidity saturated atmosphere consisted of 5% CO_2. Cells were grown for 21 days in order to form a differentiated monolayer on filters. The medium was warily aspirated (Gilson Safe Aspiration Station, Middleton, WI, USA) and replaced with fresh one every 2 days. The added volume was 0.5 mL in the apical and 1.5 mL in the basolateral compartment. Monolayer integrity was routinely checked by determining transepithelial electrical resistance (TEER) during the cell growth, before and after the transport experiment. Electrical resistance (ER) was measured with STX2 and Epithelial Volt/Ohm Meter (EVOM) (World Precision Instruments Inc., Sarasota, FL, USA). TEER, defined as ER per area, was calculated according to Equation (4).

$$\text{TEER} = (\text{R} - 120\ \Omega) \times 1.12\ \text{cm}^2 \quad (4)$$

where TEER is transepithelial electrical resistance, 120 Ω is resistance of the cell free-well (blank), 1.12 cm^2 is the filter surface.

To evaluate transepithelial permeability, medium was aspirated from both apical and basolateral chambers, and washed twice with pre-warmed PBS. Then, 0.5 mL of the sample or MIX (TS and HTS (40 μg/mL)) was added to the apical chamber and 1.5 mL of the HBSS to the basolateral chamber of each well. Samples were incubated at 100 rpm and 37 °C for 2 h in a shaker (Biosan Incubator ES-20/60, Riga, Latvia). The initial amount of HTS and TS added to a monolayer and the amount in basolateral compartment after the 2 h incubation of Caco-2 cells with the samples was determined by HPLC-FLD. The transepithelial transport of HTS and TS was expressed as % of the amount applied on cell monolayer according to Equation (5).

$$\% = \frac{\text{amount in basolateral compartment}}{\text{initial amount}} \times 100 \quad (5)$$

2.7. Statistical Analysis

All experiments were run in triplicate unless otherwise stated. Data were statistically tested by one-way analysis of variance (ANOVA), followed by Tukey's multiple comparisons test. Results were expressed as average value and standard deviation. $p \leq 0.05$ was considered statistically significant unless otherwise noted. GraphPad® Prism Software (San Diego, CA, USA) was used for statistical analysis.

3. Results and Discussion

3.1. Impact of Food-Induced Physiological Changes in Gastrointestinal System on Bioaccessibility of OPE Polyphenols

In order to assess the gastrointestinal bioaccessibility of particular compound by an in vitro approach it is essential to mimic the conditions in the gastrointestinal tract as closely as possible. There are several types of in vitro digestion methods that are commonly used for food, but static models, which use a constant ratio of food to enzymes and electrolytes, and a constant pH for each digestive phase, are used most often. However, the experimental conditions in static digestion simulation protocols differ significantly, depending on the purpose of the study and type of analyte/food matrix analyzed. This results with the large number of digestion protocols, which differ considering pH, duration of digestion phases, enzyme concentration and activity, and composition of simulated digestive fluids [26], resulting in questionable relevance of obtained data. Therefore, recently, international consensus was reached in terms of determining optimal conditions that should be applied for in vitro digestion simulation in static models. Such optimized and standardized procedure was applied in this investigation [23].

Results presented in Figure 1 show that bioaccessibility of total phenols, HTS and TS is slightly but significantly increased during gastrointestinal digestion, due to liberation of polyphenolic compounds from complex food matrix (281.0 to 357.5 mg/100g; 78.4 to 109.3 mg/100g; and 20.7 to 27.4 mg/100g, respectively). This is consistent with available literature data stating that during the gastric phase of digestion the majority of polyphenols is released from food matrix where they originally formed covalent bonds with carbohydrates of the cell wall, proteins, or one with another [10]. Our previous investigation that focused on the impact of cyclodextrin encapsulation on bioaccessibility of HTS and TS also showed that both, HTS and TS are stable in the gastrointestinal tract, and that their concentrations remain the same or increase during gastrointestinal digestion [8].

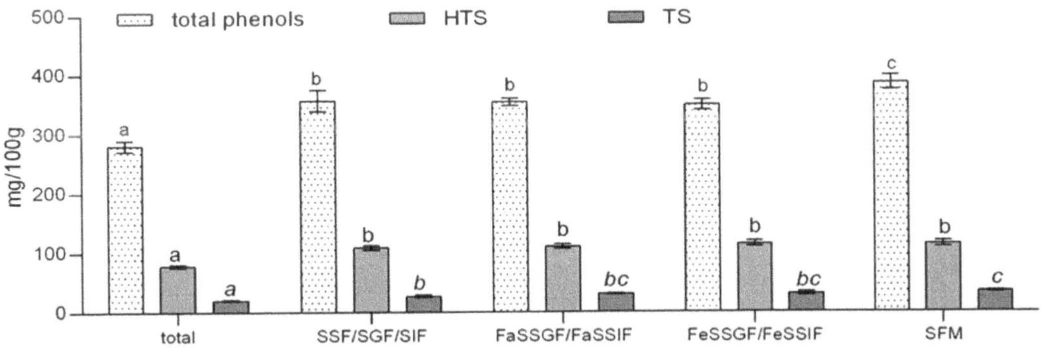

Figure 1. Impact of fed-state on gastrointestinal bioaccessibility of total polyphenols, hydroxytyrosol, and tyrosol from olive pomace extract. SSF—simulated salivary fluid; SGF—simulated gastric fluid; SIF—simulated intestinal fluid; FaSSGF—fasted state simulated gastric fluid; FaSSIF—fasted state simulated intestinal fluid; FeSSGF—fed state simulated gastric fluid; FeSSIF—fed state simulated intestinal fluid; SFM—standardized food matrix; HTS—hydroxytyrosol; TS—tyrosol. Data belonging to the same group are marked with the same letter belong to the same statistical group ($p \leq 0.05$).

As mentioned before, the effect of food on bioaccessibility of particular compounds can be assessed by several methodological approaches, including biorelevant dissolution testing. Food effects on drug absorption are generally better predicted when using biorelevant media containing bile salts and lecithin as compared to the traditional media (SGF and SIF). Namely, the presence of food in gastrointestinal tract changes the conditions in the stomach and intestines, in terms of pH, osmolarity, and composition of digestion fluids, which can significantly influence the pharmacokinetic properties and bioaccessibility of particular compounds [27]. Mentioned differences of the fed/fasted gastric/intestinal state, can be mimicked by fed–fasted state biorelevant media with sufficient accuracy, and although usually used in biorelevant dissolution testing of drugs, they can be applied in the field of nutraceutical formulation and testing. Food effects on bioaccessibility of OPE polyphenols, HTS and TS can be assessed by comparing the fasted state simulated gastric fluid (FaSSGF)/ fasted state simulated intestinal fluid (FaSSIF) and FeSSGF/FaSSIF data presented in Figure 1. Presented data clearly show that changes of pH and digestion fluid composition induced by presence of food in gastrointestinal tract do not influence the bioaccessibility of OPE polyphenols, HTS and TS. Moreover, there were no differences between results obtained by simulating digestion with SSF/SGF/SIF and biorelevant fasted state media. Considering the physicochemical characteristics of hydroxytyrosol and tyrosol, obtained results were partially expected. Namely, significant food effect can be anticipated based on both solubility and permeability of particular compound as described by the Biopharmaceutics Classification System (BCS) [28,29]. Taking into account high water solubility of HTS and TS (17.4 g/L and 25.3 g/L, respectively) and low apparent permeability assessed by predicted logP values (0.85–1.19 and 0.13–0.89, respectively) HTS and TS could be provisionally classified into class 3, according to BCS classification. BCS Class III (high solubility, low permeability) drugs tend to have negative food effects, but they can only be observed by investigating the interactions of food/food compounds with drug absorption and not biorelevant media bioaccessibility testing [30]. As mentioned before, introduction of SFM can be considered as a step forward in in vitro investigation of food effects on bioaccessibility of bioactive compounds because it takes into account wider spectra of possible bioactive compound–food matrix interactions that might affect pharmacokinetic properties of the particular compound [19]. In comparison to other applied methods, simulation of gastrointestinal digestion with SFM significantly increased bioaccessibility of OPE polyphenols in general but had no effect on HTS and TS bioaccessible fractions. This was partially expected, given the high water solubility and previously established gastrointestinal stability of HTS and TS [8]. Namely, positive food effects are usually associated with nonpolar polyphenols because the presence of fat in the food matrix enhances the formation of micelles during the intestinal digestion phase and increases polyphenol content in the soluble (bioaccessible) digest fraction [10]. Conversely to our results, absorption of tyrosol and hydroxytyrosol was positively influenced by the lipid-rich matrix (olive oil), resulting in 25% greater absorption compared to aqueous solution in the rat model [31]. However, the effect could have been achieved, not due to the lipid matrix, but the formation of HTS during gastrointestinal digestion (due to cleavage of more complex antioxidants (such as oleuropein)) and the protection of HTS and TS by other antioxidants present in the olive oil. Positive effects of food matrix on polyphenol bioavailability can also be attributed to the presence of fermentable fiber (such as pectin) that increase colonic bioavailability of particular polyphenols due to their prebiotic properties. These effects could not be monitored in our study. Therefore, observed slight, but statistically significant positive effects of SFM on phenolic bioaccessibility can likely be attributed to the impact of fat on micellization of nonpolar polyphenols present in OPE.

3.2. Gastrointestinal Interactions of HTS and TS with Particular Food

Bioavailability of olive polyphenols from food matrices other than olive oil has rarely been studied. Radić and co-workers [8] investigated the influence of olive pomace matrix and cyclodextrin encapsulation on bioavailability of olive polyphenols, and showed high bioaccessibility, but relatively low permeability, of hydroxytyrosol and tyrosol, which were both negatively affected by olive pomace matrix. Their results confirmed the previous findings of Malapert and co-workers [32], who showed that bioavailability of hydroxytyrosol was higher when it was applied as a pure compound than from Alperujo powder. They also showed that presence of foods (investigated by co-digestion with the test meal) significantly decreased hydroxytyrosol bioaccessibility and intestinal permeability (−20% and −10%, respectively). They supposed that negative food effects arise from the fact that polyphenols form complex bonds with particular food components, and that the investigation of the influence of the food matrix on the bioaccessibility of dietary plant phenols, such as HT, requires including real meal components into in vitro digestion studies [32]. This is consistent with our results (Figure 1), where the comparison of results obtained in fed/fasted biorelevant media showed that changes in pH, ionic strength, or the amount of bile during gastrointestinal digestion are not determining factors for HTS and TS bioaccessibility. However, data presented in Table S5 and Figure 2 clearly show that both bioaccessibility and relative bioaccessibility of HTS and TS can be significantly changed during co-digestion with different foods, and that the extent of observed changes depends on chemical/nutritive composition of food matrices (Table S4). Depending on the food matrix investigated, bioaccessibility of OPE polyphenols was either not affected or it was significantly reduced. The most significant impact was observed after co-digestion of OPE with soy flakes, fresh low-fat cheese, and milk formula (relative bioaccessibility of TP was 51.8%, 60.6%, and 71.9% respectively), foods with relatively high protein content (52%, 12.4%, 10.5%) Bioaccessibility of HTS and TS was also significantly reduced by some of the investigated high-protein foods: soy flakes, sauce Bolognese, breakfast cereals, and whole-grain bread, but the effect was less pronounced than in the case of TP. Observed effects were, at least partially influenced, by polyphenol–protein interactions, well described in scientific literature and reviewed recently in the work of Jakobek [14]. Polyphenols (especially polyhydroxy polyphenols) form non-covalent hydrophobic interactions with proteins, which may subsequently be stabilized by hydrogen bonding [33], and can, among other effects, change the bioavailability of polyphenols. Different authors observed negative effects of milk proteins on bioavailability of polyphenols of different origin [34–38]. The majority of observed negative interactions in literature were observed for casein, which is consistent with our results showing the stronger negative effects of foods with casein content in comparison to other high-protein foods (although total protein content was relatively low). To our knowledge, impact of proteins on bioaccessibility of hydroxytyrosol and tyrosol has not been previously investigated, but it has been shown that hydroxytyrosol can form adducts with food proteins [39]. Obtained results suggest the negative interactions between proteins and polyphenols, but additional effects of matrix components, such as lipids or carbohydrates, must also be considered. For example, despite high protein content, canned tuna or milk formula did not negatively influence bioaccessibility of hydroxytyrosol, maybe partially due to high fat content (15.5 and 27.4%, respectively). Namely, although investigations suggest that interactions between lipids and polyphenols have only a small influence on the polyphenol accessibility for absorption [14], some studies show that when lipids interact with polyphenols, they can "capture" polyphenols and protect them from degradation or forming insoluble complexes in their passage through the gastrointestinal tract [40], or increase their solubility and activity in gastrointestinal tract by forming micelles and promoting emulsification [41]. In our study, such effects were not particularly pronounced, since OPE polyphenols have been proven stable during gastrointestinal digestion and are generally soluble in water [8].

Interactions between polyphenols and available carbohydrates have been described in scientific literature because polyphenols can reduce starch digestion, possibly via amylase inhibition, and inhibit glucose uptake transporters [42]. Far fewer studies have examined the impact of carbohydrates on polyphenol bioavailability and were mostly focused on polyphenol uptake. In our investigation, corn starch and honey (100% and 80% of available carbohydrates) were selected as model foods for investigation of available carbohydrate impact on olive polyphenols bioaccessibility. Relative bioaccessibility of TF, HTS, and TS after co-digestion with corn starch/honey was 94.5/113.6%; 94.9/89.5%, and 88.7/97.8%, and observed differences were not statistically significant (Figure 2).

While the negative impacts of indigestible carbohydrates (dietary fiber) on digestibility of fat and bioaccessibility of some minerals and trace elements is well known, their influence on the bioaccessibility of polyphenolic compounds has not been thoroughly investigated. The main direct mechanisms of negative impacts of dietary fiber on polyphenol intestinal availability are an incomplete release of polyphenols from fiber rich fruit and vegetable matrices (i); presence of polyphenols bound to polysaccharides requiring enzymatic hydrolysis to be absorbed (ii); and entrapment of polyphenols by dietary fiber during digestion in the upper intestine (iii) [43]. The possibility of the formation of insoluble polyphenol–dietary fiber complexes during gastrointestinal digestion is particularly important for this investigation since it focused on the bioaccessibility of polyphenols previously isolated from its natural complex matrix. As shown in Figure 2, bioaccessibility of TP was not significantly reduced in the presence dietary fiber containing food (Table S4) except for soy flakes that contained high content of both proteins and fiber (52% and 16%, respectively). On the other hand, a negative impact of fiber was more noticeable in the case of TS and HTS. Bioaccessibility of TS was significantly reduced in the presence of breakfast cereals, wholegrain bread, apple and silver beat, ranging from 67% to 89% in relation to bioaccessibility of OPE consumed with no food. The negative effect of dietary fiber was even more pronounced in the case of HTS. Its relative bioaccessibility was significantly reduced in the presence of all fiber containing foods and ranged from 54.8% up to 84.2%. Pronounced negative effects on hydroxytyrosol bioaccessibility might be explained by the additional hydroxyl group in HTS structure since dietary fiber–polyphenol interactions were observed to appear through non-covalent bonds as electrostatic forces and hydrogen bonds as Van der Waals forces between hydroxyl groups of phenolic compounds and various components of dietary fibers [44]. The negative impact on HTS/TS bioaccessibility was not proportional to the content of dietary fiber in the food matrix probably because it is the consequence of complex interactions of all matrix components and also the chemical composition of the fiber. In order to investigate the gastrointestinal polyphenol–dietary fiber interactions more thoroughly, we additionally simulated gastrointestinal digestion of OPE in the presence of cellulose, pectin and inulin and assessed the impact on the relative bioaccessibility of OPE antioxidants (Figure 3). Presented data show that the impact of dietary fiber on polyphenol bioaccessibility depends on both types of dietary fiber and chemical characteristics of particular polyphenols. All investigated fiber significantly reduced relative bioaccessibility of TP from OPE (69.8–79%), and cellulose showed the strongest negative impact. Relative bioaccessibility of HTS was reduced to 88.1% by cellulose and to 93.2% by pectin and was not influenced by the presence of inulin in the reaction mixture. TS relative bioaccessibility was reduced to 87.4% by cellulose and was not affected by the presence of other dietary fiber. The comparison of fiber-in-food-matrix–polyphenol interactions to pure fiber–polyphenol interactions (Figures 2 and 3, respectively) indicate the significant effect of the food matrix on the type and extent of polyphenol–dietary fiber interactions. Therefore, data on the effect of fiber-rich food on polyphenol bioaccessibility cannot be extrapolated from the data obtained by in vitro digestion of polyphenols with pure dietary fiber. Therefore, in order to guide the design of functional foods enriched with phenolic substances, we should significantly increase the number of in vitro and in vivo studies on the bioavailability of particular phenolic substances in contact with particular foods. This is consistent with the conclusions of Pinarli and co-workers [45], stating that, due to complexity of interactions within the food matrix, every food material and component should be evaluated individually with respect to its interacting phenolic compound. Although HTS/TS-dietary fiber interactions have hardly been investigated, our observations are consistent with the recent findings of Bermúdez-Oria and co-authors [46], who confirmed the formation of predominant hydrogen–bonding interactions between HTS and strawberry dietary fiber. Tomas and co-authors [47] noticed modulation of polyphenols profile of blackberry purees by soluble dietary fiber (inulin or pectin), during a simulated in vitro gastrointestinal digestion and large intestine fermentation process, and explained it by the interactions of dietary fiber and polyphenols.

3.3. *Impact of Food on Intestinal Permeability of TP, HTS, and TS*

The influence of MIX and investigated food components on the viability of human epithelial colorectal adenocarcinoma cells Caco-2 was determined by using the MTT assay (Figure 4a) and by measuring TEER values, before and after the experiment (Figure 4b), as previously described. The results presented in Figure 4 show that cell viability was significantly decreased when cells were treated with the MIX and HPB, which is consistent with previously obtained data [48]. Although significantly decreased in relation to positive control (CTR+), viability of monolayers treated with MIX and HPB was above 80% (81.4 and 80.3%, respectively) and, therefore, suitable for further analysis. Moreover, it is evident from Figure 4b that, even though tested food matrices do not produce significant cytotoxic effects, they can significantly affect the intestinal barrier, and may increase bilayer permeability or promote barrier integrity. Those effects are achieved through different mechanisms: affecting mucus permeation, paracellular permeation, bilayer permeability, or active transport and efflux transport [12,49]. As shown previously, food matrix can significantly affect intestinal permeability of polyphenols through formation of soluble or insoluble complexes, resulting with positive or negative effects on bioaccessibility. Therefore, the actual intestinal permeability of a particular compound is the result of all of the above-mentioned interactions and, because of that, it is very hard to predict.

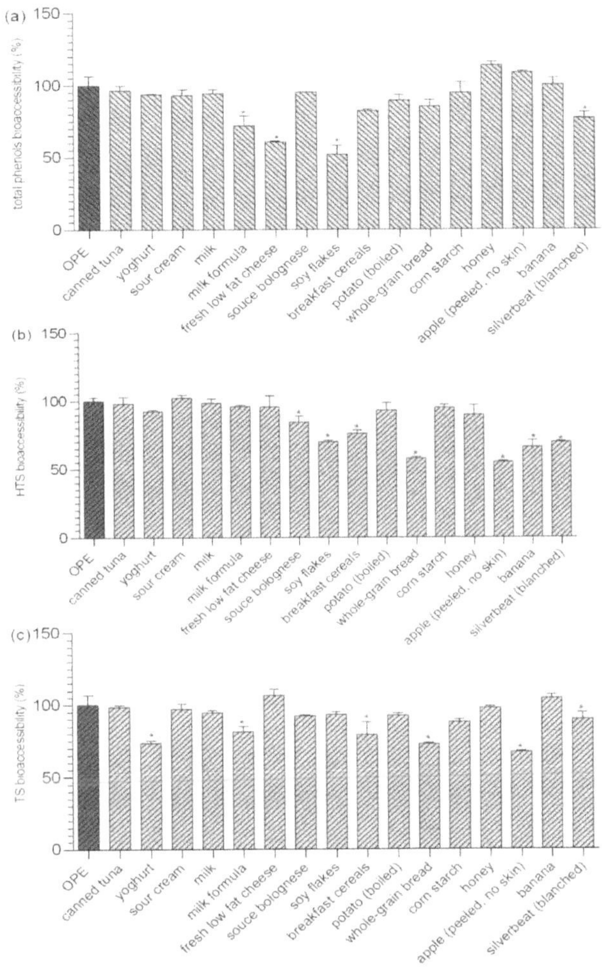

Figure 2. Impact of different foods on relative bioaccessibility* of total polyphenols (**a**), HTS) (**b**) and TS (**c**) from OPE. * Relative bioaccessibility was calculated in relation to in vitro bioaccessibility of total phenols, HTS, and TS from OPE obtained after simulation of gastrointestinal digestion using FaSSIF/FeSSIF. Columns marked with * differ significantly from OPE ($p \leq 0.05$). OPE—olive pomace extract; FaSSGF—fasted state simulated gastric fluid; FaSSIF—fasted state simulated intestinal fluid; HTS—hydroxytyrosol; TS—tyrosol.

At the moment, available data on the impact of food matrix/nutrients on intestinal permeability of polyphenols are scarce. Recently, Nogueira Mendes and co-authors [50] showed that intestinal permeability of guarana catechins and procyanidins was not significantly affected by macronutrients (casein, starch and oil). On the other hand, transepithelial transport of indicaxanthin and betanin was negatively affected by particular food matrix components while intestinal transport of green tea catechins was positively affected by milk proteins, probably due to impact of milk on tight junction permeability [51,52]. The mentioned results point out the significance of chemical characteristics of targeted molecules and the exact composition of the food matrix in predicting food matrix effects, as well as the necessity of focused and tailored research.

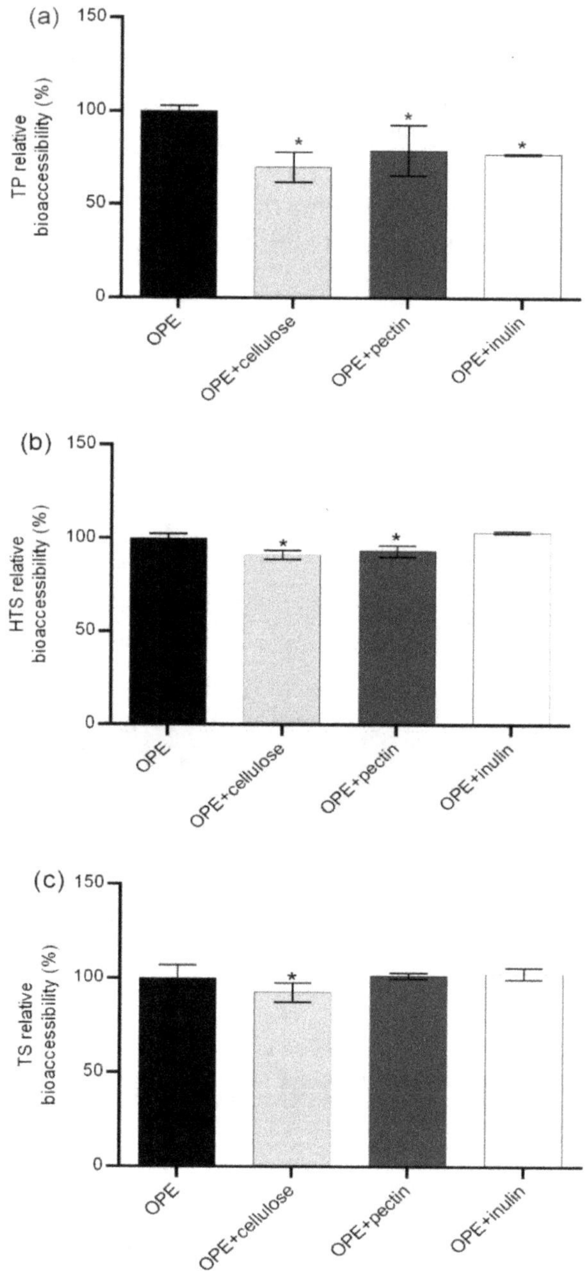

Figure 3. Impact of cellulose, pectin and inulin on relative bioaccessibility* of TP, HTS, and TS from OPE. * Relative bioaccessibility was calculated in relation to in vitro bioaccessibility of TP, HTS, and TS from OPE obtained after simulation of gastrointestinal digestion using FaSSIF/FeSSIF. Columns marked with * differ significantly from OPE ($p \leq 0.05$). OPE—olive pomace extract; FaSSGF—fasted state simulated gastric fluid; FaSSIF—fasted state simulated intestinal fluid; TP—total phenols; HTS—hydroxytyrosol; TS—tyrosol.

In order to investigate the impact of glucose, amino acids, dietary fiber (inulin and apple fiber), and HPB (excipient often used in nutraceutical production) on transepithelial permeability of HTS and TS, they were applied to Caco-2 monolayers in combination, and their permeability was compared to permeability of HTS and TS from pure mixture (MIX). As presented in Figure 5, permeability of HTS and TS was mostly unaffected by tested compounds, with few exceptions. First, glucose significantly improved permeability of both HTS and TS. The mechanisms of such interaction are unknown and beyond the scope of this investigation, but certain assumptions can be made based on available literature data. DeSouza and co-authors [53] investigated Caco-2 cell permeability was evaluated in isotonic media containing high (25 mM) or physiological (5.5 mM) glucose concentrations, and concluded that high extracellular glucose concentration in isotonic media significantly alters physical barrier properties of Caco-2 cell monolayers, which predominantly affects transepithelial transport of solutes permeating the cell barrier by paracellular and transcellular passive diffusion through decreasing TEER of cell monolayers, increasing membrane fluidity. Their results are in consistence with data presented in Figure 4B showing that glucose significantly decreased TERR of Caco-2cell monolayers (20%).

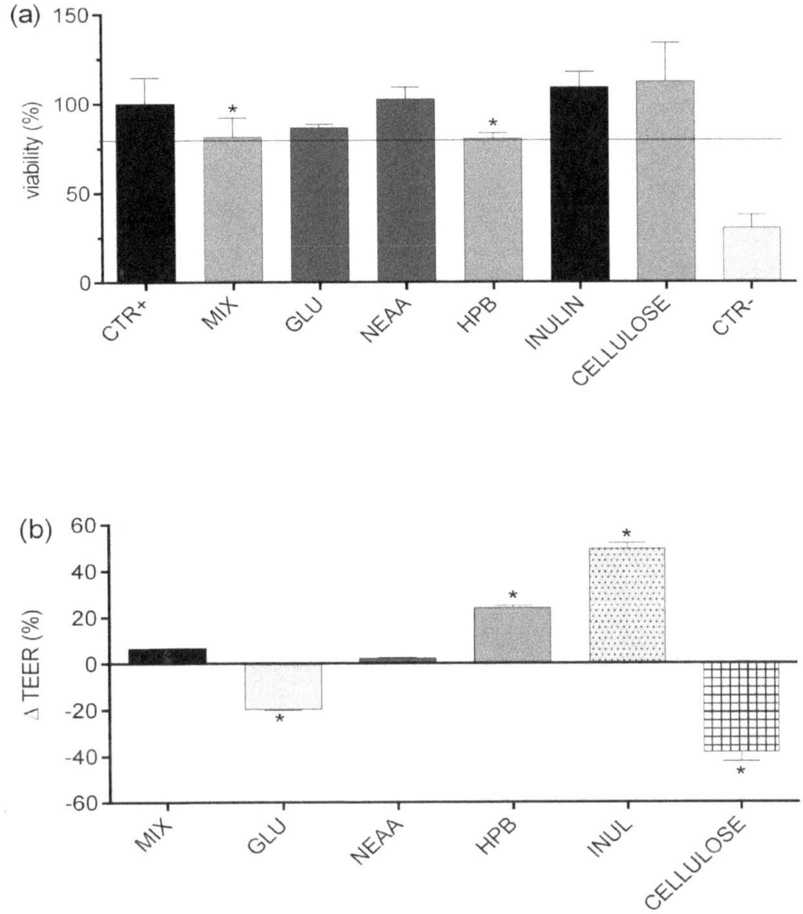

Figure 4. Viability (%) of Caco-2 cell monolayer determined by MTT test after exposure to analyzed food fractions (**a**). Relative change (%) of TEER values during the experiment (**b**). positive control (CTR+)—HBSS; MIX—TS + HTS (40 mg/L); EDTA (10μM); GLU—glucose (10 mM); NEAA—non-essential amino acids (0.25%); HPB—hydroxypropyl beta-cyclodextrin (2.4 g/L); CELLULOSE—cellulose (1%); INULIN—inulin (1%); CTR¯tBOOH (350 μM); TEER—transepithelial electrical resistance. Columns marked with * differ significantly from the reference column: (CTR+ (**a**); MIX (**b**)).

The TEER of cell monolayers was also negatively affected by cellulose (40%, but it did not result in increased permeability of HTS/TS. This is probably due to formation of insoluble complexes with HTS/TS, as shown in Figure 3, where cellulose decreased bioaccessibility of both investigated phenolic compounds. These observations are consistent with data obtained by Bermudez-Oria and co-authors [46], who showed that olive polyphenols form insoluble complexes with dietary fibers. On the other hand, inulin had the opposite effects on HTS and TS intestinal permeability. As shown in Figure 4B, it significantly increased TEER (40%). This observation is consistent with available literature data showing that fructooligosaccharides can improve intestinal barrier function through short fatty acid formation [54,55], but such effects could not have been noticed in our investigation (that did not include the step of microbial fermentation of fermentable fiber). However, our data show that inulin can have additional, direct impacts on Caco-2 cell permeability, and it resulted in a significant reduction of HTS transepithelial permeability.

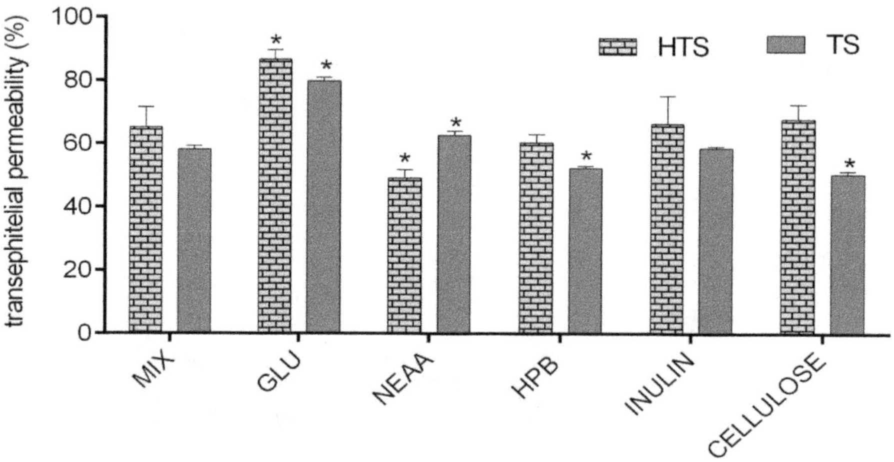

Figure 5. Permeability (%) of HTS and TS in Caco-2 cell monolayer (the amount of TS/HTS in basolateral compartment was expressed as the percentage of the amount applied to Caco-2 cell monolayer). MIX-TS + HTS (40 mg/L); GLU—glucose (10 mM); NEAA—non-essential amino acids (0.25%); HPB—hydroxypropyl beta-cyclodextrin (2.4 g/L); APPLE FIBRE—apple fiber (1%); INULIN (1%). Columns belonging to the same series marked with * differ significantly ($p \leq 0.05$) from the reference column (MIX).

4. Conclusions

Changes in pH, ionic strength, enzyme activity, or the amount of bile due to presence of food in digestive system, are not determining factors for HTS and TS bioaccessibility, but can slightly improve bioaccessibility of other OPE polyphenols. Soy, milk formula, cheese, and breakfast cereals exerted negative effects on HTS and TS bioaccessibility, probably due to negative HTS/TS-casein and HTS/TS-dietary fiber interactions. Particular nutrients significantly influenced the permeability of Caco-2 cell monolayer (without exerting cytotoxic effects); it was increased by glucose and cellulose while inulin improved monolayer barrier function. Those effects significantly affected transepithelial transport of HTS and TS. Our results provide new insights into factors affecting bioaccessibility and transepithelial permeability of HTS and TS and point out the complexity of polyphenol interactions within the food matrix. Therefore, in the process of formulating functional foods enriched with phenolic substances, every food matrix should be evaluated individually, with respect to its interacting phenolic compounds.

Supplementary Materials: Table S1. Composition of simulated salivary fluid (SSF), simulated gastric fluid (SGF) and simulated intestinal fluid (SIF); Table S2. Composition of standardized food model (SFM); Table S3. Chemical composition of OPE; Table S4. Macronutritive composition of food matrices used for investigations of gastrointestinal interactions with hydroxytyrosol and tyrosol; Table S5. Impact of different foods and dietary fibre on relative bioaccessibility* of HTS, TS and total polyphenols from OPE.

Author Contributions: Conceptualization, D.V.Č.; methodology, D.V.Č. and K.R.; formal analysis, D.A., B.K., and M.Š.; investigation, P.T. and K.R.; resources, D.V.Č.; data curation, P.T.; writing—original draft preparation, P.T. and K.R.; writing—review and editing, D.V.Č.; visualization, D.V.Č. and K.R.; supervision, D.V.Č.; project administration, K.R.; funding acquisition, D.V.Č. All authors have read and agreed to the published version of the manuscript.

Acknowledgments: The authors would like to thank Jelena Filipović Grčić and Jasmina Lovrić from the Department of Pharmaceutical Technology, Faculty of Pharmacy and Biochemistry, University of Zagreb, for their support during the research.

References

1. EFSA Panel on Dietetic Products, Nutrition and Allergies (NDA). Scientific Opinion on the substantiation of health claims related to polyphenols in olive and protection of LDL particles from oxidative damage (ID 1333, 1638, 1639, 1696, 2865), maintenance of normal blood HDL cholesterol concentrations (ID 1639), mainte. *EFSA J.* **2011**, *9*, 2033. [CrossRef]
2. Servili, M.; Sordini, B.; Esposto, S.; Urbani, S.; Veneziani, G.; Di Maio, I.; Selvaggini, R.; Taticchi, A. Biological Activities of Phenolic Compounds of Extra Virgin Olive Oil. *Antioxidants* **2013**, *3*, 1–23. [CrossRef] [PubMed]
3. Chanioti, S.; Tzia, C. Extraction of phenolic compounds from olive pomace by using natural deep eutectic solvents and innovative extraction techniques. *Innov. Food Sci. Emerg. Technol.* **2018**, *48*, 228–239. [CrossRef]
4. Goldsmith, C.D.; Vuong, Q.V.; Stathopoulos, C.E.; Roach, P.; Scarlett, C.J. Ultrasound increases the aqueous extraction of phenolic compounds with high antioxidant activity from olive pomace. *LWT* **2018**, *89*, 284–290. [CrossRef]
5. Jurmanović, S.; Jug, M.; Safner, T.; Radić, K.; Domijan, A.-M.; Pedisić, S.; Šimić, S.; Jablan, J.; Vitali Čepo, D. Utilization of olive pomace as the source of polyphenols: Optimization of microwave-assisted extraction and characterization of spray-dried extract. *J. Food Nutr. Res.* **2019**, *58*, 51–62.
6. Albahari, P.; Jug, M.; Radić, K.; Jurmanović, S.; Brnčić, M.; Brnčić, S.R.; Vitali Čepo, D. Characterization of olive pomace extract obtained by cyclodextrin-enhanced pulsed ultrasound assisted extraction. *LWT* **2018**, *92*, 22–31. [CrossRef]
7. Vitali Čepo, D.; Radić, K.; Jurmanović, S.; Jug, M.; Rajković, M.G.; Pedisić, S.; Moslavac, T.; Albahari, P. Valorization of olive pomace-based nutraceuticals as antioxidants in chemical, food, and biological models. *Molecules* **2018**, *23*, 2070. [CrossRef]
8. Radić, K.; Jurišić Dukovski, B.; Vitali Čepo, D. Influence of pomace matrix and cyclodextrin encapsulation on olive pomace polyphenols' bioaccessibility and intestinal permeability. *Nutrients* **2020**, *12*, 669. [CrossRef]
9. D'Archivio, M.; Filesi, C.; Varì, R.; Scazzocchio, B.; Masella, R. Bioavailability of the Polyphenols: Status and Controversies. *Int. J. Mol. Sci.* **2010**, *11*, 1321–1342. [CrossRef]
10. Bohn, T. Dietary factors affecting polyphenol bioavailability. *Nutr. Rev.* **2014**, *72*, 429–452. [CrossRef]
11. Ting, Y.; Jiang, Y.; Ho, C.-T.; Huang, Q. Common delivery systems for enhancing in vivo bioavailability and biological efficacy of nutraceuticals. *J. Funct. Foods* **2014**, *7*, 112–128. [CrossRef]
12. McClements, D.J. Enhancing nutraceutical bioavailability through food matrix design. *Curr. Opin. Food Sci.* **2015**, *4*, 1–6. [CrossRef]
13. Koziolek, M.; Alcaro, S.; Augustijns, P.; Basit, A.W.; Grimm, M.; Hens, B.; Hoad, C.L.; Jedamzik, P.; Madla, C.M.; Maliepaard, M.; et al. The mechanisms of pharmacokinetic food-drug interactions—A perspective from the UNGAP group. *Eur. J. Pharm. Sci.* **2019**, *134*, 31–59. [CrossRef] [PubMed]
14. Jakobek, L. Interactions of polyphenols with carbohydrates, lipids and proteins. *Food Chem.* **2015**, *175*, 556–567. [CrossRef]
15. Bermúdez-Oria, A.; Rodríguez-Gutiérrez, G.; África, F.-P.; Knicker, H.; Fernández-Bolaños, J. Confirmation by solid-state NMR spectroscopy of a strong complex phenol-dietary fiber with retention of antioxidant activity in vitro. *Food Hydrocoll.* **2020**, *102*, 105584. [CrossRef]
16. Fitó, M.; De La Torre, R.; Farré-Albaladejo, M.; Khymenetz, O.; Marrugat, J.; Covas, M.I. Bioavailability and antioxidant effects of olive oil phenolic compounds in humans: A review. *Ann. Ist. Super. Sanità* **2007**, *43*, 374–381.
17. García-Villalba, R.; Larrosa, M.; Possemiers, S.; Tomás-Barberán, F.A.; Espín, J.C. Bioavailability of phenolics from an oleuropein-rich olive (Olea europaea) leaf extract and its acute effect on plasma antioxidant status: Comparison between pre- and postmenopausal women. *Eur. J. Nutr.* **2014**, *53*, 1015–1027. [CrossRef]
18. Serra, A.; Rubió, L.; Borràs, X.; Macià, A.; Romero, M.-P.; Motilva, M.-J. Distribution of olive oil phenolic compounds in rat tissues after administration of a phenolic extract from olive cake. *Mol. Nutr. Food Res.* **2012**, *56*, 486–496. [CrossRef]
19. Zhang, Z.; Zhang, R.; McClements, D.J. Establishing the impact of food matrix effects on the bioaccessibility of nutraceuticals and pesticides using a standardized food model. *Food Funct.* **2019**, *10*, 1375–1385. [CrossRef]

20. Antonić Degač, K.; Hrabak-Žerjavić, V.; Kaić-Rak, A.; Matasović, D.; Maver, H.; Mesaroš Kanjski, E.; Petrović, Z.; Reiner, Z.; Strnad, M.; Šerman, D. *Prehrambene smjernice za odrasle*; Hrvatski Zavod za Javno Zdravstvo: Zagreb, Croatia; Akademija Medicinskih Znanosti Hrvatske: Zagreb, Croatia, 2002; Volume 8, pp. 1–16.
21. Ainsworth, E.A.; Gillespie, K.M. Estimation of total phenolic content and other oxidation substrates in plant tissues using Folin–Ciocalteu reagent. *Nat. Protoc.* **2007**, *2*, 875–877. [CrossRef] [PubMed]
22. Tsarbopoulos, A.; Gikas, E.; Papadopoulos, N.; Aligiannis, N.; Kafatos, A. Simultaneous determination of oleuropein and its metabolites in plasma by high-performance liquid chromatography. *J. Chromatogr. B* **2003**, *785*, 157–164. [CrossRef]
23. Brodkorb, A.; Egger, L.; Alminger, M.; Alvito, P.; Assunção, R.; Ballance, S.; Bohn, T.; Bourlieu-Lacanal, C.; Boutrou, R.; Carrière, F.; et al. INFOGEST static in vitro simulation of gastrointestinal food digestion. *Nat. Protoc.* **2019**, *14*, 991–1014. [CrossRef] [PubMed]
24. Riss, T.L.; Moravec, R.A.; Niles, A.L.; Duellman, S.; Benink, H.A.; Worzella, T.J.; Minor, L. *Cell Viability Assays*; Eli Lilly and Company: Indianapolis, IN, USA; National Center for Advancing Translational Sciences: Bethesda, MA, USA, 2004.
25. Hubatsch, I.; Ragnarsson, E.G.E.; Artursson, P. Determination of drug permeability and prediction of drug absorption in Caco-2 monolayers. *Nat. Protoc.* **2007**, *2*, 2111–2119. [CrossRef]
26. Hur, S.J.; Lim, B.O.; Decker, E.A.; McClements, D.J. In vitro human digestion models for food applications. *Food Chem.* **2011**, *125*, 1–12. [CrossRef]
27. Jones, H.M.; Parrott, N.; Ohlenbusch, G.; Lavé, T. Predicting Pharmacokinetic Food Effects Using Biorelevant Solubility Media and Physiologically Based Modelling. *Clin. Pharmacokinet.* **2006**, *45*, 1213–1226. [CrossRef]
28. Wu, C.-Y.; Benet, L.Z. Predicting Drug Disposition via Application of BCS: Transport/Absorption/Elimination Interplay and Development of a Biopharmaceutics Drug Disposition Classification System. *Pharm. Res.* **2005**, *22*, 11–23. [CrossRef]
29. Benet, L.Z. The Role of BCS (Biopharmaceutics Classification System) and BDDCS (Biopharmaceutics Drug Disposition Classification System) in Drug Development. *J. Pharm. Sci.* **2013**, *102*, 34–42. [CrossRef]
30. Lentz, K.A. Current Methods for Predicting Human Food Effect. *AAPS J.* **2008**, *10*, 282–288. [CrossRef]
31. Tuck, K.L.; Freeman, M.P.; Hayball, P.J.; Stretch, G.L.; Stupans, I. The In Vivo Fate of Hydroxytyrosol and Tyrosol, Antioxidant Phenolic Constituents of Olive Oil, after Intravenous and Oral Dosing of Labeled Compounds to Rats. *J. Nutr.* **2001**, *131*, 1993–1996. [CrossRef]
32. Malapert, A.; Tomao, V.; Dangles, O.; Reboul, E. Effect of Foods and β-Cyclodextrin on the Bioaccessibility and the Uptake by Caco-2 Cells of Hydroxytyrosol from Either a Pure Standard or Alperujo. *J. Agric. Food Chem.* **2018**, *66*, 4614–4620. [CrossRef] [PubMed]
33. Yuksel, Z.; Avci, E.; Erdem, Y.K. Characterization of binding interactions between green tea flavanoids and milk proteins. *Food Chem.* **2010**, *121*, 450–456. [CrossRef]
34. Duarte, G.S.; Farah, A. Effect of Simultaneous Consumption of Milk and Coffee on Chlorogenic Acids' Bioavailability in Humans. *J. Agric. Food Chem.* **2011**, *59*, 7925–7931. [CrossRef] [PubMed]
35. Mullen, W.; Borges, G.; Donovan, J.L.; Edwards, C.A.; Serafini, M.; Lean, M.E.; Crozier, A. Milk decreases urinary excretion but not plasma pharmacokinetics of cocoa flavan-3-ol metabolites in humans. *Am. J. Clin. Nutr.* **2009**, *89*, 1784–1791. [CrossRef]
36. Urpi-Sarda, M.; Llorach, R.; Khan, N.; Monagas, M.; Rotches-Ribalta, M.; Lamuela-Raventós, R.M.; Estruch, R.; Tinahones, F.J.; Andres-Lacueva, C. Effect of Milk on the Urinary Excretion of Microbial Phenolic Acids after Cocoa Powder Consumption in Humans. *J. Agric. Food Chem.* **2010**, *58*, 4706–4711. [CrossRef]
37. Serafini, M.; Testa, M.F.; Villaño, D.; Pecorari, M.; Van Wieren, K.; Azzini, E.; Brambilla, A.; Maiani, G. Antioxidant activity of blueberry fruit is impaired by association with milk. *Free Radic. Biol. Med.* **2009**, *46*, 769–774. [CrossRef]
38. Roowi, S.; Mullen, W.; Edwards, C.A.; Crozier, A. Yoghurt impacts on the excretion of phenolic acids derived from colonic breakdown of orange juice flavanones in humans. *Mol. Nutr. Food Res.* **2009**, *53*, S68–S75. [CrossRef]
39. Pham, L.B.; Wang, B.; Zisu, B.; Adhikari, B. Covalent modification of flaxseed protein isolate by phenolic compounds and the structure and functional properties of the adducts. *Food Chem.* **2019**, *293*, 463–471. [CrossRef]
40. Ortega, N.; Reguant, J.; Romero, M.-P.; Macià, A.; Motilva, M.-J. Effect of Fat Content on the Digestibility and Bioaccessibility of Cocoa Polyphenol by an In Vitro Digestion Model. *J. Agric. Food Chem.* **2009**, *57*, 5743–5749. [CrossRef]

41. Lu, W.; Kelly, A.L.; Miao, S. Emulsion-based encapsulation and delivery systems for polyphenols. *Trends Food Sci. Technol.* **2016**, *47*, 1–9. [CrossRef]
42. Shimizu, M. Interaction between Food Substances and the Intestinal Epithelium. *Biosci. Biotechnol. Biochem.* **2010**, *74*, 232–241. [CrossRef] [PubMed]
43. Palafox-Carlos, H.; Ayala-Zavala, J.F.; González-Aguilar, G.A. The Role of Dietary Fiber in the Bioaccessibility and Bioavailability of Fruit and Vegetable Antioxidants. *J. Food Sci.* **2011**, *76*, R6–R15. [CrossRef] [PubMed]
44. Velderrain-Rodríguez, G.; Quirós-Sauceda, A.; Mercado-Mercado, G.; Ayala-Zavala, J.F.; Astiazarán-García, H.; Robles-Sánchez, R.M.; Wall-Medrano, A.; Sayago-Ayerdi, S.; González-Aguilar, G.A. Effect of dietary fiber on the bioaccessibility of phenolic compounds of mango, papaya and pineapple fruits by an in vitro digestion model. *Food Sci. Technol.* **2016**, *36*, 188–194. [CrossRef]
45. Pinarli, B.; Karliga, E.S.; Ozkan, G.; Capanoglu, E. Interaction of phenolics with food matrix: In vitro and in vivo approaches. *Mediterr. J. Nutr. Metab.* **2020**, *13*, 63–74. [CrossRef]
46. Bermúdez-Oria, A.; Rodríguez-Gutiérrez, G.; Fernández-Prior, A.; Vioque, B.; Fernández-Bolaños, J. Strawberry dietary fiber functionalized with phenolic antioxidants from olives. Interactions between polysaccharides and phenolic compounds. *Food Chem.* **2019**, *280*, 310–320. [CrossRef]
47. Tomas, M.; Rocchetti, G.; Ghisoni, S.; Giuberti, G.; Capanoglu, E.; Lucini, L. Effect of different soluble dietary fibres on the phenolic profile of blackberry puree subjected to in vitro gastrointestinal digestion and large intestine fermentation. *Food Res. Int.* **2020**, *130*, 108954. [CrossRef]
48. Radić, K.; Vinković Vrček, I.; Pavičić, I.; Čepo, D.V. Cellular Antioxidant Activity of Olive Pomace Extracts: Impact of Gastrointestinal Digestion and Cyclodextrin Encapsulation. *Molecules* **2020**, *25*, 5027. [CrossRef]
49. Santis, S.E.; Cavalcanti, E.; Mastronardi, M.; Jirillo, E.; Chieppa, M. Nutritional Keys for Intestinal Barrier Modulation. *Front. Immunol.* **2015**, *6*, 612. [CrossRef]
50. Mendes, T.M.N.; Murayama, Y.; Yamaguchi, N.; Sampaio, G.R.; Fontes, L.C.B.; Torres, E.A.F.D.S.; Tamura, H.; Tamura, H. Guaraná (Paullinia cupana) catechins and procyanidins: Gastrointestinal/colonic bioaccessibility, Caco-2 cell permeability and the impact of macronutrients. *J. Funct. Foods* **2019**, *55*, 352–361. [CrossRef]
51. Tesoriere, L.; Gentile, C.; Angileri, F.; Attanzio, A.; Tutone, M.; Allegra, M.; Livrea, M.A. Trans-epithelial transport of the betalain pigments indicaxanthin and betanin across Caco-2 cell monolayers and influence of food matrix. *Eur. J. Nutr.* **2012**, *52*, 1077–1087. [CrossRef]
52. Xie, P.-J.; Huang, L.-X.; Zhang, C.-H.; Zhang, Y.-L. Phenolic compositions, and antioxidant performance of olive leaf and fruit (Olea europaea L.) extracts and their structure–activity relationships. *J. Funct. Foods* **2015**, *16*, 460–471. [CrossRef]
53. Souza, V.M.D.; Shertzer, H.G.; Menon, A.G.; Pauletti, G.M. High glucose concentration in isotonic media alters Caco-2 cell permeability. *AAPS Pharmsci.* **2003**, *5*, 17–25. [CrossRef] [PubMed]
54. Chen, T.; Kim, C.Y.; Kaur, A.; Lamothe, L.; Shaikh, M.; Keshavarzian, A.; Hamaker, B.R. Dietary fibre-based SCFA mixtures promote both protection and repair of intestinal epithelial barrier function in a Caco-2 cell model. *Food Funct.* **2017**, *8*, 1166–1173. [CrossRef] [PubMed]
55. Feng, Y.; Wang, Y.; Wang, P.; Huang, Y.; Wang, F. Short-Chain Fatty Acids Manifest Stimulative and Protective Effects on Intestinal Barrier Function Through the Inhibition of NLRP3 Inflammasome and Autophagy. *Cell. Physiol. Biochem.* **2018**, *49*, 190–205. [CrossRef] [PubMed]

5

Functional Food from Endangered Ecosystems: *Atriplex portulacoides* as a Case Study

Lorenzo Zanella and Fabio Vianello *

Department of Comparative Biomedicine and Food Science, University of Padua, Viale dell'Università 16, 35020 Legnaro, Italy; lorenzo.zanella@libero.it
* Correspondence: fabio.vianello@unipd.it

Abstract: Biodiversity is a reservoir of potential sources of novel food and feed ingredients with suitable compositions for the improvement of the diet and well-being of humans and farmed animals. The halophyte *Atriplex portulacoides* occurs in habitats that are exposed to seawater inundations, and shows biochemical adaptations to saline and oxidative stresses. Its composition includes long chain lipids, sterols, phenolic compounds, glutathione and carotenoids. These organic compounds and micronutrients, such as Fe, Zn, Co and Cu, make this plant suitable as an optimal functional food that is potentially able to reduce oxidative stress and inflammatory processes in humans and animals. Indeed, many of these compounds have a protective activity in humans against cardiovascular pathologies, cancer, and degenerative processes related to aging. The analysis of its history as food and forage, which dates back thousands of years, attests that it can be safely consumed. Here, the limits of its chemical and microbiological contamination are suggested in order to comply with the European regulations. The productivity of *A. portulacoides* in natural environments, and its adaptability to non-saline soils, make it a potential crop of high economic interest.

Keywords: halophyte; *Atriplex portulacoides*; food supplement; functional food; antioxidants; sustainable food production

1. Introduction

Brackish wetlands and salt marshes are endangered habitats of great ecological interest, and have therefore been identified as special protection areas pursuant to Council Directive 92/43/EEC, also known as the Habitats Directive. The biodiversity occurring in these environments is characterized by peculiar adaptations to tolerate soil salinity and periodic tidal flood, especially in the case of sessile organisms, such as halophytes.

These vascular plants are endowed with uncommon biochemical defenses to protect against oxidative stress, which make them potential sources of secondary metabolites of nutritional, medical and pharmaceutical interest [1–5]. *Atriplex portulacoides*, commonly called sea purslane, is an edible halophyte that shows these traits and is potentially suitable to be cultivated for human and animal nutrition.

The introduction of innovative crops into European agrosystems is becoming an urgent need in order to counteract the heavy loss of agro-biodiversity [6], which is related to many pivotal sustainability issues, e.g., the precipitous decline of terrestrial European insects [7]. Field-based investigations have shown that biodiversity also affects the forage quality, with important economic benefits for farmers and graziers [8]. The identification of plants with high-value biochemical composition, adaptability to climate changes, and an intrinsic potential to reconnect croplands with endangered natural ecosystems is a challenging issue. Intriguingly, *A. portulacoides* shows all of these characteristics.

The present work is aimed at the revision and discussion of the scientific literature concerning the composition and productivity of *A. portulacoides*, in order to point out its potential exploitation as functional food. Although this plant has been consumed by some populations since ancient times, it is not currently included in any official list of species intended for human consumption, and falls within novel foods according to European legislation. The present review, therefore, besides the analysis of its functional properties to favor human health, also considers historical uses and other aspects in support of its authorization as food. Consistently, issues concerning safety, toxicology and contamination limits in the case of commercialisation as food or fodder are analysed as well.

The use as forage, in addition to favoring animal welfare and promoting significant productions of this currently-uncultivated species, could allow the vehiculation of some functional compounds through food products of daily consumption, such as milk and dairy products. Importantly, *A. portulacoides* can be cultivated in saline and arid lands, and is thus an optimal plant for a sustainable agriculture.

2. Morphology and Systematics of *Atriplex portulacoides*

Atriplex portulacoides L. 1753 is a small perennial, halophile shrub, which is common along the European coasts and occurs in North Africa, Asia minor, and Western Cape province (South Africa), and has been introduced to North America [9]. Its branches are initially woody and decumbent, then soft and erected up to 20–50 cm height [10] (Figure 1), and are characterised by opposite leaves, slightly fleshy, linear-lanceolate with a full margin, and a glaucous silvery-gray colour. Its flowering period is between June and July.

A. portulacoides belongs to the Chenopodiacee family, whose phylogeny is complex and the object of disputed interpretations. In fact, some botanists consider Chenopodiaceae to be monophyletic because of some molecular markers [11], whereas others interpret this family as paraphyletic to Amaranthaceae, and include it therein [12].

Linnaeus described *Atriplex portulacoides* in 1753, but the position of this taxon was then revised by Moquin-Tandon [13], placing it under the genus *Obione*, and finally it was separated into the new genus *Halimione* by Aellen [14]. The genus name *Halimione*, which derives from the Greek 'halimos' (ἅλιμος) and means 'seashore' [15], is the most frequently used in literature, and is still considered valid by many authors. However, Kühn et al. [16] synonymized both *O. portulacoides* (L.) Moq. and *H. portulacoides* (L.) Aellen with *Atriplex portulacoides* L., re-establishing the original nomenclatorial act by Linnaeus. Even more recently, Kadereit et al. [17] resurrected the genus *Halimione* because of some molecular and morphological markers that are distinctive from *Atriplex*, which is the largest genus of the Chenopodiaceae family, with about 300 species. In this controversial background, *Atriplex portulacoides* is acknowledged as a senior synonym of *Halimione* in the International Plant Names Index, and this taxon name will be therefore adopted in the present work.

Interestingly, the species name *portulacoides* is obtained by combining 'Portulaca', a genus name of a species belonging to the family Portulacaceae, with 'eidos' (εἶδος), a Greek word that means 'appearance' [15]. The species name, therefore, means 'similar to Portulaca', recalling the leaf similarity with the common purslane (*Portulaca oleracea* L.), which belongs to another family of the order Caryophyllales. Importantly, this morphological resemblance and nomenclatorial assonance have induced some non-specialists (for instance, in patent applications) to include *A. portulacoides* between the plants of the so-called 'purslane family' (see Bair et al. [18] for a correct interpretation of this group), but this association in erroneous, and is a potential source of relevant mistakes.

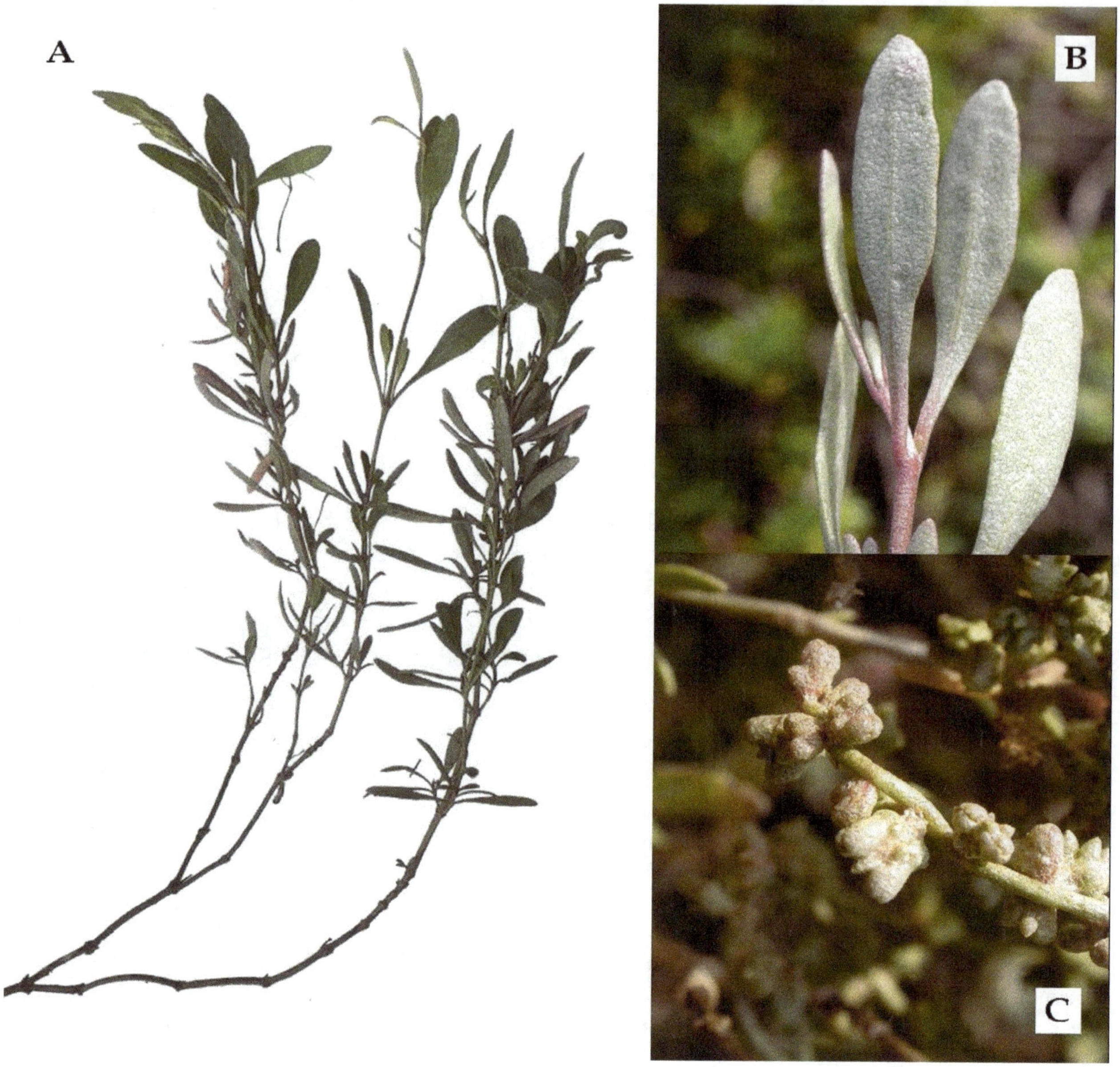

Figure 1. Morphology of *A. portulacoides*: (**A**) branching and decumbent habit; (**B**) leaf close up; (**C**) freshly formed fruits in autumn.

3. Use History of *A. portulacoides*

A. portulacoides can be eaten both raw and cooked [19]. The dietary use of halophytes by coastal populations dates to the late Neolithic period, as evidenced by the discovery of *A. portulacoides* amongst ancient charred remains of food in northern Holland [20]. These findings show that this halophyte was habitually consumed, and perhaps cultivated, around 2500 cal BC.

According to Custódio et al. [21], *A. portulacoides* is collected from the wild by professional foragers, and is sold in specialised online platforms for local restaurants and gourmet cuisine. In Italy, this herb was traditionally eaten in salads, or boiled. In the Marche and Sardinia regions, it entered into some recipes based on fish [22]. Its buds can be preserved in vinegar, as occurs for capers [10]. An ancient Sardinian recipe adopted by fishermen inhabiting the lagoon area of Cabras, locally called '*mreca*', is based on mullet (*Mugil cephalus*) boiled in brackish water and then wrapped with fronds of *A. portulacoides* to make a sort of 'cocoon'. This preparation shows preservative properties for a few days, and was traditionally used as a ready-to-eat fish during fishery trips [23].

4. Eco-Physiology of *A. portulacoides* and the Implications for Its Chemical Composition

The knowledge of the ecophysiology of this plant is important not only to explain its high content of biologically active compounds, but also to evaluate its cultivability for food purposes.

A. portulacoides is adapted to live in soils with varying degrees of salinity, and can survive short periods of submersion in saltwater [24,25]. It can occupy salt marsh and coastal habitats where other species cannot survive or are competitively less efficient. Crain et al. [26] showed that many halophilous plants do not necessarily require saline soil to live, but they are able to adapt to saline environments and prevail over most potential competitors. This is the case for *A. portulacoides*, which finds optimal conditions in moderately saline environments but can successfully develop in non-saline soils, as inferred from several studies. Under controlled conditions, the net organic matter production (ash-free dry weight) of plants cultivated in the absence of salt showed a productivity not far from the best performances of others treated with 85–170 mM NaCl (about 5 to 10 PSU (Practical Salinity Unit)), whereas it decreased exceeding 200 mM NaCl (about 12 PSU), with a relevant impact from 500 mM NaCl (about 29 PSU) [25]. In another experiment, groups of plants were treated for 2 weeks with different salt concentrations (0–15 PSU), and the best growth was recorded at 5 PSU [19]. Finally, Redondo-Gómez et al. [27], recorded the maximum relative growth rate (RGR) at 200 mM NaCl.

In order to overcome the negative osmotic pressure due to the salty environment, halophytes accumulate various metabolites, including quaternary ammonium compounds; ternary sulfonium compounds; proline; and soluble carbohydrates, such as sucrose, sorbitol, mannitol, and pinitol, etc. [28]. The production of osmolytes varies among different halophytes, regarding both the chemical species and relative concentrations. Glycine-betaine (a quaternary ammonium compound, also called simply 'betaine') and proline are organic osmolytes that are dominant in Chenopodiacee and Graminee [29]. The betaine concentration can reach 238 μmol/g dry weight (DW) in epigean biomass, corresponding to 27.9 mg/g DW, and about an 85:1 molar ratio with respect to proline, according to Storey et al. [29]. Betaine is an electrically neutral compound at pH 7.0 (zwitterion), is very soluble, and is suitable to form hydrogen bonds with a high number of water molecules (solvation sphere). For this reason, it is very effective in retaining tissue water, and an excellent moisturizing ingredient for cosmetic use [30].

A. portulacoides also reacts to mild saline stress (10 PSU) by increasing its content of proline and antioxidants within a few hours, then decreasing to low values in the subsequent days [19].

In addition to organic osmolytes, salts passively introduced with water contribute to enhance the tissue's osmotic pressure. Some plants developed in soils with $\pi = 450$ mOsm presented a lymph with a calculated osmotic pressure of $\pi = 1087$ mOsm, to which K contributed 72 meq/l, Na contributed 532 meq/L, Cl contributed 433 meq/L, and Ca and Mg were not detectable [29]. Redondo-Gómez et al. [27] found that NaCl is compartmentalised according to the following concentration gradient: leaves > stems > roots. In the leaves, Na and Cl accumulate at increasing concentrations with aging, whereas Mg and Ca show the opposite trend [24,29]. Plants treated with increasing salinities for 40 days showed that Na and Cl increased mainly in the leaves, whereas K and Ca decreased, the latter to a lesser extent [31]. Plant composition and saline content can vary significantly in relation to the season, the geographical locations and the morphology of the development environment.

Some adaptations to salinity have similarities with those aimed at resisting drought, as—in both cases—the plant needs to absorb and retain water under the conditions of an adverse gradient. Therefore, it is not surprising that *A. portulacoides* tolerates temporary water shortage, despite the fact that it develops in salt marshes and other coastal humid environments. Indeed, its zonation in the typical environment reflects its preference for well drained soils and limited exposure to prolonged flooding [24,32]. This trait is consistent with the absence of aerenchyma in its roots, which presupposes a well oxygenated soil, unlike other halophytes which, instead, occupy the lower salt marsh and contribute to the substrate aeration, thanks to their radical aerenchyma [32].

Metabolism of Heavy Metals

An adaptive trait related with the accumulation of mineral osmolytes is the capacity of *A. portulacoides* to concentrate seawater metal cations, which is of interest for some micronutritional applications. However, in addition to naturally occurring metals, halophytes are currently exposed to toxic metals derived from anthropogenic pollution [33]. Therefore, attention must be paid to the site from which plants intended for food use are harvested. Several studies have shown that the high levels of heavy metals present in some European estuarine and lagoon environments have an impact on the composition of *A. portulacoides*, and on its lipid profile. For instance, linolenic acid content decreased in favour of palmitic acid and a reduction of mono- and di-galactosyldiacylglycerol was observed as effects of chronic exposure to environmental pollutants, mainly heavy metals with oxidizing activity [34]. Interestingly, *A. portulacoides* can sequester and/or compartmentalise metals, binding most of them to the structural components of the cell wall (pectins, lignin, cellulose, other polysaccharides), or to special proteins [33,35–37] according to the following affinity scale: Zn > Pb > Cu > Ni > Co > Cd [35]. Due to this trait, the use of halophytes for the phytoremediation of heavily polluted wet areas has been proposed [35,38]. A case study of the accumulation/repartition of metals in the different parts of the plant and cell compartments is shown in Figure 2.

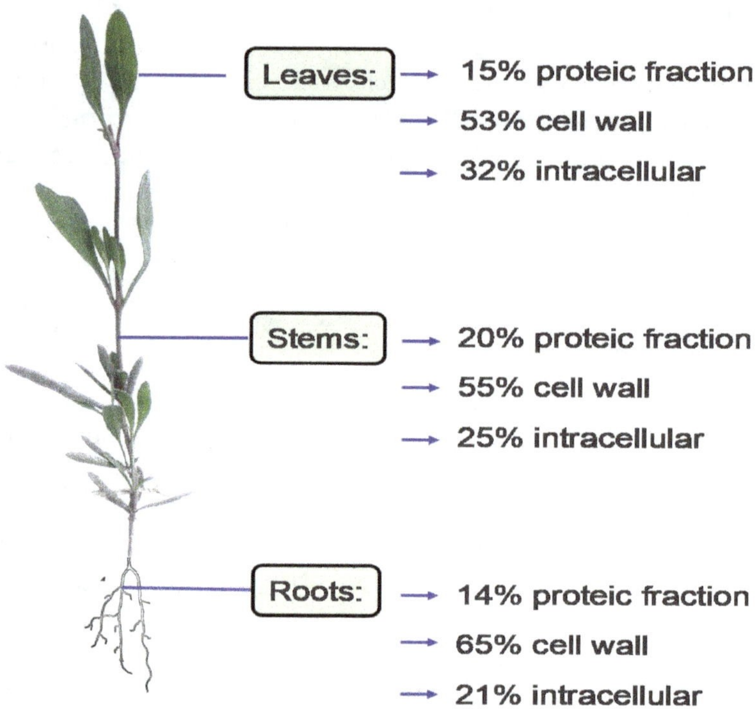

Figure 2. Metal distribution (leaves, stems, and roots) and compartmentation (cell wall, proteic fraction, and intracellular location) in *A. portulacoides* (redrawn and modified from Sousa et al. [35]).

Phytochelatins are amongst the inducible metabolites that are suitable for metal binding. These compounds are peptides that are rich in cysteine, with general structure of (γ-Glu-Cys)$_n$-Gly, in which 'n' usually varies between 2 and 5 [39]. Phytochelatins can bind ions by means of coordination bonds with the thiol functional groups, as occurs with other abundant mono-thiol compounds, i.e., glutathione (GSH), γ-glutamyl-cysteine and cysteine molecules [39]. These functional groups are also extremely active in the broad-spectrum prevention of damage from oxidative stress.

5. Chemical Biomass Composition and Related Nutritional Value

The leaves are the most interesting plant compartment for nutritional purposes and—despite the fact that they are only 2.3% of the total dry biomass due to their high content in water— they show the highest content of nitrogen, which is indicative of their protein content (Table 1).

Table 1. Dry biomass and approximate composition values of *A. portulacoides* biomass (FW = fresh weight, DW = dry weight).

	Leaves	Stems	Shoots (Leaves + Stems)	Roots	Reference
Biomass (g/m²)	212.8	1345.6		7686.1	[40]
Nitrogen (% DW)	1.63	1.23		0.75	[40]
Carbon (% DW)	30.7	40.0		15.0	[40]
Moisture (% FW)	87.5–90.9 *				[31]
			85.9–86.8 *	61.5–80.3 *	[41]
			85.9		[29]
Protein (% DW)	5.6–9.4 **	3.1–4.4 **		6.0–7.5 **	[42]
	10.2% **	7.7 **		4.7 **	[40]
	10–11.2	6.6		3.5	[33,43]
Lipid (% DW)	2.1	1.7		3.2	[44]
Ash (% DW)	32–40 *	12–15 *		12–24 *	[27]
			30–35 *	10–12 *	[41]
			27–49	9–42	[25]

* approximate value extrapolated from graph. Data from [41] selected for plants treated with 0–25% seawater; ** the reference provided only the N content, from which the protein value was estimated here using a 6.25 nitrogen-to-protein conversion factor.

A. portulacoides has been extensively studied with regard to ecology and physiology, but insufficient data are available concerning its quantitative and qualitative protein content. Some crude protein data, inferred from their total N content, and other approximate composition values are shown in Table 1, from which it can be deduced that the leaves' crude proteins range from 5 to 11% DW, with a modal value around 10%, whereas the lipids vary from 1.7 to 3.2% DW, depending on the plant compartment being considered. Boughalleb et al. [45] quantified the lipids that are extractable with different solvents, obtaining yields on DW biomass of 1.8% with petroleum ether, 2.1% with acetone, and 3.1% with methanol. An indicative crude lipid content of about 2% DW is therefore plausible as a general case.

Fresh epigeal biomass generally comprises > 80% moisture, with an average value around 87.5%, whereas ashes increase with environmental salinity, ranging from 27 to 49% in the shoots' dry biomass [25]. The high ash content is directly related to the mineral concentration of the tissue, which in turn depends on what the plant needs to counteract the environmental osmotic pressure.

5.1. Lipids

The lipid fraction of the biomass is of special interest for human and animal nutrition, as it comprises many active compounds, such as long chain polyunsaturated fatty acids (PUFAs), carotenoids, and sterols, etc.

An important contribution in this regard was disclosed by Vilela et al. [44], who worked on samples from estuarine environments of Portugal (Table 2). The roots showed the highest lipid content (3.2% DW), followed by the leaves (2.1% DW) and the stems (1.7% DW) [44]. The main lipids detected in the leaves were saturated fatty acids (0.062% DW), whereas unsaturated fatty acids were 0.018% DW, and were almost totally composed of oleic acid (0.012% DW) and linoleic acid (0.006% DW). However, Maciel et al. [46] obtained a leaf fatty acid profile composed of 60% PUFAs, of which 43.5% were due to linolenic acid and 14% linoleic acid, and a n-6/n-3 fatty acids ratio equal to 0.32, which is particularly favorable for nutrition purposes. Small fractions of uncommon long chain saturated fatty acids, containing up to 24 carbon atoms, were also present. The same study showed the appreciable presence of phospholipids and glycolipids of high biological value.

It seems that the ratio between the unsaturated and saturated fatty acids is affected by environmental contaminants, especially sedimentary heavy metals, and other generators of reactive oxygen species. Thus, this ratio has been proposed as a biomarker of pollution [34]. Amongst the compounds of interest shown in Table 2, long chain aliphatic alcohols (LCAA) appeared, which are generally constituents of epicuticular waxes. In leaves, about 46% of these were represented by 1-octacosanol ($C_{28}H_{58}O$), 24% by 1-hexacosanol ($C_{26}H_{54}O$), and 22% by 1-triacontanol ($C_{30}H_{62}O$).

Amongst sterols, β-sitosterol and its hydrogenated derivative, β-sitostanol, prevailed; both are known as anti-cholesterolemic agents. The roots showed a higher content of sterols/triterpenoids than epigeal compartments, which can amount to about 3.2 g/kg DW, of which about 87% was hop-17(21)-en-3-one, as a sum of both the ketone and enolic form.

Table 2. Main compounds (mg/kg DW) identified in extracts from the leaves, stems and roots of *A. portulacoides* (from Vilela et al. [44], modified).

Lipidic Compounds (mg/kg of Dry Material)		**Leaves**	**Stems**	**Roots**
Fatty acids		798	252	374
Saturated		619	193	316
	Hexadecanoic acid	99	81	75
	Hexacosanoic acid	66	13	18
	Octacosanoic acid (montanoic ac.)	230	32	70
	Triacontanoic acid (melissic ac.)	147	20	90
	Other saturated fatty acids	77	47	63
Unsaturated		179	59	58
	Octadec-9-enoic acid (oleic ac.)	115	32	38
	Octadeca-9,12-dienoic acid (linoleic ac.)	64	27	20
Long chain aliphatic alcohols		546	82	274
	1-Hexacosanol	132	18	53
	1-Octacosanol	252	33	98
	1-Triacontanol	122	8	31
	Other long chain aliphatic alcohols	40	23	92
Long chain n-alkanes		106	9	15
Sterols/triterpenoids		323	609	3245
	Cholesterol	66	5	19
	Campesterol	37	4	9
	Stigmasterol	20	169	n.d.
	β-Sitosterol + β-Sitostanol	148	n.d.	291
	Spinasterol + β-Sitosterol + β-Sitostanol	n.d.	122	n.d.
	Schottenol	52	30	108
	Hop-17(21)-en-3-one	n.d.	169	2102
	Hop-17(21)-en-3-one (enolic form)	n.d.	110	716
Other identified and unidentified compounds		273	130	243
Total detected compounds		**2066**	**1084**	**4151**
Phenolic Content (mg/kg of Dry Material)		**Leaves**	**Stems**	**Roots**
Isorhamnetin-glucosyl-rhamnosyl-glucuronide isomer		457	–	–
Isorhamnetin-sulphate-pentoside isomer		67	–	–
Isorhamnetin-sulphate-glucosyl-rhamnoside		1190	–	–
Diosmetin-sulphate-glucuronide		422	19	–
Isorhamnetin-sulphate-pentoside isomer		384	18	–
Isorhamnetin-glucosyl-rhamnoside isomer		107	38	–
Isorhamnetin-sulphate-glucosyl-rhamnosyl-glucuronide		782	–	–
Diosmetin-hexoside		77	–	–
Isorhamnetin-glucosyl-rhamnoside isomer		514	–	–
Isorhamnetin-pentoside		89	–	–
Isorhamnetin-glucosyl-rhamnosyl-glucuronide isomer		185	–	–
Diosmetin-sulphate		243	–	–
Diosmetin		61	–	–
Total detected compounds		**4578**	**76**	**–**

n.d., not detectable. The determinations were carried out by UHPLC–MS (ultra-high performance liquid chromatography-mass spectrometry). The results are the average of the concordant values obtained (less than a 5% variation between injections) for two aliquots of each sample injected in triplicate.

Amongst Chenopodiaceae, *A. portulacoides* stands out for its high content of ecdysone-related compounds, which are not degraded by cooking and can produce an anabolic effect in vertebrates [47,48]. The prevalence of 20-hydroxyecdisone in the epigean parts was found, whereas its derivative 20-hydroxyecdisone-septanoside was in roots [49]. The adaptive meaning of ecdysteroids is related to their interfering action on the metamorphosis and moulting of potentially harmful phytophagous arthropods [47].

5.2. Carotenoids

Carotenoids are accessory pigments that enhance the absorbance of radiant energy in the chloroplast, but also protect the structural integrity of thylacoids from oxidative damage [50]. They can be ingested by humans alongside their normal diet for health improvements [51].

Anjum et al. [52] quantified the carotenoids of *A. portulacoides* leaves in 5 μg/g fresh weigh (FW), corresponding to 40 μg/g DW if a moisture of 87.5% is assumed. The same study showed an increase of carotenoids in some plants grown in highly contaminated soils, in response to mercury toxicity, up to more than twice than that of the controls. Higher contents of carotenoids (around 50 μg/g FW) were detected by Duarte et al. [53] in plants maintained under favourable conditions, which decreased drastically following the exposure to saline stress. This was partially counterbalanced by an increase in anthocyanins and beta-cyanins.

Carotenoids from 30 to 100 μg/g FW (approximate values estimated from graphical representations) were reported by Duarte et al. [54] in plants stressed by frequent tidal floods, which decreased with the reduction of the flood frequency. In another study, Duarte et al. [55] quantified the leaf carotenoids in about 109–230 μg/g FW, indicatively corresponding to 0.87–1.84 mg/g DW, assuming a moisture of 87.5%, amongst which zeaxanthin was the most abundant. Intense changes of temperature produced relevant variations of some carotenoids, with different effects depending on the compound and the treatment considered [55]. The most abundant carotenoids were β-carotene, auroxanthin, antheraxanthin, lutein, violaxanthin, and zeaxanthin [53,55].

5.3. Phenolic Compounds

A. portulacoides synthesizes numerous phenolic compounds, and in higher amounts if exposed to environmental stresses [56]. According to data published by Vilela et al. [44], total phenols were more abundant in root extracts (142.1 mgGAE, (gallic acid equivalent)/g dry extract) than in extracts from the stems and leaves (52.1 and 48.3 mgGAE/g dry extract, respectively), but the leaves showed the highest amount of phenolic compounds per DW of extracted biomass (19.9 mgGAE/g DW). Sulphonated and/or glucuronated derivatives of isorhamnetin were the main compounds detected (Table 2). Phenolic compounds conjugated with sulphate groups were about 3.0 g/kg DW in leaves, which is an extremely high value when compared to other plant sources [44].

Ethyl acetate, methanol and water extracts of epigeal parts of *A. portulacoides* were studied by Zengoin et al. [57]. The authors recorded a total phenolic and total flavonoid content in ethyl acetate extract of 14.59 ± 0.21 mgGAE/g of extract and 6.19 ± 0.06 mgGAE/g of extract, respectively. Furthermore, this study disclosed the presence in the methanol extract of an amount of quinic acid that was even higher than rhamnetin, followed by other minor compounds, such as p-coumaric acid, 4-OH benzoic acid, salicylic acid, malic acid, tr-caffeic acid, vanillin, hesperidin, rutin, rosmarinic acid, chlorogenic acid, and gallic acid [57].

6. Productivity and Cultivability

The availability of wild plants is generally limited, especially if they develop in environments that are at risk of disappearance. Thus, their potential economic exploitation depends on the option of a profitable cultivation. Some field studies in natural environments showed that the primary productivity of *A. portulacoides* could be of interest for agricultural exploitation. Jensen [25] studied the ash-free DW relative growth rate (RGR) in experimental hydroponics under different salinities, from seedlings until the second pair of leaves had emerged. In a 9 week treatment, the RGR ranged between 43 and 53 mg/g/day, with a salinity between 0 and 515 mM NaCl (about 30 PSU), while it decreased to 27 mg/g/day at 690 mM NaCl (about 40 PSU). Under different experimental conditions, Redondo-Gómez et al. [27] detected an ash-free RGR between 20 mg/g/day (control in the absence of salt) and 40 mg/g/day at 200 mM NaCl (about 12 PSU), which dropped to about 5 mg/g/day at 700 mM NaCl (about 41 PSU) (values estimated from graphic representations).

As a whole, although they were recorded under different experimental conditions, these data are not far from the RGR performances of some alfalfa cultivars, which showed RGR between 20 and 30 mg/g/day [58]. Importantly, the RGR of *A. portulacoides* was also high in the absence of NaCl, thus resulting in its being adaptable to conventional agricultural lands.

Some biomass density and productivity data were estimated in the wild using different methods, amongst which the following were obtained with the Smalley method, which is the most frequently adopted method. Data concerning the epigean biomass can range between 598 g/m^2 DW [42] and 1363 g/m^2 DW [59], whereas (in Portugal) the values of RGR were estimated to be more favourable in winter–spring, with 7.9 mg/g/day, or 0.8% per day [42]. The productivity data were assessed in the salt marshes of some European countries: 952 g/m^2/year DW was found in the Cantabrian Sea (Biscay Gulf, Spain) [60]; 790–1434 g/m^2/year DW was found in a Danish salt marsh (Krabbendijke) [61].

Overall, the above reported data suggest that, under natural conditions, an approximate primary productivity of 1000 g/m^2/year, or 10 t/ha/year DW, might be calculated. This estimation is consistent with the most conservative data reported for other halophyte cultivations investigated within projects aimed at the agricultural development of arid or saline regions. Sardo [62] reported on productivity values of 24 t/ha DW for a generic *Atriplex* sp. Le Houérou [63] reported on halophyte forage productions of about 20 t/ha/year DW in irrigated saline environments, which dropped to 2–10 t/ha/year DW in semi-arid environments (rainfalls of 400–800 mm/year). Yields of 18 t/ha/year DW were reported for *Atriplex lentiformis* grown at a salinity of 500 mM, and 21.3 t/ha/year DW were reported for *Atriplex triangularis* at salinity of 150 mM [64].

6.1. Exploitation as Forage

The extensive grazing of livestock, mainly sheep, on extensive areas vegetated by halophytes has been practiced since ancient times in some European salt marshes. In the Wadden Sea (the coast of the North Sea), natural salt marsh has been exploited as grazing lands since 2600 years ago [65]. In Mont Saint-Michel bay (France), three-quarters of the salt marsh area (30–32 km^2) were grazed by 17,000 sheep in recent times [66]. In natural wetlands, not only sheep and cows graze halophytes comprising *A. portulacoides*, but also wild species, such as wild boars [67], geese and hares [68,69].

These investigations attest that halophytes can be used as pasture, but were focused on the ecological impact of grazing, whereas nothing was reported about the quality of the breeding products. The latter is expected to be increased due to the active compounds comprised in the *A. portulacoides* biomass. Some nutritional criticalities can arise for the high content of ash and salts, the low metabolisable energy, and the possible presence of undesired secondary metabolites [70]. Nonetheless, the use of halophytes for animal nutrition has long been considered an important opportunity for economic development [3], especially for arid geographical areas or in the need to irrigate using salty water [62,63,71,72]. The nutritional value as forage can be inferred by comparing some data of a hypothetical production of *A. portulacoides* with those of alfalfa and other fodders (Table 3). Assuming a conservative yield estimation of 10 t/ha DW, based on the data discussed above, *A. portulacoides* shows productive parameters close to alfalfa, which is the most productive grassland crop in terms of dry matter and proteins [73]. The protein content is obviously lower than the comparative legume, which shows the highest value of this parameter, i.e., two times higher in soy and three times in pea sown in the fall [73]. However, the protein intake provided by *A. portulacoides* is higher than the minimum required for weight maintenance by sheep or cows, i.e., 7–9% [3], and is in line with the highest content of alternative forages considered in Table 3. Importantly, the protein content is lower than the minimum required for lactating animals, equal to 14–18% [3].

The lipid content of *A. portulacoides* is higher or comparable to that of fodder alternatives (Table 3), but with a more interesting quality profile (Section 5).

Table 3. Comparison of the productivity and composition of *A. portulacoides* and some typical forage crops.

	Productivity DW (t/ha)	Ash %	Protein %	Lipid %
Atriplex portulacoides	10 [a]	27 [c]	10–11.2 [e]	2.1 [f]
Medicago sativa hay	11 [b]	10.3 [d]	17 [d]	2.1 [g]
Forage grasses (Graminaceae)		9.9 [b]	8.8 [b]	1.6 [b]
Polyphitic meadows		9.7 [b]	8.9 [b]	1.6 [b]
Wheat		7.7 [b]	8.9 [b]	2.1 [b]

[a] This review (estimation); [b] 4 year cycle average [73]; [c] refers to shoots in the absence of salinity [25]; [d] harvest following the first year [74]; [e] refers to leaves [43]; [f] refers to leaves [44]; [g] refers to leaves [75].

Chenopodiacee are a good source of protein, sulfur and minerals, while providing insufficient metabolisable energy [3]. The nitrogen deriving from betaine, which assumes relevance in *A. portulacoides*, is generally metabolised up to 50% by the rumen microbiome, and this fraction can increase in diets with low metabolisable energy, whereas proline can be easily absorbed at the ileum level [3]. The high ash content is mainly due to salts and metal ions, which contribute to the micronutritional value, and make *A. portulacoides* an optimal ingredient for the improvement of the nutritional profile of mixed forages [76]. In Table 4, some essential minerals required by sheep and cattle are compared with the composition of *A. portulacoides* and some other plants that are used to feed animal husbandry. Whenever possible, data on *A. portulacoides* were chosen from those referring to plants grown in the absence of salt, since they are considered more representative of potential cultivated crops. As is consistent with its high content of ashes and its metal storage capacity, *A. portulacoides* is rich in some elements of which other forages are deficient with respect to animal needs. Therefore, if used in proper proportions in the formulation of forage blends, this halophyte can be a useful dietary supplement for livestock nutrition. In particular, the content in S can support the requirement of sheep reared for wool production. Among metals, *A. portulacoides* is a valid source of Fe, Zn, Co and Cu.

Table 4. Recommended dietary intake (in g/kg DW) of the minerals that are considered essential for animal nutrition (from CSIRO [77]), and estimations of their intake provided by *A. portulacoides* (stems and/or leaves) and other forage plants.

	Sheep		Cattle		*Atriplex portulacoides*	Corn-Silage	Polyphitic Meadows	Alfalfa
Mineral	Maintenance Requirement (g/kg DW)	Growing, Pregnant, or Lactating Animals (g/kg DW)	Maintenance Requirement (g/kg DW)	Growing, Pregnant, or Lactating Animals (g/kg DW)	(g/kg DW)	(g/kg DW)	(g/kg DW)	(g/kg DW)
Calcium	1.4	7.0	2.0	11.0	7–9 [a]	2.7 [h]	6.8 [f]	15.3 [f]
Phosphorus	0.9	3.0	1.0	3.8	1.1–1.4 [a]	2.3 [h]	2.6 [f]	2.6 [f]
Chlorine	0.3	1.0	0.7	2.4	21–31 [d]	-	-	-
Magnesium	0.9	1.2	1.3	2.2	7–10 [a]	1.8 [h]	1.7 [f]	2.4 [f]
Potassium	5.0	5.0	5.0	5.0	43–37 [d]	10.7 [h]	23.3 [f]	26.2 [f]
Sodium	0.7	1.0	0.8	1.2	34–41 [d]	0.05 [h]	0.14 [h]	-
Sulfur	2.0	2.0	1.5	1.5	2 [e]	1.4 [h]	2.0 [h]	-
Cobalt	0.00008	0.00015	0.00007	0.00015	0.008–0.010 [c]	-	-	-
Copper	0.004	0.014	0.004	0.014	0.012–0.015 [c]	0.0081 [h]	0.0129 [h]	0.011 [i]
Iodine	0.0005	0.0005	0.0005	0.0005	-	-	-	-
Iron	0.040	0.040	0.040	0.040	0.194–0.715 [g]	0.200 [h]	0.184 [h]	0.382 [i]
Manganese	0.020	0.025	0.020	0.025	0–0.02 [a]	0.0381 [h]	0.0764 [h]	-
Selenium	0.00005	0.00005	0.00004	0.00004	-	-	-	-
Zinc	0.009	0.020	0.009	0.020	0.045–0.108 [b]	0.0308 [h]	0.0276 [h]	0.029 [i]

[a] Ref. [42] leaf content is approximate from the graph; [b] Ref. [33], the first value is from stems, and the second value is from leaves; [c] Ref. [35], the first value is from leaves, and the second value is from stems; [d] Ref. [31], the first value (in the absence of salinity) is from stems, and the second value is from leaves, as approximated from the graph; [e] Ref. [78], value from leaves; [f] Ref. [73]; [g] Ref. [43] the first value is from cultivated plants irrigated with freshwater, and the second value is the average from the natural habitat; [h] Ref. [79] the first value is from stems, and the second is from leaves; [i] Ref. [80].

6.2. Human Nutrition

A. portulacoides, although it is considered an almost-forgotten traditional food, still appears in culinary cookbooks dedicated to alimurgical plants, in some gourmet preparations, and among the proposals of chefs dedicated to creative reinterpretations of traditional cuisine. Its biochemical composition comprises many molecules that are useful for the promotion of human health, although important information is still missing concerning, for instance, the composition and digestibility of its plant proteins.

The lipid fraction is dominated by oleic and linolenic acid [44,46], both of which have antioxidant, antinflammatory and anti-trombotic activities [81,82]. Among the lipophilic active molecules, attention should be paid to LCAAs, sterols and ecdysone-derived steroids. Indeed, 1-octacosanol showed beneficial activities, such as antiradical activity, protection from parkinsonism by regulating the proNGF (precursor of nerve growth factor) and NGF (nerve growth factor) signals [83], the stimulation of the activity of creatine phosphokinase in plasma and citrate synthetase in the muscle of rats subjected to stress [84], and the reduction of plasma triglycerides [85]. Another LCAA, 1-triacontanol ($C_{30}H_{62}O$), showed anti-inflammatory properties following topical skin applications [86]. Sterols and stanols, β-sitosterol and β-sitostanol, exert an anti-cholesterolemic action due to their low intestinal absorption, combined with a cholesterol sequestering ability, which increases fecal cholesterol and bile acid excretion [87]. According to the European Food Safety Authority (EFSA) a consumption of 1.5–2.4 g/day of phytosterols and/or stanols is recommended in the order to reduce blood cholesterol [88]. Long-term feeding tests showed that β-sitostanol is more active than β-sitosterol [89], but the latter is by far the most abundant phytosterol in the human diet, and is credited with numerous beneficial effects, although not all have been sufficiently demonstrated. Amongst the most relevant are: cardiovascular protection, immune system modulation, the prevention of some types of cancer and rheumatoid arthritis, and the prevention of hair loss [88]. Hopenone is an uncommon triterpenoid ketone with an anti-proliferative action, which is deemed potentially useful for cancer prevention [90,91]. Amongst steroids, ecdysone septanoside-derivatives showed antioxidant activity, the inhibition of cholinesterase (potentially functional for preventing hypertension and related heart disease) and a mild inhibiting activity against some bacteria strains of interest [49].

The useful compounds for human health also include carotenoids, which reduce the incidence of cardiovascular diseases and the risk of cancer in some organs: breast, lung, various compartments of the female genital system, the prostate and the colon [92]. Amongst the most represented xanthophylls are lutein, zeaxanthin, violaxanthin and antheroxanthin [53], all of which are strong antioxidants, the first two of which are active in the protection of the eye retina [93]. The polyphenol content is quite relevant, and is characterized by uncommon sulphated flavonoids, mainly isoramnetin derivatives, which showed antithrombotic activities [44], colon–rectal anti-carcinogenic properties [94], anti-inflammatory activity by COX2 (cyclooxygenase-2) inhibition, the activation of the Nrf2 factor (NF-E2 p45-related factor 2) [95], and the inhibition of the inflammatory signalling mediated by NF-kB (nuclear factor kappa-light-chain-enhancer of activated B cells) and MAPKs (mitogen-activated protein kinases) [96].

Other compounds of interest are glycolipids, which are also in sulphate form, e.g., mono- and di-galactosyldiacylglycerol, sulfoquinovosyldiacylglycerol and hexosylceramide [46], which disclose a significant anti-inflammatory activity [97,98].

Amongst the hydrophilic antioxidants are glutathione, other monothiol compounds and phytochelatins, which in turn could be decomposed to single- or oligo-peptides by digestion. GSH, and probably also γ-glutamyl-cysteine, can be absorbed through the gastrointestinal tract by Na-dependent and Na-independent carriers, especially at the level of the small intestine, despite some doubts which remain on the absorption of GSH [99]. However, GSH absorption through the oral mucosa was shown using oral mucosa models, while plasma GSH levels increased significantly in a clinical trial conducted with rapid/slow release GSH preparations [100].

The antioxidant phytocomplex of *A. portulacoides* is consistent with its anti-inflammatory properties, which it is one of the strengths of this food. Extracts of this plant have been shown to reduce the nitric oxide release by human macrophages stimulated with sulphate lipopolysaccharides [101]. Besides this, topical treatments with hydroalcoholic and aqueous extracts of this plant significantly reduced the release of interleukin IL-1α in human skin samples stimulated with 2% sodium dodecyl sulphate [102]. In vitro tests with shoot extracts showed an inhibitory activity on some enzymes, such as butyrylcholinesterase, tyrosinase, amylase and glucosidase [57], with potential effects on the production of acetylcholine, melanin, and on the glycaemic control, respectively.

All of these properties are of interest for human nutrition, especially because this plant can be eaten raw, without undesired compositional modifications due to cooking processes. Furthermore, *A. portulacoides* is a source of some important minerals for micro-nutritional purposes, namely Mg, K, Ca, Fe, Zn, Cu and Mn. The bioavailability of these elements for humans has not been assessed yet, and metals bound to phytochelatins and other peptides could be released following protein digestion. Table 5 shows the mineral intake levels recommended for the adult Italian population, while the last line shows the related intake provided by 100 g FW *A. portulacoides*. It should be noted that this modest ration takes at least 10% of the recommended intake of most minerals, exceeding 40% in some cases, e.g., Fe and Mg.

Table 5. Recommended Dietary Allowance (RDA in bold) and Adequate Intake (AI in italics) of minerals for the Italian adult population, and the mineral intake provided by 100 g FW of *A. portulacoides*.

	Age (Years)	Ca (g)	P (g)	Mg (mg)	Na (g)	K (g)	Cl (g)	Fe (mg)	Zn (mg)	Cu (mg)	Se (μg)	I (mg)	Mn (mg)	Mo (μg)	Cr (μg)	F (mg)
Males	30–59	**1**	**0.7**	**0.24**	*1.5*	*3.9*	*2.3*	**10**	**12**	**0.9**	**55**	*0.15*	*2.7*	*65*	*35*	*3.5*
Females	30–59	**1**	**0.7**	**0.24**	*1.5*	*3.9*	*2.3*	**18/10**	**9**	**0.9**	**55**	*0.15*	*2.3*	*65*	*25*	*3.0*
	FW (g)	**Ca (g)**	**P (g)**	**Mg (mg)**	**Na (g)**	**K (g)**	**Cl (g)**	**Fe (mg)**	**Zn (mg)**	**Cu (mg)**	**Se (μg)**	**I (mg)**	**Mn (mg)**	**Mo (μg)**	**Cr (μg)**	**F (mg)**
A. portulac.	100	0.1	0.016	0.11	0.47	0.5	0.33	5.7	1.0	0.17	-	-	0.13	-	-	-

Values on a daily basis (from http://www.sinu.it, modified). With regard to Fe, in females aged 39–59, the second RDA value refers to postmenopausal women. The assumption of the minerals provided by 100 g FW of *A. portulacoides* were estimated from the averages of the intervals shown in Table 4, assuming a dry weight equal to 12.5% of the fresh biomass: contributions that are ≥ 40% RDA are highlighted in dark grey; those that are ≥ 10% are highlighted in light grey.

7. Safety Specifications and Recommendations

A. portulacoides is a perennial plant that has edible parts, mostly represented by the leaves and tender stems, which are assimilable to many other vegetables for safety concerns. However, its prerogative to absorb and concentrate some substances, especially metals, makes it potentially dangerous if collected from contaminated environments. Microbiological contaminations should also be considered, as this plant is suitable to be eaten raw. Table 6 shows some chemical and microbiological limits provided by the current legislation for some foods that are comparable to *A. portulacoides*. Microbiological analyses performed by Mangia et al. [23] on *A. portulacoides* that was freshly collected and then used for the preparation of a traditional *mreca* (Section 3) showed quite high microbiological loads, which were possibly related to the soil microbiome and/or inadequate handling, confirming the importance of carefully assessing the site of cultivation and the need to implement adequate hygiene conditions throughout the product's processing.

Table 6. Permissible limit of heavy metals and microbiological criteria for edible plants.

Chemical Hazard			
Code	**Element**	**Limit (mg/kg FW)**	**Law Reference**
3.1.11	Lead	0.30	Commission Regulation (EC) n. 1881/2006 of 19 December 2006
3.2.17	Cadmium	0.20	Commission Regulation (EC) n. 629/2008 of 2 July 2008

Biological Hazard					
Food Category	**Microorganism**	**Limit (cfu/g)**	**Analytical Reference Method**	**Stage Where the Criterion Applies**	**Law Ref.**
1.2. Ready-to-eat foods able to support the growth of *L. monocytogenes*, other than those intended for infants and for special medical purposes	*Listeria monocytogenes*	*n* = 5 c = 0 absent in 25 g or < 100 cfu/g	EN/ISO 11290-2	Products placed on the market during their shelf-life	(A)
1.19. Pre-cut fruit and vegetables (ready-to-eat)	*Salmonella*	*n* = 5 c = 0 absent in 25 g	EN/ISO 6579	Products placed on the market during their shelf-life	(A)
2.5.1. Pre-cut fruit and vegetables (ready-to-eat)	*E. coli*	*n* = 5 c = 2 m = 100 M = 1000	ISO 16649-1 or 16649-2	Manufacturing process	(A)
1.29. Sprouts	Shiga toxin producing *E. coli* (STEC)	*n* = 5 c = 0 absent in 25 g	CEN/ISO TS 13136	Products placed on the market during their shelf-life	(B)
other spices and herbs	Enterobacter	*n* = 5 c = 1 m = 10 M = 100	ISO 5552	Import or production/packaging or wholesale/establishment/retail	(C)
other spices and herbs	*Clostridium perfrigens*	*n* = 5 c = 1 m = 100 M = 1000	ISO 7937	Import or production/packaging or wholesale/establishment/retail	(C)
other spices and herbs	*Bacillus cereus*	*n* = 5 c = 1 m = 1000 M = 10,000	ISO 7932	Import or production/packaging or wholesale/establishment/retail	(C)

n, samples required; c, samples admitted with acceptable counts; m, lower limit; M, maximum limit. Criteria: satisfactory, if all of the values observed are < m; acceptable, if a maximum of c/n values are between m and M, and the rest of the values observed are ≤ m; unsatisfactory, if one or more of the values observed are > M, or more than c/n values are between m and M. (A) Commission Regulation (EC) n. 2073/2005 of 15 November 2005; (B) Commission Regulation (EC) n. 209/2013 of 11 March 2013; (C) Commission Recommendation of 19 Dec 2003 (2004/24/EC).

The nitrate content also deserves a special comment due to the relevance it assumes in some leafy vegetables. Some studies have shown that *A. portulacoides* probably transforms nitrates into organic osmolytes, such as betaine [25,29], and thus their concentration in the leaves varied inversely to salinity. This peculiar metabolic trait should also prevent problems concerning high nitrate levels under conditions of fertilised cultivation. In any case, the nitrate concentration must respect the limit of 2500–3000 mg/kg FW prescribed for spinach and lettuce in summer crops by the Commission Regulation (EC) No. 1881/2006, and the subsequent amendments of the Regulation (EC) No. 629/2008.

Betaine is the main organic osmolyte in *A. portulacoides*, and the possible end metabolite of nitrate exceeding protein synthesis requirements. Rats treated with high betaine doses (426 to 2442 mg/kg body weight (BW) per day), for 12 months, resulted in the lowest mean corpuscular haemoglobin and mean corpuscular volume, whereas their blood platelets were increased [103]. Obese human subjects with metabolic syndromes treated with 4 g/day betaine showed an increase of blood total cholesterol and LDL (low density lipoprotein) levels; however, the same dosage did not produce any adverse effect in healthy subjects, nor at intakes of 3 g/day [103]. Therefore, considering 4 g/day betaine as a reference point, and applying a cautelative 10 factor decrement, an amount of 400 mg/day betaine (i.e., about 6 mg/kg BW per day for adults), in addition to the background exposure (830 mg/day for the adult European population), was considered to be safe by EFSA [103]. Interestingly, the choline intake must also be taken into account, since over 50% of this compound is irreversibly oxidized to betaine in the human body.

Storey et al. [29] estimated a betaine content of 27.9 mg/g DW in *A. portulacoides* which was developed in a natural saline environment, whereas values of about 1.7 mg/g FW are reported in the absence of salt, according to graphic results by Benzarti et al. [31]. Consuming a ration of 100 g FW (assuming 87.5% moisture), the betaine intake would vary from 349 mg/100 g FW to 170 mg/100 g FW, respectively, i.e., values that are by far within the limits recommended by the EFSA.

8. Toxicology

The edibility of *A. portulacoides* is supported by its use history as a traditional food, although it is limited to some coastal populations and is currently almost abandoned, and as pasture for sheep and cattle (Section 6.1). Furthermore, cytotoxicity tests carried out for 72 h with aqueous, methanolic and chloroform extracts of *A. portulacoides* by Rodrigues et al. [101] on hepatocellular carcinoma HepG2 cell cultures, showed the total absence of toxicity. The same study also comprised highly lipophilic extracts (ether or hexane), which reduced the cell survival to 20–30% following the strongest treatment, i.e., 125 μg/mL. A cell survival of < 70% is required for the consideration of a compound as potentially toxic [104], and this did not occur despite the protracted treatment period (72 h).

Some rough transpositions are proposed here, which are aimed at the estimation of the food intake necessary to reproduce, in vivo, an equivalent treatment of highly lipophilic compounds. If we express the treatment in terms of the biomass from which the highly lipophilic extracts are obtained (assuming a yield < 5% of DW biomass, according to the personal experience of one of the authors), 125 μg/mL might correspond to a dose that is not lower than 2.5 mg/mL as DW biomass, or 20 mg/mL as FW biomass (calculated on 87.5% moisture). In order to expose the human body to an equivalent treatment, an intake of *A. portulacoides* FW biomass of at least 20 g/kg BW might be estimated, i.e., a value that is more than tenfold the suggested 100 g food ration. In light of these results, it is reasonable to state that there is no evidence of toxicity for *A. portulacoides*.

9. Conclusions and Perspectives

Modern nutrition science is always looking for novel ingredients and foods that are suitable to improve human (and animal) diets, not only in order to meet the energy and essential nutrient needs, but also to preserve and enhance the state of our health. The latter issue is related with the intake of biologically active compounds for the prevention or delay of cell damage due to environmental stresses or the physiological aging processes. In this context, the research is focused on foods that are rich in vitamins, antioxidants, immunostimulants, anti-inflammatory substances, and natural regulators of blood glucose and lipemic metabolism, etc. Moreover, in accordance with the principles of sustainable development and the green economy, food sources should respect the natural environment, and should not contribute to climate change. Halophytes, as with many organisms that have adapted to stressing environments, have developed ecophysiological adaptations based on antioxidant bioactives [4], and on the ability to concentrate some minerals of nutritional interest. *A. portulacoides* shows the properties typical of halophytes, but—in addition—it can grow in non-saline soils, and is therefore suitable to be cultivated in conventional agricultural lands. In the latter case, this plant seems to have the potentiality to develop under poor irrigation, allowing the exploitation of arid and even marginal saline lands. Thus, in view of the ongoing climate change, its production could offer an interesting opportunity for agricultural diversification, both for production aimed at the human diet, and to be used in properly balanced forages.

Concerning the composition of *A. portulacoides*, particular attention should be paid to its content in PUFAs, sterols and phenolic compounds. These active molecules appear to be suitable for being assimilated by dairy animals, and—at least partly—are transferred into milk, fortifying this food which is widely consumed on a daily basis. The impact on human nutrition deriving from the use of this fodder could, therefore, be even greater than the direct consumption of the plant carried out on an occasional basis. The improvement of the lipid profile of milk obtained by integrating bovine feed with non-traditional ingredients has already been demonstrated. For instance, the decrease of the n-6/n-3 fatty acid ratio of milk and ripened cheese was successfully obtained by supplementing the cows' diet with extruded flaxseed [105].

The present review highlights that *A. portulacoides* possesses the characteristics to become a functional food which is useful for improving human well-being and for the diversification of agricultural productions in a sustainable way. This justifies further investments in research, which are necessary because several nutritional and functional issues of *A. portulacoides* have not been investigated yet, including its protein quality and composition, vitamin content, fruit composition, the bioavailability of the compounds of interest, its overall digestibility, and its effect on mammalian metabolism and serum parameters, etc. Many results that were obtained from in vitro experimental models need to be confirmed in in vivo tests, especially for phytocomplexes that are rich in compounds, whose metabolic responses depend on the sum of their activities. For instance, extracts tested on ex vivo skin samples produced an increase of melanogenesis [102], in spite of the inhibiting activity on tyrosinase shown in vitro [57].

Furthermore, cultivation trials and the assessment of the related yields have not been carried out yet. As this plant is perennial, the harvest should therefore be performed by taking only the upper part of the canopy, preserving the roots and most woody part of the stems in a vital state for new shoot production. The actual productivity, seasonality and composition of the harvested biomass, which would include the fruit—if the harvest is carried out in the autumn—are still unknown.

Abbreviations

BW	body weight
DW	dry weight
EFSA	European Food Safety Authority
FW	fresh weight
GSH	glutathione
LCAA	long chain aliphatic alcohol
PSU	practical salinity unit
PUFA	Polyunsaturated fatty acid

References

1. Ksouri, R.; Ksouri, W.M.; Jallali, I.; Debez, A.; Magné, C.; Hiroko, I.; Abdelly, C. Medicinal halophytes: Potent source of health promoting biomolecules with medical, nutraceutical and food applications. *Crit. Rev. Biotechnol.* **2012**, *32*, 289–326. [CrossRef] [PubMed]
2. Ventura, Y.; Wuddineh, W.A.; Myrzabayeva, M.; Alikulov, Z.; Khozin-Goldberg, I.; Shpigel, M.; Samocha, T.M.; Sagi, M. Effect of seawater concentration on the productivity and nutritional value of annual *Salicornia* and perennial *Sarcocornia* halophytes as leafy vegetable crops. *Sci. Hortic.* **2011**, *128*, 189–196. [CrossRef]
3. Norman, H.C.; Masters, D.G.; Barrett-Lennard, E.G. Halophytes as forages in saline landscapes: Interactions between plant genotype and environment change their feeding value to ruminants. *Environ. Exp. Bot.* **2013**, *92*, 96–109. [CrossRef]
4. Maciel, E.; Leal, M.; Lillebø, A.; Domingues, P.; Domingues, M.; Calado, R. Bioprospecting of marine macrophytes using MS-based lipidomics as a new approach. *Mar. Drugs* **2016**, *14*, 49. [CrossRef] [PubMed]
5. Barreira, L.; Resek, E.; Rodrigues, M.J.; Rocha, M.I.; Pereira, H.; Bandarra, N.; da Silva, M.M.; Varela, J.; Custódio, L. Halophytes: Gourmet food with nutritional health benefits? *J. Food Compos. Anal.* **2017**, *59*, 35–42. [CrossRef]

6. Pacicco, L.; Bodesmo, M.; Torricelli, R.; Negri, V. A methodological approach to identify agro-biodiversity hotspots for priority in situ conservation of plant genetic resources. *PLoS ONE* **2018**, *13*, e0197709. [CrossRef] [PubMed]
7. Habel, J.C.; Samways, M.J.; Schmitt, T. Mitigating the precipitous decline of terrestrial European insects: Requirements for a new strategy. *Biodivers. Conserv.* **2019**, *28*, 1343–1360. [CrossRef]
8. French, K.E. Species composition determines forage quality and medicinal value of high diversity grasslands in lowland England. *Agric. Ecosyst. Environ.* **2017**, *241*, 193–204. [CrossRef]
9. Chapman, V.J. Halimione portulacoides (L.). *Aell. J. Ecol.* **1950**, *38*, 214–222. [CrossRef]
10. Anoè, N.; Calzavara, D.; Salviato, L.; Zanaboni, A. Flora e vegetazione delle barene. In *Gli Ambienti Salmastri della Laguna di Venezia*; Soc Veneziana di Scienze Naturali: Venezia, Italy, 2001; Volume 26, pp. 9–84.
11. Kadereit, G.; Borsch, T.; Weising, K.; Freitag, H. Phylogeny of Amaranthaceae and Chenopodiaceae and the evolution of C4 photosynthesis. *Int. J. Plant Sci.* **2003**, *164*, 959–986. [CrossRef]
12. APG (Angiosperm Phylogeny Group) An update of the Angiosperm Phylogeny Group classification for the orders and families of flowering plants: APG IV. *Bot. J. Linn. Soc.* **2016**, *181*, 1–20. [CrossRef]
13. Moquin-Tandon, A. *Chenopodearum Monographica Enumeratio*; Loss: Paris, France, 1840; 182p.
14. Aellen, P. Revision der australischen und neuseelandischen Chenopodiaceae. *Bot. Jahrb. Syst.* **1938**, *68*, 345–435.
15. Acta Plantarum, from 2007+ Etimologia dei Nomi Botanici e Micologici. Available online: http://www.actaplantarum.org/etimologia/etimologia.php (accessed on 6 March 2020).
16. Kühn, U.; Bittrich, V.; Carolin, R.; Freitag, H.; Hedge, I.C.; Uotila, P.; Wilson, P.G. Chenopodiaceae. In *The Families and Genera of Vascular Plants*; Kubitzki, K., Rohwer, J.G., Bittrich, V., Eds.; Springer: Berlin/Heidelberg, Germany, 1993; Volume 2, pp. 253–281.
17. Kadereit, G.; Mavrodiev, E.V.; Zacharias, E.H.; Sukhorukov, A.P. Molecular phylogeny of Atripliceae (Chenopodioideae, Chenopodiaceae): Implications for systematics, biogeography, flower and fruit evolution, and the origin of C4 photosynthesis. *Am. J. Bot.* **2010**, *97*, 1664–1687. [CrossRef] [PubMed]
18. Bair, A.; Howe, M.; Roth, D.; Taylor, R.; Ayers, T.; Kiger, R.W. Vascular Plants of Arizona: Portulacaceae. *Canotia* **2006**, *2*, 1–22.
19. Boestfleisch, C.; Papenbrock, J. Changes in secondary metabolites in the halophytic putative crop species *Crithmum maritimum* L., *Triglochin maritima* L. and *Halimione portulacoides* (L.) Aellen as reaction to mild salinity. *PLoS ONE* **2017**, *12*, e0176303. [CrossRef]
20. Kubiak-Martens, L.; Brinkkemper, O.; Oudemans, T.F. What's for dinner? Processed food in the coastal area of the northern Netherlands in the Late Neolithic. *Veg. Hist. Archaeobot.* **2015**, *24*, 47–62. [CrossRef]
21. Custódio, M.; Villasante, S.; Cremades, J.; Calado, R.; Lillebø, A.I. Unravelling the potential of halophytes for marine integrated multi-trophic aquaculture (IMTA) a perspective on performance, opportunities and challenges. *Aquac. Environ. Interact.* **2017**, *9*, 445–460. [CrossRef]
22. Guarrera, P.M.; Savo, V. Wild food plants used in traditional vegetable mixtures in Italy. *J. Ethnopharmacol.* **2016**, *185*, 202–234. [CrossRef]
23. Mangia, N.P.; Murgia, M.A.; Fancello, F.; Mouannes, E.; Deiana, P. Tecnologia e controllo microbiologico della mreca, alimento tradizionale a base di *Mugil cephalus*. *Ind. Aliment.* **2014**, *547*, 21–24.
24. Stienstra, A.W. Mineral composition of *Halimione portulacoides* (L.) Aellen leaves. *Hydrobiologia* **1977**, *52*, 89–91. [CrossRef]
25. Jensen, A. On the ecophysiology of *Halimione portulacoides*. *Vegetatio* **1985**, *61*, 231–240. [CrossRef]
26. Crain, C.M.; Silliman, B.R.; Bertness, S.L.; Bertness, M.D. Physical and Biotic Drivers of Plant Distribution across Estuarine Salinity Gradients. *Ecology* **2004**, *85*, 2539–2549. [CrossRef]
27. Redondo-Gómez, S.; Mateos-Naranjo, E.; Davy, A.J.; Fernández-Muñoz, F.; Castellanos, E.M.; Luque, T.; Figueroa, M.E. Growth and photosynthetic responses to salinity of the salt-marsh shrub *Atriplex portulacoides*. *Ann. Bot.* **2007**, *100*, 555–563.
28. Bessieres, M.A.; Gibon, Y.; Lefeuvre, J.C.; Larher, F. A single-step purification for glycine betaine determination in plant extracts by isocratic HPLC. *J. Agric. Food Chem.* **1999**, *47*, 3718–3722. [CrossRef] [PubMed]
29. Storey, R.; Ahma, N.; Jones, R.W. Taxonomic and ecological aspects of the distribution of glycinebetaine and related compounds in plants. *Oecologia* **1977**, *27*, 319–332. [CrossRef]
30. Rabbani, G.; Choi, I. Roles of osmolytes in protein folding and aggregation in cells and their biotechnological applications. *Int. J. Biol. Macromol.* **2018**, *109*, 483–491. [CrossRef]

31. Benzarti, M.; Rejeb, K.B.; Messedi, D.; Mna, A.B.; Hessini, K.; Ksontini, M.; Abdelly, C.; Debez, A. Effect of high salinity on *Atriplex portulacoides*: Growth, leaf water relations and solute accumulation in relation with osmotic adjustment. *S. Afr. J. Bot.* **2014**, *95*, 70–77. [CrossRef]
32. Cott, G.M.; Reidy, D.T.; Chapman, D.V.; Jansen, M.A. Waterlogging affects the distribution of the saltmarsh plant *Atriplex portulacoides* (L.) Aellen. *Flora Morphol. Distrib. Funct. Ecol. Plants* **2013**, *208*, 336–342. [CrossRef]
33. Reboredo, F. Zinc compartmentation in *Halimione portulacoides* (L.) Aellen and some effects on leaf ultrastructure. *Environ. Sci. Pollut. Res.* **2012**, *19*, 2644–2657. [CrossRef]
34. Duarte, B.; Carreiras, J.; Pérez-Romero, J.A.; Mateos-Naranjo, E.; Redondo-Gómez, S.; Matos, A.R.; Marques, S.C.; Caçador, I. Halophyte fatty acids as biomarkers of anthropogenic-driven contamination in Mediterranean marshes: Sentinel species survey and development of an integrated biomarker response (IBR) index. *Ecol. Indic.* **2018**, *87*, 86–96. [CrossRef]
35. Sousa, A.I.; Caçador, I.; Lillebø, A.I.; Pardal, M.A. Heavy metal accumulation in *Halimione portulacoides*: Intra-and extra-cellular metal binding sites. *Chemosphere* **2008**, *70*, 850–857. [CrossRef] [PubMed]
36. Castro, R.; Pereira, S.; Lima, A.; Corticeiro, S.; Válega, M.; Pereira, E.; Duarte, A.; Figueira, E. Accumulation, distribution and cellular partitioning of mercury in several halophytes of a contaminated salt marsh. *Chemosphere* **2009**, *76*, 1348–1355. [CrossRef] [PubMed]
37. Válega, M.; Lima, A.I.G.; Figueira, E.M.A.P.; Pereira, E.; Pardal, M.A.; Duarte, A.C. Mercury intracellular partitioning and chelation in a salt marsh plant, *Halimione portulacoides* (L.) Aellen: Strategies underlying tolerance in environmental exposure. *Chemosphere* **2009**, *74*, 530–536.
38. Válega, M.; Lillebø, A.I.; Pereira, M.E.; Caçador, I.; Duarte, A.C.; Pardal, M.A. Mercury in salt marshes ecosystems: *Halimione portulacoides* as biomonitor. *Chemosphere* **2008**, *73*, 1224–1229. [CrossRef]
39. Negrin, V.L.; Teixeira, B.; Godinho, R.M.; Mendes, R.; Vale, C. Phytochelatins and monothiols in salt marsh plants and their relation with metal tolerance. *Mar. Pollut. Bull.* **2017**, *121*, 78–84. [CrossRef]
40. Cartaxana, P.; Catarino, F. Allocation of nitrogen and carbon in an estuarine salt marsh in Portugal. *J. Coast. Conserv.* **1997**, *3*, 27–34. [CrossRef]
41. Harrouni, M.C.; Daoud, S.; Koyro, H.W. Effect of Seawater Irrigation on Biomass Production and Ion Composition of Seven Halophytic Species in Morocco. In *Cash Crop Halophytes: Recent Studies*; Kratochwil, A., Lieth, H., Eds.; Springer: Dordrecht, The Netherlands, 2003; pp. 59–70.
42. Neves, J.P.; Ferreira, L.F.; Simões, M.P.; Gazarini, L.C. Primary production and nutrient content in two salt marsh species, *Atriplex portulacoides* L. and *Limoniastrum monopetalum* L., in Southern Portugal. *Estuaries Coasts* **2007**, *30*, 459–468. [CrossRef]
43. Reboredo, F. Some observations on the effects of iron on the leaf ultrastructure of *Halimione portulacoides*. *J. Plant Physiol.* **1997**, *151*, 581–589. [CrossRef]
44. Vilela, C.; Santos, S.A.; Coelho, D.; Silva, A.M.; Freire, C.S.; Neto, C.P.; Silvestre, A.J. Screening of lipophilic and phenolic extractives from different morphological parts of *Halimione portulacoides*. *Ind. Crop. Prod.* **2014**, *52*, 373–379. [CrossRef]
45. Boughalleb, N.; Trabelsi, L.; Harzallah-Skhiri, F. Antifungal activity from polar and non-polar extracts of some Chenopodiaceae wild species growing in Tunisia. *Nat. Prod. Res.* **2009**, *23*, 988–997. [CrossRef]
46. Maciel, E.; Lillebø, A.; Domingues, P.; Da Costa, E.; Calado, R.; Domingues, M.R.M. Polar lipidome profiling of *Salicornia ramosissima* and *Halimione portulacoides* and the relevance of lipidomics for the valorization of halophytes. *Phytochemistry* **2018**, *153*, 94–101. [CrossRef] [PubMed]
47. Dinan, L.; Whiting, P.; Scott, A.J. Taxonomic distribution of phytoecdysteroids in seeds of members of the Chenopodiaceae. *Biochem. Syst. Ecol.* **1998**, *26*, 553–576. [CrossRef]
48. Parr, M.K.; Botrè, F.; Naß, A.; Hengevoss, J.; Diel, P.; Wolber, G. Ecdysteroids: A novel class of anabolic agents? *Biol. Sport* **2015**, *32*, 169–173. [CrossRef]
49. Ben Nejma, A.B.; Nguir, A.; Jannet, H.B.; Daïch, A.; Othman, M.; Lawson, A.M. New septanoside and 20-hydroxyecdysone septanoside derivative from *Atriplex portulacoides* roots with preliminary biological activities. *Bioorg. Med. Chem. Lett.* **2015**, *25*, 1665–1670. [CrossRef] [PubMed]
50. Zakar, T.; Laczko-Dobos, H.; Toth, T.N.; Gombos, Z. Carotenoids assist in cyanobacterial photosystem II assembly and function. *Front. Plant Sci.* **2016**, *7*, 295. [CrossRef] [PubMed]
51. Zhang, J.; Sun, Z.; Sun, P.; Chen, T.; Chen, F. Microalgal carotenoids: Beneficial effects and potential in human health. *Food Funct.* **2014**, *5*, 413–425. [CrossRef] [PubMed]

52. Anjum, N.A.; Israr, M.; Duarte, A.C.; Pereira, M.E.; Ahmad, I. *Halimione portulacoides* (L.) physiological/biochemical characterization for its adaptive responses to environmental mercury exposure. *Environ. Res.* **2014**, *131*, 39–49. [CrossRef]
53. Duarte, B.; Santos, D.; Marques, J.C.; Caçador, I. Ecophysiological adaptations of two halophytes to salt stress: Photosynthesis, PS II photochemistry and anti-oxidant feedback–implications for resilience in climate change. *Plant Physiol. Biochem.* **2013**, *67*, 178–188. [CrossRef]
54. Duarte, B.; Silva, H.; Dias, J.M.; Sleimi, N.; Marques, J.C.; Caçador, I. Functional and ecophysiological traits of *Halimione portulacoides* and *Sarcocornia perennis* ecotypes in Mediterranean salt marshes under different tidal exposures. *Ecol. Res.* **2018**, *33*, 1145–1156. [CrossRef]
55. Duarte, B.; Santos, D.; Marques, J.C.; Caçador, I. Impact of heat and cold events on the energetic metabolism of the C3 halophyte *Halimione portulacoides*. *Estuarine Coast. Shelf Sci.* **2015**, *167*, 166–177. [CrossRef]
56. Benzarti, M.; Rejeb, K.B.; Debez, A.; Messedi, D.; Abdelly, C. Photosynthetic activity and leaf antioxidative responses of *Atriplex portulacoides* subjected to extreme salinity. *Acta Physiol. Plant.* **2012**, *34*, 1679–1688. [CrossRef]
57. Zengin, G.; Aumeeruddy-Elalfi, Z.; Mollica, A.; Yilmaz, M.A.; Mahomoodally, M.F. In vitro and in silico perspectives on biological and phytochemical profile of three halophyte species—A source of innovative phytopharmaceuticals from nature. *Phytomedicine* **2018**, *38*, 35–44. [CrossRef] [PubMed]
58. Seker, H.; Yolcu, H.; Acikgoz, E. Primary growth parameters of three alfalfa cultivars adapted to highland climatic conditions. *J. Agron. Crop Sci.* **2015**, *201*, 219–227. [CrossRef]
59. Jensen, A. Seasonal changes in near infrared reflectance ratio and sanding crop biomass in a salt marsh community dominated by *Halimione portulacoides* (L.) AELLEN. *New Phytol.* **1980**, *86*, 57–67. [CrossRef]
60. Benito, I.; Onaindia, M. Biomass and aboveground production of four angiosperms in Cantabrian (N. Spain) salt marshes. *Vegetatio* **1991**, *96*, 165–175. [CrossRef]
61. Groenendijk, A.M. Primary production of four dominant salt-marsh angiosperms in the SW Netherlands. *Vegetatio* **1984**, *57*, 143–152. [CrossRef]
62. Sardo, V. Halophytes and Salt-Tolerant Glycophytes a Potential Resource. In *The Use of non-Conventional Water Resources*; CIHEAM/EU DG Research: Bari, Italy, 2005; pp. 87–98.
63. Le Houérou, H.N. Forage Halophytes and Salt-Tolerant Fodder Crops in the Mediterranean Basin. In *Halophytes as a Resource for Livestock and for Rehabilitation of Degraded Lands*; Squires, V.R., Ayoub, A.T., Eds.; Springer: Dordrecht, The Netherlands, 1994; pp. 123–137.
64. Ventura, Y.; Sagi, M. Halophyte crop cultivation: The case for *Salicornia* and *Sarcocornia*. *Environ. Exp. Bot.* **2013**, *92*, 144–153. [CrossRef]
65. Bakker, J.P.; Bos, D.; De Vries, Y. To Graze or not to Graze: That is the Question. In Proceedings of the 10th International Scientific Wadden Sea Symposium, Groningen, The Netherlands, 31 October–3 November 2000; Wolff, W.J., Essink, K., Kellermann, A., Van Leeuwe, M.A., Eds.; University of Groningen: Groningen, The Netherlands, 2003.
66. Laffaille, P.; Lefeuvre, J.C.; Feunteun, E. Impact of sheep grazing on juvenile sea bass, *Dicentrarchus labrax* L., in tidal salt marshes. *Biol. Conserv.* **2000**, *96*, 271–277. [CrossRef]
67. Giménez-Anaya, A.; Herrero, J.; Rosell, C.; Couto, S.; García-Serrano, A. Food habits of wild boars (*Sus scrofa*) in a Mediterranean coastal wetland. *Wetlands* **2008**, *28*, 197–203. [CrossRef]
68. Bos, D.; Loonen, M.J.; Stock, M.; Hofeditz, F.; Van der Graaf, A.J.; Bakker, J.P. Utilisation of Wadden Sea salt marshes by geese in relation to livestock grazing. *J. Nat. Conserv.* **2005**, *13*, 1–15. [CrossRef]
69. Kuijper, D.P.J.; Bakker, J.P. Top-down control of small herbivores on salt-marsh vegetation along a productivity gradient. *Ecology* **2005**, *86*, 914–923. [CrossRef]
70. Attia-Ismail, S.A. Halophytes as Forages. In *New Perspectives in Forage Crops*; Loiola Edvan, R., Rocha Bezerra, L., Eds.; IntechOpen: London, UK, 2018; pp. 69–87. [CrossRef]
71. Gihad, E.A.; Shaer, H.E. Utilization of Halophytes by Livestock on Rangelands. Problems and Prospects. In *Halophytes as a Resource for Livestock and for Rehabilitation of Degraded Lands*; Squires, V.R., Ayoub, A.T., Eds.; Springer: Dordrecht, The Netherlands, 1994; pp. 77–96.
72. Miyamoto, S.; Glenn, E.P.; Singh, N.T. Utilization of Halophytic Plants for Fodder Production with Brackish Water in Subtropic Deserts. In *Halophytes as a Resource for Livestock and for Rehabilitation of Degraded Lands*; Squires, V.R., Ayoub, A.T., Eds.; Springer: Dordrecht, The Netherlands, 1994; pp. 43–75.

73. Pacchioli, M.T.; Fattori, G. *Gli Alimenti per la Vacca da Latte: I Foraggi*; Centro Ricerche Produzioni Animali—C.R.P.A.: Reggio Emilia, Italy, 2014; 81p.
74. Bortolazzo, E.; Dal Prà, A.; Davolio, R.; Ruozzi, F. Produttività e composizione dell'erba medica. In *L'informatore Agrario*; Edizioni L'Informatore Agrario Srl: Verona, Italy, 2016; pp. 40–43.
75. Hojilla-Evangelista, M.P.; Selling, G.W.; Hatfield, R.; Digman, M. Extraction, composition, and functional properties of dried alfalfa (*Medicago sativa* L.) leaf protein. *J. Sci. Food Agric.* **2017**, *97*, 882–888. [CrossRef] [PubMed]
76. Swingle, R.S.; Glenn, E.P.; Riley, J.J. Halophytes in Mixed Feeds for Livestock. In *Halophytes as a Resource for Livestock and for Rehabilitation of Degraded Lands*; Squires, V.R., Ayoub, A.T., Eds.; Springer: Dordrecht, The Netherlands, 1994; pp. 97–100.
77. CSIRO. *Nutrient Requirements of Domesticated Ruminants*; CSIRO Publishing: Collingwood, Australia, 2007; 270p.
78. Cambrollé, J.; Mancilla-Leytón, J.M.; Muñoz-Vallés, S.; Luque, T.; Figueroa, M.E. Tolerance and accumulation of copper in the salt-marsh shrub *Halimione portulacoides*. *Mar. Pollut. Bull.* **2012**, *64*, 721–728. [CrossRef] [PubMed]
79. Adams, R.S. Variability in mineral and trace element content of dairy cattle feeds. *J. Dairy Sci.* **1975**, *58*, 1538–1548. [CrossRef]
80. Kincaid, R.L.; Cronrath, J.D. Amounts and distribution of minerals in Washington forages. *J. Dairy Sci.* **1983**, *66*, 821–824. [CrossRef]
81. Massaro, M.; De Caterina, R. Vasculoprotective effects of oleic acid: Epidemiological background and direct vascular antiatherogenic properties. *Nutr. Metab. Cardiovasc. Dis.* **2002**, *12*, 42–51.
82. Fleming, J.A.; Kris-Etherton, P.M. The evidence for α-linolenic acid and cardiovascular disease benefits: Comparisons with eicosapentaenoic acid and docosahexaenoic acid. *Adv. Nutr.* **2014**, *5*, 863S–876S. [CrossRef]
83. Wang, T.; Liu, Y.Y.; Wang, X.; Yang, N.; Zhu, H.B.; Zuo, P.P. Protective effects of octacosanol on 6-hydroxydopamine-induced Parkinsonism in rats via regulation of ProNGF and NGF signaling. *Acta Pharmacol. Sin.* **2010**, *31*, 765–774. [CrossRef]
84. Kim, H.; Park, S.; Han, D.S.; Park, T. Octacosanol supplementation increases running endurance time and improves biochemical parameters after exhaustion in trained rats. *J. Med. Food* **2003**, *6*, 345–351. [CrossRef]
85. Xu, Z.; Fitz, E.; Riediger, N.; Moghadasian, M.H. Dietary octacosanol reduces plasma triacylglycerol levels but not atherogenesis in apolipoprotein E–knockout mice. *Nutr. Res.* **2007**, *27*, 212–217. [CrossRef]
86. McBride, P.T.; Clark, L.; Krueger, G. Evaluation of triacontanol-containing compounds as anti-inflammatory agents using guinea pig models. *J. Investig. Dermatol.* **1987**, *89*, 380–383. [CrossRef]
87. Sugano, M.; Morioka, H.; Ikeda, I. A comparison of hypocholesterolemic activity of β-sitosterol and β-sitostanol in rats. *J. Nutr.* **1977**, *107*, 2011–2019. [CrossRef] [PubMed]
88. Saeidnia, S.; Manayi, A.; Gohari, A.R.; Abdollahi, M. The story of Beta-sitosterol—A review. *Eur. J. Med. Plants* **2014**, *4*, 590–609. [CrossRef]
89. Ikeda, I.; Morioka, H.; Sugano, M. The effect of dietary β-sitosterol and β-sitostanol on the metabolism of cholesterol in rats. *Agric. Biol. Chem.* **1979**, *43*, 1927–1933. [CrossRef]
90. Samarakoon, S.R.; Fernando, N.; Ediriweera, M.K.; Adhikari, A.; Wijayabandara, L.; de Silva, E.D.; Tennekoon, K.H. Isolation of hopenone-I from the leaves of mangrove plant *Scyphiphora hydrophyllacea* and its cytotoxic properties. *Br. J. Pharm. Res.* **2016**, *10*, 1–6. [CrossRef]
91. Perera, L.M.S.; Veloz, A.I.R.; GoisRuiz, A.L.T.; Foglio, M.A.; de Oliveira Sousa, I.M.; Tinti, S.V.; Possenti, A.; de Carvalho, J.E. In vitro and In vivo Antiproliferative activity of extracts and fractions of leaves and stem from *Tabebuia hypoleuca* (C. Wright). *Urb. Drug Discov.* **2019**, *13*, 10–21.
92. Merhan, O. Biochemistry and Antioxidant Properties of Carotenoids. In *Carotenoids*; Cvetkovic, D., Nikolic, G., Eds.; IntechOpen: London, UK, 2017; pp. 51–66.
93. Nakajima, Y.; Shimazawa, M.; Otsubo, K.; Ishibashi, T.; Hara, H. Zeaxanthin, a retinal carotenoid, protects retinal cells against oxidative stress. *Curr. Eye Res.* **2009**, *34*, 311–318. [CrossRef]
94. Saud, S.M.; Young, M.R.; Jones-Hall, Y.L.; Ileva, L.; Evbuomwan, M.O.; Wise, J.; Colburn, N.H.; Kim, Y.S.; Bobe, G. Chemopreventive activity of plant flavonoid isorhamnetin in colorectal cancer is mediated by oncogenic Src and β-catenin. *Cancer Res.* **2013**, *73*, 5473–5484. [CrossRef]
95. Chirumbolo, S. Anti-inflammatory action of isorhamnetin. *Inflammation* **2014**, *37*, 1200–1201. [CrossRef]

96. Chi, G.; Zhong, W.; Liu, Y.; Lu, G.; Lü, H.; Wang, D.; Sun, F. Isorhamnetin protects mice from lipopolysaccharide-induced acute lung injury via the inhibition of inflammatory responses. *Inflamm. Res.* **2016**, *65*, 33–41. [CrossRef]
97. Bruno, A.; Rossi, C.; Marcolongo, G.; Di Lena, A.; Venzo, A.; Berrie, C.P.; Corda, D. Selective in vivo anti-inflammatory action of the galactolipid monogalactosyldiacylglycerol. *Eur. J. Pharmacol.* **2005**, *524*, 159–168. [CrossRef]
98. Banskota, A.H.; Gallant, P.; Stefanova, R.; Melanson, R.; O'Leary, S.J. Monogalactosyldiacylglycerols, potent nitric oxide inhibitors from the marine microalga *Tetraselmis chui*. *Nat. Prod. Res.* **2013**, *27*, 1084–1090. [CrossRef]
99. Valencia, E.; Hardy, G. Practicalities of glutathione supplementation in nutritional support. *Curr. Opin. Clin. Nutr. Metab. Care* **2002**, *5*, 321–326. [CrossRef] [PubMed]
100. Buonocore, D.; Grosini, M.; Giardina, S.; Michelotti, A.; Carrabetta, M.; Seneci, A.; Verri, M.; Dossena, M.; Marzatico, F. Bioavailability study of an innovative orobuccal formulation of glutathione. *Oxidative Med. Cell. Longev.* **2016**. [CrossRef] [PubMed]
101. Rodrigues, M.; Gangadhar, K.; Vizetto-Duarte, C.; Wubshet, S.; Nyberg, N.; Barreira, L.; Varela, J.; Custódio, L. Maritime halophyte species from southern Portugal as sources of bioactive molecules. *Mar. Drugs* **2014**, *12*, 2228–2244. [CrossRef] [PubMed]
102. Zanella, L.; Pertile, P. Extracts of Halimione Portulacoides and Their Application. U.S. Patent WO2015/040010A1, 26 March 2015.
103. EFSA-NDA panel. Safety of betaine as a novel food pursuant to Regulation (EC) No 258/97. Scientific opinion adopted on 17 October 2017. *EFSA J.* **2017**, *15*, 5057. [CrossRef]
104. Srivastava, G.K.; Alonso-Alonso, M.L.; Fernandez-Bueno, I.; Garcia-Gutierrez, M.T.; Rull, F.; Medina, J.; Coco, R.M.; Pastor, J.C. Comparison between direct contact and extract exposure methods for PFO cytotoxicity evaluation. *Sci. Rep.* **2018**, *8*, 1495. [CrossRef]
105. Cattani, M.; Mantovani, R.; Schiavon, S.; Bittante, G.; Bailoni, L. Recovery of n-3 polyunsaturated fatty acids and conjugated linoleic acids in ripened cheese obtained from milk of cows fed different levels of extruded flaxseed. *J. Dairy Sci.* **2014**, *97*, 123–135. [CrossRef]

6

Botanicals in Functional Foods and Food Supplements: Tradition, Efficacy and Regulatory Aspects

Francesca Colombo [1], Patrizia Restani [1,2,*], Simone Biella [1] and Chiara Di Lorenzo [1]

[1] Department of Pharmacological and Biomolecular Sciences, Università degli Studi di Milano, 20133 Milan, Italy; francesca.colombo1@unimi.it (F.C.); simone.biella@unimi.it (S.B.); chiara.dilorenzo@unimi.it (C.D.L.)

[2] CRC "Innovation for Well-Being and Environment", Università degli Studi di Milano, 20122 Milan, Italy

* Correspondence: patrizia.restani@unimi.it

Featured Application: The review aims to provide guidance on the definitions and regulation of products containing botanical ingredients, which are at present quite complex.

Abstract: In recent decades, the interest in products containing botanicals and claiming "functional" properties has increased exponentially. Functional foods, novel foods and food supplements have a special impact on the consumers, who show significant expectation for their well-being. Food supplements with botanical ingredients are the food area that has witnessed the greatest development, in terms of the number of available products, budget, and consumer acceptability. This review refers to and discusses some open points, such as: (1) the definitions and regulation of products containing botanicals; (2) the difficulty in obtaining nutritional and functional claims (botanical ingredients obtaining claims in the EU are listed and summarized); (3) the safety aspects of these products; and (4) the poor harmonization between international legislations. The availability of these "new" products can positively influence the well-being of the population, but it is essential to provide the consumers with the necessary recommendations to guide them in their purchase and use.

Keywords: botanicals; food supplements; nutritional claims; functional food

---

1. Introduction

The sentence "Let thy food be thy medicine and medicine be thy food", commonly attributed to Hippocrates (400 BC), indicates the importance that nutrition has always had in the concept of health and prevention of disease. This relationship has obviously undergone changes and historical recurrences with an evolution parallel to that of human civilization with its variable habits in social behavior and diet. More than 2500 years after Hippocrates' claim, the concept of diet has evolved to include aspects based on research in the field of nutrition and on knowledge relating to active molecules contained in foods with potential benefit to human health.

The vegetables entered massively in the diet of humans with the Agricultural Revolution that occurred about 12,000 years ago. Cereals, only rarely consumed in the Paleolithic era, have become the basis of human nutrition with milk derivatives [1]. However, considering the use of plants for their healing properties, archaeological excavations place their use up to 60,000 years ago. These were plants not commonly consumed as food: poppy (opium), ephedra and cannabis.

The possible placement of the plants among food and products with therapeutic properties is therefore ancient history and reappears, with its contradictions, in the current legislation, as described below. The aim of this review was the clarification and relative discussion of the most critical aspects regarding products containing botanicals, in order to promote the correct use of plant food supplements among consumers.

2. Definitions and Regulation

There is no internationally shared definition of the term "botanical". However, it is possible to cite what was defined by European Food Safety Authority (EFSA) in its guidelines published in 2009 [2]. The term *botanical* includes whole, fragmented or cut plants, plant parts, fungi and lichens. The term *botanical preparations* include all preparations obtained from botanicals by various processes, such as pressing, squeezing, extraction, fractionation, distillation, concentration, drying up and fermentation. A similar definition is reported by a group of food and beverage producers: "*botanicals* are fresh or dried plants, plant parts or plants' isolated or collective chemical components, extracted in water, ethanol, or other organic solvents, plus essential oils, oleoresins, and other extractives used for flavoring, fragrance, functional health benefits, medicine, or other uses" [3].

Based on the definitions listed above, it is clear that botanicals include numerous possible ingredients with extremely variable composition and characteristics. First of all, the presence and concentration of active molecules can vary greatly, with possible effects on the beneficial effect expected on the consumers' health.

Hundreds of plants are ingredients commonly used in the food industry as such or derivatives, or food additives (flavorings, colorings, preservatives, etc.), and botanicals can be included in different types of products regulated by the food law as illustrated in Figure 1.

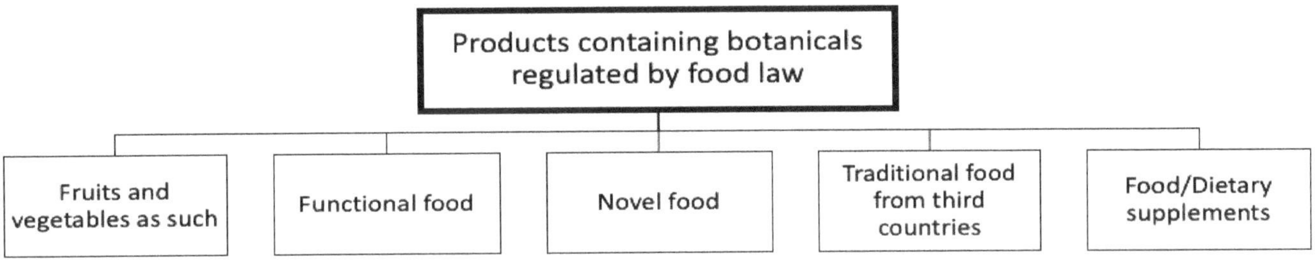

Figure 1. Categories of food containing botanicals.

2.1. *Fruits and Vegetables*

Fruits and vegetables have been included in the diet of humans since ancient times; they can be consumed as such or as household or industrial derivatives (jams, juice, purée, etc.). Fruits and vegetables are included in the EC Regulation N. 178/2002, which defines any unprocessed or processed substances or product designed for human consumption [4]. Generally speaking, consumers prefer products from the geographical area of belonging, but with the increasing globalization it is possible to expand the choice to imported products.

2.2. *Enriched or Functional Food*

Although there is no international agreement, according to the consensus document on "Scientific Concepts of Functional Foods in Europe" of the European Commission Concerted Action on Functional Food Science in Europe (FUFOSE), functional food is usually considered a product to which one or more ingredients have been added (or more rarely subtracted) with a positive consequence on the functionality of human organs or systems [5]. It is, therefore, a food that has not only the function of providing calories and nutrients but intends to carry out a favorable action on the consumer's health. This effect must be reached with the quantity of food normally consumed, it must be in "traditional" form (and not in pharmaceutical form) and must guarantee the safety of the subjects taking the product, even if they present common pathologies. As an example, the prebiotic ingredients are frequently added to food; they are soluble fibers capable to promote the growth of the positive intestinal microbiota; among others, the most important fibers in this field are inulin and fructo-oligosaccharides (from chicory or Jerusalem artichoke). Further details will be reported in Section 4.1.2.

2.3. *Novel Food and Traditional Food from Third Countries*

At the European level the regulation of new food, or novel food, was amended in 2015 (EU Regulation 2015/2283). Compared to the previous regulations, the definition of this products was maintained: "novel food means any food that was not used for human consumption to a significant degree within the Union before 15 May 1997". Some of the categories listed in novel food include botanicals: (1) food consisting of, isolated from or produced from microorganisms, fungi or algae; (2) food consisting of, isolated from or produced from plants or their parts. Novel food category also includes products obtained with new technologies. Before marketing them, appropriate documentation must be provided in order to demonstrate their safety. Examples of novel food include: new sources of vitamin K (menaquinone) or some extracts from existing food (Antarctic krill oil rich in phospholipids from *Euphausia superba*) [6].

The aforementioned regulation has introduced a new authorization procedure for "traditional foods deriving from Third Countries", where a food with proven tradition of safe use in a third country for at least 25 years is included. Compared to the novel food procedure, this new category must present less documentation for their approval. Examples of foods belonging to this category are the dried aerial parts from *Hoodia parviflora* N.E.Br. (hoodia) and seeds from *Salvia hispanica* L. (chia) [6].

2.4. *Food/Dietary Supplements*

Botanicals are widely used in the formulation of food (or dietary in US) supplements, that can be defined as "products intended to supplement the common diet and which constitute a concentrated source of nutrients, such as vitamins and minerals, or other substances having a nutritional or physiological effect, in particular, but not exclusively, amino acids, essential fatty acids, fibers and extracts of vegetable origin, both single- and multi-compound, in pre-dosed forms" [7]. The role of food supplements is limited to correcting nutritional deficiencies, maintaining the recommended intake of some essential nutrients and supporting specific nutritional needs such as pregnancy, breastfeeding and menopause. They must not show therapeutic activity or significantly modify the physiological functions [8]. Among the most frequently botanical ingredients used in food supplements, there are *Ginkgo biloba* L. (ginkgo), *Oenothera biennis* L. (evening primrose), *Cynara scolymus* L. (artichoke) and *Panax ginseng* C.A. Meyer (ginseng) [9].

2.5. *Other Categories*

Botanicals can be regulated by drug law. In fact, their use can enter into conventional medicine, or, as in some European countries (e.g., Germany), in "Traditional Herbal Medicinal Products (THMPs)". THMPs must guarantee their safety in the expected conditions of use and their biological activity/efficacy must be plausible on the basis of a chronic use and of available experience [10].

Botanicals can also be ingredients of products belonging to the category of medical devices; among others: (1) ophthalmic solutions containing chamomile (*Matricaria recutita* L.), calendula (*Calendula officinalis* L.), cornflower (*Centaurea cyanus* L.), etc.; (2) some liquids used in contact lens care, which include arabinogalactans and plant extracts; (3) some solutions used for oral hygiene containing mainly chamomile, aloe (*Aloe vera* (L.) Burm.f.) and marshmallow (*Althaea officinalis* L.). Since this chapter is about food, only examples of the use of botanicals in functional foods and food supplements will be described.

3. Claims

One of the most interesting aspects associated with functional food and food supplements is the possibility to boast on the label their health properties, the so-called "claims".

The European Commission allows health claims when they can be supported by the scientific literature and if they can be understood by consumers. In the EU, the European Food Safety Authority (EFSA) is in charge of evaluating the scientific evidence [11] and provides the guidelines, which describes in detail the studies required for the approval of nutritional/physiological claims [2,12].

There are two types of health sentences, those related to art. 13, and those relating to art. 14 of the European Regulation 1924/2006. Article 13 claims refer to: (1) growth, development and functions of the body; (2) psychological and behavioral functions; (3) slimming or weight control. Article 14 claims are associated with: (1) a reduction of risk factors in the development of diseases; (2) support of normal children's development and health. Table 1 lists the most important health claims allowed for vegetable/botanical ingredients in the EU [13].

Table 1. List of main claims allowed in the EU for plant (botanical) ingredients contained in, or added to, functional food or food supplements [13].

Claim Type	Botanical Ingredients	Claim	Condition of Use of the Claim Restrictions of Use
Art.13(1)	Arabinoxylan produced from wheat endosperm	Consumption of arabinoxylan as part of a meal contributes to a reduction of the blood glucose rise after that meal	Food must contain at least 8 g of arabinoxylan-rich fibre/100 g of bioavailable carbohydrate. The consumer should be informed that the ingredient must be part of meal.
Art.13(1)	Barley grain fibre	Barley grain fibre contributes to an increase in faecal bulk	Refer to products included in the claim "high fibre" as listed in the Annex to Regulation (EC) No 1924/2006.
Art.13(1)	Beta-glucans from oats, oat bran, barley, barley bran, or from mixtures of these sources	Beta-glucans contribute to the maintenance of normal blood cholesterol levels	Food must contain at least 1 g of beta-glucans per quantified portion. Consumers must be informed that the healthy effect is obtained with a daily intake of 3 g of beta-glucans.
Art.13(1)	Beta-glucans from oats and barley	Consumption of beta-glucans from oats or barley as part of a meal contributes to the reduction of the blood glucose rise after that meal	Food must contain at least 4 g of beta-glucans/30 g of bioavailable carbohydrates. The ingredient must be part of meal.
Art.13(5)	Cocoa flavanols	Cocoa flavanols help maintain the elasticity of blood vessels, which contributes to normal blood flow	The positive effect is due to a daily intake of 200 mg of cocoa flavanols having a degree of polymerization 1-10. Products included: cocoa beverages (with cocoa powder) or dark chocolate.
Art.13(1)	Dried plums of 'prune' cultivars (*Prunus domestica* L.)	Dried plums/prunes contribute to normal bowel function	The "active" daily intake is 100 g of dried plums (prunes).
Art.13(1)	Glucomannan (konjac mannan)	Glucomannan contributes to the maintenance of normal blood cholesterol levels	Consumer must be informed that the healthy effect is associated with the intake of three doses of 1 g each, together with 1-2 glasses of water, before meals and during an energy-restricted diet. Recommendation about an adequate fluid intake to ensure ingredient reaches the stomach must be added.
Art.13(1)	Glucomannan (konjac mannan)	Glucomannan in the context of an energy restricted diet contributes to weight loss	
Art.13(1)	Guar Gum	Guar gum contributes to the maintenance of normal blood cholesterol levels	Claim is allowed for foods containing 10 g of guar gum/daily dose recommending an adequate fluid intake to ensure ingredient reaches the stomach.
Art.13(1)	Hydroxypropyl methylcellulose (HPMC)	Consumption of hydroxypropyl methylcellulose with a meal contributes to a reduction in the blood glucose rise after that meal	Claim is allowed for foods containing 4 g of HPMC/per portion during meal. Recommendation about an adequate fluid intake to ensure ingredient reaches the stomach must be added.
Art.13(1)	Hydroxypropyl methylcellulose (HPMC)	Hydroxypropyl methylcellulose contributes to the maintenance of normal blood cholesterol levels	Claim is allowed for foods providing 5 g of HPMC/day. Recommendation about an adequate fluid intake to ensure ingredient reaches the stomach must be added.
Art.13(1)	*Monascus purpureus* (red yeast rice)	Monacolin K from red yeast rice contributes to the maintenance of normal blood cholesterol levels	Claim is allowed for foods providing 10 mg of monacolin K/day.
Art.13(5)	Native chicory inulin	Chicory inulin contributes to normal bowel function by increasing stool frequency	Claim is allowed for foods providing at least 12 g of inulin/day. It must contain non-fractionated mixture of monosaccharide (<10%), disaccharide, inulin-type fructans and inulin, with a mean degree of polymerization > or = 9.

Table 1. *Cont.*

Claim Type	Botanical Ingredients	Claim	Condition of Use of the Claim Restrictions of Use
Art.13(1)	Oat grain fibre	Oat grain fibre contributes to an increase in faecal bulk	Refer to products included in the claim "high fibre" as listed in the Annex to Regulation (EC) No 1924/2006.
Art.13(1)	Olive oil polyphenols	Olive oil polyphenols contribute to the protection of blood lipids from oxidative stress	Claim is allowed for olive oils providing at least 5 mg of hydroxytyrosol and its derivatives in the daily dose, corresponding to 20 g.
Art.13(1)	Pectins	Consumption of pectins with a meal contributes to the reduction of the blood glucose rise after that meal	Claim is allowed for foods providing 10 g of pectins/portion during meal. Recommendation about an adequate fluid intake to ensure ingredient reaches the stomach must be added.
Art.13(1)	Pectins	Pectins contribute to the maintenance of normal blood cholesterol levels	The claim can be used only when the product provides 6 g of pectins/daily dose. Recommendation about an adequate fluid intake to ensure ingredient reaches the stomach must be added.
Art.13(1)	Plant sterols and plant stanols	Plant sterols/stanols contribute to the maintenance of normal blood cholesterol levels	Claim is allowed for foods providing at least 0.8 g of plant sterols/stanols with the daily portion.
Art.13(1)	Rye fibre	Rye fibre contributes to normal bowel function	Refer to products included in the claim "high fibre" as listed in the Annex to Regulation (EC) No 1924/2006.
Art.13(5)	Sugar beet fibre	Sugar beet fibre contributes to increase faecal bulk	Refer to products included in the claim "high fibre" as listed in the Annex to Regulation (EC) No 1924/2006.
Art.13(1)	Walnuts	Walnuts contribute to the improvement of the elasticity of blood vessels	Claim is allowed only for food providing with the daily portion 30 g of walnuts.
Art.13(5)	Water-soluble tomato concentrate (WSTC) I and II	Water-soluble tomato concentrate (WSTC) I and II helps to maintain contributes to healthy blood flow	Consumer must be informed that healthy effect is obtained with a daily dose of 3 g of WSTC I or 150 mg of WSTYC II in: (1) up to 250 mL of liquid products or (2) food supplements. Liquid products include fruit juices, flavoured drinks or yogurt drinks; food supplements require a glass of liquid.
Art.13(1)	Wheat bran fibre	Wheat bran fibre contributes to an acceleration of intestinal transit	Refer to products included in the claim "high fibre" as listed in the Annex to Regulation (EC) No 1924/2006. Claim is allowed only for food providing a daily intake of at least 10 g of bran fibre.
Art.13(1)	Wheat bran fibre	Wheat bran fibre contributes to an increase in faecal bulk	Refer to products included in the claim "high fibre" as listed in the Annex to Regulation (EC) No 1924/2006.
Art.14(1)(a)	Barley beta-glucans	Barley beta-glucans has been shown to lower/reduce blood cholesterol. High cholesterol is a risk factor in the development of coronary heart disease.	Claim is allowed only for foods providing 3 g of beta-glucan/daily portion.
Art.14(1)(a)	Oat beta-glucan	Oat beta-glucan has been shown to lower/reduce blood cholesterol. High cholesterol is a risk factor in the development of coronary heart disease	Claim is allowed only for foods providing 3 g of beta-glucan/daily portion.

Table 1. *Cont.*

Claim Type	Botanical Ingredients	Claim	Condition of Use of the Claim Restrictions of Use
Art.14(1)(a)	Plant sterols/Plant stanol esters	Plant sterols and plant stanol esters have been shown to lower/reduce blood cholesterol. High cholesterol is a risk factor in the development of coronary heart disease.	Claim is allowed only for foods providing a daily intake of 1,5-3 g plant sterols/stanols. Food categories included: yellow fat spreads, dairy products, mayonnaise and salad dressings. Reduction of blood cholesterol is estimated: 7–10% with a daily intake of 1.5–2.4 g or 10–12.5% with 2,5-3 g plant sterols/stanols. The effect appears after 2 to 3 weeks.
Art.14(1)(a)	Plant sterols: Sterols extracted from plants, free or esterified with food grade fatty acids.	Plant sterols have been shown to lower/reduce blood cholesterol. High cholesterol is a risk factor in the development of coronary heart disease.	
Art.14(1)(a)	Plant stanol esters	Plant stanol esters have been shown to lower/reduce blood cholesterol. High cholesterol is a risk factor in the development of coronary heart disease.	

4. Botanicals in Functional Foods

Some botanical derivatives have been successfully included in functional food for their healthy properties. Among others, soluble and insoluble fibers, beta glucans and phytosterols/phytostanols deserve a more in-depth description.

4.1. Soluble and Insoluble Fibers

The beneficial properties of dietary fiber intake have been known for a long time and have been publicized since the 1920s. Over the years, the importance of fiber for human health has been fluctuating to be re-evaluated in the second half of the 20th century [14]. With the progress of knowledge, dietary fiber has been classified in various ways; the first subdivision concerns the difference between fiber, which are soluble or insoluble in aqueous medium. In addition to the obvious difference in "chemical" behavior, the solubility (or less) of the fiber in water greatly conditions the activity on humans' health. Insoluble fiber acts mainly on the intestinal transit, while the soluble fibers mediate beneficial properties based on different biological mechanisms.

4.1.1. Insoluble Fiber

Insoluble fiber includes mainly cellulose, hemicellulose and lignin, and it is characterized by its "inertia" at the level of human organism. In other words, it does not undergo any metabolic modification during the transit in the gastro-intestinal tract. Products containing insoluble fiber from different plant sources can use the health claim "the fiber contributes: (1) to normal bowel function; or (2) to increase faecal bulk; or (3) to an acceleration of intestinal transit" (see barley, oat, rye, sugar beet, and wheat fiber in Table 1). Insoluble fiber increases fecal bulk, that leads to a speeding of intestinal transit with the consequent beneficial effects (elimination of waste containing toxic molecules, less contact of fecal waste with the intestinal mucosa, etc.). These effects have been recognized as protective factors versus some cancers including the colon cancer.

4.1.2. Prebiotic Fibers

The prebiotic fibers fall into the category of soluble fibers. The definition of the term "prebiotic" has undergone a certain number of changes since the 1990s, a period in which they were identified as beneficial ingredients of the human diet. In agreement with the International Scientific Association for Prebiotics and Probiotics, a prebiotic fiber is "a substrate, that is selectively used by host microorganisms conferring a health benefit" [15]. Similarly, the Food and Agriculture Organization of the United Nations (FAO) published the following definition in 2008: "a nonviable food component that confers a health benefit on the host associated with modulation of the microbiota" [16].

In recent decades, the awareness of the critical role played by the intestinal microbiota on human health has progressively grown. Studies to support this knowledge have stimulated the formulation of food products capable to contribute to the modulation of microbiota towards positive bacterial strains (mainly lactic bacteria) at the expense of pathogenic ones. These foods, mostly milk-based, contain particular strains of live bacteria (probiotics) or soluble fibers capable of promoting their growth. In functional foods, the most commonly used prebiotic fibers are: inulin, fructo-oligosaccharides (FOS) and galacto-oligosaccharides (GOS); the latter are mostly included in products for infants. Inulin is a linear polymer of 2-60 fructose molecules linked by β-(2-1)-bonds.

The nature of chemical bonds prevents inulin from the usual digestion of caloric sugars. FOS are similar to inulin for chemical bonds, but the number of units ranges between 2 and 10 [17]. Inulin and FOS are storage carbohydrates contained in several plants; the most important sources are chicory, sugar beet, leeks, asparagus, and Jerusalem artichokes. Inulin and FOS reach the colon undigested where they are fermented by the "positive" microbiota. A health claim for "native chicory inulin" is allowed in EU; it states that "chicory inulin contributes to normal bowel function by increasing stool frequency". This claim must be associated with those products, providing at least a daily intake of 12 g of inulin, as a non-fractionated mixture of monosaccharides (<10%), disaccharide, inulin-type fructans and inulin, with an average of polymerization $\geq$ 9 (see Table 1).

Although from animal origin, galacto-oligosaccharides (GOS) are considered here to describe the possible healthy effect due to prebiotic fiber. GOS are oligosaccharides containing 2-10 molecules of galactose and one molecule of glucose. The purity and degree of polymerization largely influence the prebiotic properties of these oligosaccharides, as shown in clinical studies [18,19]. GOS are widely used in lactating formulas to improve the microbiota colonization and modulate the intestinal disorders such as colic. The effects of GOS added to infant formulas were evaluated in a randomized, double-blind, controlled, parallel-group clinical trial including healthy term infants [20]. Three groups were considered: breastfed, formula-fed, and GOS-supplemented formula-fed infants. The effects of supplemented formula were assessed considering four bacterial targets: *Bifidobacterium*, *Lactobacillus*, *Clostridium*, and *Escherichia coli*. The effect of the prebiotic-supplemented formula was very close to that of breast-feeding in stimulating *Bifidobacterium* and *Lactobacillus* growth and in inhibiting *Clostridium* growth. The whole result was a significantly lower incidence of colic [20].

4.1.3. Beta-Glucans

Beta-glucans are soluble fibers contained in cereals, such as barley, oat, rye, wheat and some mushrooms [21]. They are linear polymers of glucose linked by β-(1-4) and β-(1-3) bounds. Two claims for beta-glucans received positive opinion by EFSA and were included in the list of wordings allowed in the EU (Table 1) [22].

The first claim is "consumption of beta-glucans from oats or barley as part of a meal contributes to the reduction of the blood glucose rise after that meal" (Table 1). In fact, beta-glucans modulate the post-prandial glycemic response by increasing the meal bolus viscosity, with a consequent delayed absorption of nutrients (including glucose) in the small intestine [23].

On the basis of intervention studies performed in healthy subjects, EFSA concluded that quantities of about 4 g of beta-glucans/30 g of available carbohydrates are capable to decrease the post-prandial glycemic response without modifying the insulin release [22]. The claim must be associated with the recommendation to use beta glucans during meals.

The EFSA received from the European Commission a second request for an opinion regarding the claim associating beta-glucans with the positive modulation of normal blood cholesterol levels [24]. On the basis of a certain number of randomized-controlled trials in adults with normal or mildly increased cholesterolemia, the EFSA Panel formulated the following wording "regular consumption of beta-glucans contributes to the maintenance of normal blood cholesterol levels". The beneficial effect is linked to a daily consumption of 3 g of beta-glucans in one or more servings. The proposed mechanism of action is based on the fact that dietary beta-glucan forms, in the small intestine, a viscous mixture that reduces the intestinal absorption of dietary cholesterol and the re-uptake of bile acids. As a consequence, new bile acids are synthetized from circulating cholesterol [25].

4.2. Phytosterols/Phytostanols

Phytosterols and phytostanols are compounds of plant origin, which are commonly part of the human diet. Phytosterols can be transformed in phytostanols by hydrogenation and both class of molecules can be esterified with fatty acids from vegetable origin to the corresponding esters [26,27]. Phytosterols and phytostanols are structurally similar to cholesterol, apart from their side chain. The most common phytosterols and phytostanols are sitosterol, sitostanol, campesterol, campestanol, stigmasterol and brassicasterol [26].

In the EU, the use of phytosterols, phytostanols and their esters in foods refers to the Regulation (EC) No. 258/97 of the European Parliament and of the Council of 27 January 1997 concerning novel foods/novel food ingredients.

These molecules reduce the intestinal absorption of cholesterol and, as a consequence, cause a decrease in blood cholesterol levels. For this property, phytosterols and phytostanols, in free or esterified form, can be added to foods for their properties to maintain normal (claim under Art. 13) or reduce blood cholesterol levels (claim under Art. 14). The first wording is allowed for food providing 0.8 g of plant sterols/stanols with the daily dose and the second for daily doses ranging from 1.5 to 3 g. Doses of 1.5–2.4 g/day are associated with a cholesterol level reduction of 7–10%, while 2.4–3 g/day can produce a decrease of 10–12.5% [28].

5. Botanicals in Food Supplements

The category of food/dietary supplements is that in which the presence of ingredients from plant origin is more frequent (botanicals). Food supplements containing plants or derivatives have found an increasing diffusion and acceptance by the consumers, which consider the word "natural" synonymous with "non-chemical" and for association with safe. This belief explains the success of these products and therefore their consistent market presence.

The plants contained in food supplements are many and most of them derive from the tradition of use, that is the preparation of infusions or decoctions. The same plants have been then used by the industries to prepare extracts, in order to enrich the products in active molecules and enhance the expected positive properties. Supplements may contain a single plant ingredient or a mixture of them. It is clear that the greater the number of botanicals present in the finished product, the greater the problems in the correct use by the consumer and in the quality control especially when the product is already on sale.

Another critical aspect derives from the fact that there is no harmonization at the international level (even in Europe) as regards the lists of plants allowed in food supplements. Many countries of the European Union, but also of other continents, have published positive and/or negative lists of botanical ingredients, which are allowed or prohibited in food/dietary supplements. Unfortunately, there is few correlations between them.

The inconsistent situation of the European market of products with botanical ingredients (presence both in products regulated by food or drug laws, see Section 2) leads to several consequences, including the difficulty in discriminating "healthy" or "therapeutic" information for the same plant used in different product classes. As the researchers well know, the dose makes the difference, but discriminating the dose with physiological effects from the one that is suitable for clinical applications is a complex objective even for plants of more ancient tradition. These difficulties were reflected in the very small number of claims approved by EFSA in the field of botanicals.

To boast a nutritional or health claim as a guide for the consumer, it is necessary to refer to the European Regulation n. 1924/2006, according to which: "Scientific substantiation should be the main aspect to be taken into account for the use of nutrition and health claims and the food business operators using claims should justify them". To obtain authorization to associate a nutrition/health claim with a botanical in EU, the manufacturer must submit a dossier to EFSA, which evaluates the scientific evidence of the studies provided and publishes the relative opinion. The guidelines provided by EFSA [2,8] describe in detail the studies required for the approval of nutritional/physiological claims.

The guidelines published by EFSA, although extremely well-articulated, have nevertheless led to immediate difficulties in the creation of a dossier that could meet all the listed requirements. Among the most critical and important aspects:

(a) speaking of dietary supplements, food industries cannot claim any therapeutic effect, but only physiological ones; as a consequence, apart from few exceptions, it is very difficult to prove a healthy activity that aims to maintain homeostasis or reducing disease risk factors in the long term;

(b) to obtain statistical significance, it is necessary to recruit a very large "healthy" population that is willing to take a certain product for very long periods. All this is economically unsustainable, and the results could still be affected by the dietary habits (and not only) of the subjects considered;

(c) it seems unreasonable that the tradition of use has been accepted for traditional medicine drugs and not for food supplements.

Considering the list of claims listed in Table 1, only one case can be clearly associated with food supplements: *Monascus purpureus* (red yeast rice); in the remaining cases, claims are related to ingredients generally used in all foods.

Red Yeast Rice (RYR) is a rice fermented by the red yeast *Monascus purpureus*, which contain a certain number of active polyketides named monacolins, that are secondary metabolites deriving from the fermentation process [29]. The most abundant active molecule is monacolin K.

RYR obtained the approval of the claim: "Monacolin K from red yeast rice contributes to the maintenance of normal blood cholesterol levels" [30]. This wording was supported by two randomized controlled studies, where RYR preparations providing 10 mg of monacolin K (with the daily dose) were responsible of a reduction of blood Low-Density Lipoprotein- cholesterol (LDL-cholesterol) level in subjects suffering from hypercholesterolemia. EFSA considered also the fact that the effect of pure monacolin K (chemically identical to the drug lovastatin) on blood LDL-cholesterol concentration was well known and based on the inhibition of HMG-CoA (3-Hydroxy-3-Methyl-Glutaryl-Coenzyme A) reductase [31].

6. Safety Aspects

This chapter deals with food, the safety of which should be able to be taken for granted. Actually, when botanicals are food supplement ingredients, some distinction has to be made. Compared to common or functional food, food supplements containing botanicals have no or little role from the nutritional point of view, as these do not contribute significantly to the intake of calories and nutrients. In fact, normally these products do not contain caloric nutrients (sugars, fats and proteins) and the presence of vitamins and minerals (not mandatory) covers, with a few exceptions, very limited percentages of the recommended daily dose. On the other hands, food supplements with botanicals are frequently promoted for their possible healthy properties, leading the consumer to prolonged use over time. Furthermore, as mentioned above, the growing popularity among consumers of "natural products" has led to an increasing number of producers and thousands of food supplements on the international market, without certainties relating their composition, activity and safety. While biological activity may be at least partly based on the "tradition of use", the risk/benefit assessment still remains orphaned of sufficiently reliable scientific data.

Botanicals, especially if in their extract form, can have biological effects which, in relation to the dose and quality of the ingredient, can be functional, therapeutic and also toxic [32]. Different factors could be involved in the incidence of adverse effects such as the quality of the raw botanical material, the presence of environmental contaminants, the specific technological process applied (extraction and concentration), misidentifications of the plant ingredients, adulterations, counterfeits. The phytochemical fingerprint of a botanical can vary significantly, when the biological variability or the different processes applied are considered. Different factors (extractant solvent, the temperature and time, the time from harvesting, etc.) can modulate the quality of botanical ingredients, with consequent changes in the relative abundance of active molecules present in the final product. Consumer's age and gender, unsuitable use of botanical food supplements, genetic factors and specific pathological or physiological conditions are further possible sources of unexpected adverse reactions.

Confirming the particularity of the supplements with respect to usual food, there are cases in which limits on the content of molecules naturally present in botanicals are regulated by national and international directives. The established values must also be indicated on the label, such as in the case of bitter orange (*Citrus aurantium* L.) for which it is necessary to declare the content of synephrine and other active amines with the daily dose (Figure 2). Limits are established for molecules that can lead to unwanted side effects at high levels and therefore for which safe daily doses for consumers need to be "standardized".

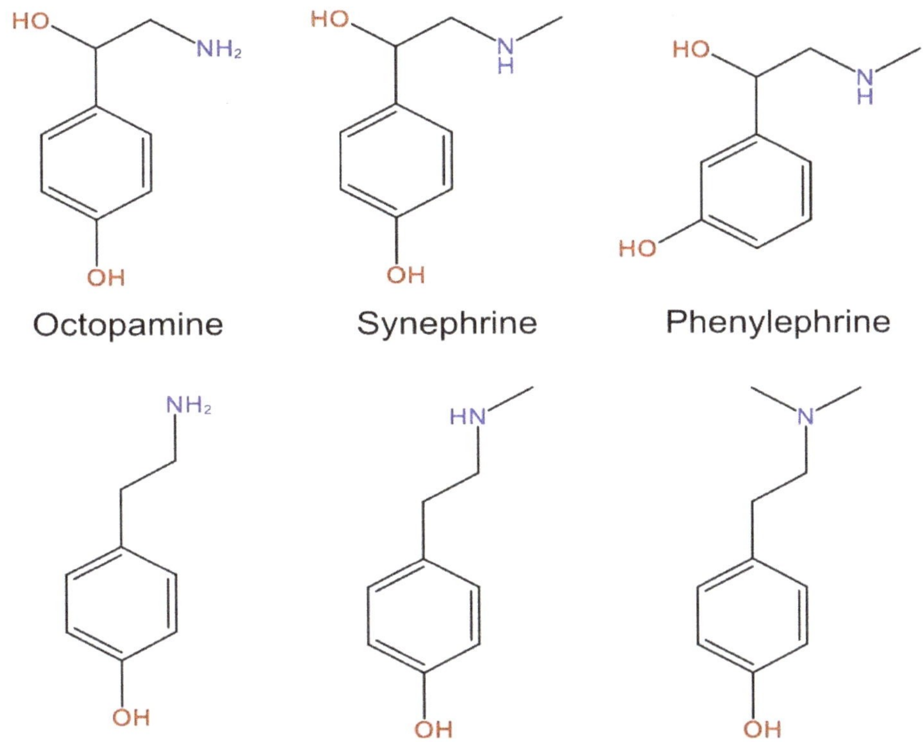

Figure 2. Active amines of *Citrus aurantium* L. regulated for their content in food supplements.

6.1. Adverse Events

Even in the case of adverse events, supplements containing botanicals show specific characteristics. Excluding the accidental presence of toxic xenobiotics, the adverse events associated with common foods are mostly due to allergies and intolerances, which concern restricted groups of at-risk populations. On the contrary, in the case of supplements with botanicals, the consumer must be informed that adverse events can occur. Moreover, pregnant, lactating women and children should avoid food supplements or strictly follow the doctor's/pediatrician's indications.

Since botanicals are "natural", the average consumer considers them safe and rarely communicates their use to doctors in the case of short- or long-term therapy. This point is probably the most important factor leading to unexpected adverse effects. Botanicals could modify the efficacy of other molecules (pharmaceutical drugs or other dietetic compounds) reducing or increasing their plasmatic concentration. To give an example of the possible adverse events to supplements containing botanicals, the case of RYR is described here.

6.2. The Case of RYR

As described previously (see Section 5), in 2011 RYR received a positive opinion for the claim supporting the reduction of LDL-cholesterol plasma level, if the daily intake of monacolin K was 10 mg. In 2018, the EFSA was asked a second time in relation to RYR, with the request being to evaluate the safety of the monacolins contained in it and to provide advice on the daily dose of monacolins that does not give rise to concerns for harmful effects [33]. Since the lactonic form of monacolin K has the same chemical structure of lovastatin (a pharmaceutical drug), the EFSA, after consulting the scientific material provided, concluded that the intake of 10 mg of monacolin K with a food supplement would lead to the intake of a therapeutic dose. Moreover, the evaluation of the data presented showed that several adverse events were reported following the consumption of RYR. These adverse events involved musculoskeletal system (the most severe clinical event associated was rhabdomyolysis) and liver. The clinical symptoms appeared after consumption of RYR, with an intake of 3–10 mg/day of monacolin K.

Two problems have therefore been highlighted for RYR:

1. the dose of monacolin K required to boast the claim about the LDL-cholesterol reduction corresponded to the lower therapeutic dose of the drug lovastatin, chemically identical to the lactonic form of monacolin K. This fact is not acceptable due to the legal definition of a dietary supplement, which must not show pharmacological activity.
2. EFSA "was unable to identify a dietary intake of monacolins from RYR that does not give rise to concerns about harmful effects to health, for the general population, and as appropriate, for vulnerable subgroups of the population" [33]. This fact makes uncertain the marketing of RYR as food supplement, products that do not require medical supervision.

7. Conclusions

Since the last century, a progressive lengthening of the average life of the population has been observed; this social phenomenon is in itself a positive fact, but inevitably entails an increase in the occurrence of chronic-generative diseases more frequent in elderly: cardiovascular diseases, tumors, dementias, etc. At the same time, new data on the role of nutrition in human health has stimulated important international researches and industrial activities:

1. the tables of nutritional requirements (RDA) have been prepared which, with some differences, indicate to consumers all over the world the quantity of calories and nutrients necessary to maintain health;
2. the possible protective role of some components present in foods (antioxidants are the most popular) against the chronic-degenerative diseases described above has been highlighted.

These premises explain the great interest of the food industry for products that present, in addition to nutritional ingredients (proteins, carbohydrates and fats), new "functional" properties, which have special impact on the consumer. In this area, particular interest has been paid to ingredients of vegetable origin, the botanicals. Most products containing botanicals are regulated by food law: fruits and vegetables, functional foods, novel foods, traditional foods from third countries, and food supplements. Some botanical ingredients have received positive opinion by EFSA to support their health claims; fibers, beta glucans and phytosterols/phytostanols are among the most known functional ingredients. Food supplements with botanical ingredients are the sector that has witnessed the greatest development, in terms of both the number of products on the market and consumer acceptability. The availability of these "new" functional products can positively influence the well-being of the population, but it is essential to provide the consumer with the necessary information to guide him in the purchase and use of food supplements.

The difficulties in demonstrating scientifically the supposed physiological/healthy properties of botanicals are the reasons of the limited number of claims approved by EFSA. In addition, safety aspects should be considered in relation to the high number of products available on the market and their growing popularity among consumers: among other things, the quality of raw materials, possible adulterations, presence of active molecules regulated by national/international directives and factors associated with consumers (age, gender, concomitant diseases/drugs). These factors can contribute to adverse effects occurring, underlying the need for tools and intervention to promote consumers safety.

In conclusion, this review provides an overview on the actual knowledge about products containing botanicals aimed to promote consumers' wellbeing. The main purpose is to provide useful information to consumers in order to guide their choices. In fact, although much progress has been made in the field of botanicals, there is still a lack of data, information, and guidelines to ensure the suitable use of these products.

Author Contributions: Investigation, F.C. and S.B.; Writing-Original Draft Preparation, P.R.; Data curation, S.B. and F.C.; Writing-Review & Editing, C.D.L. All authors have read and agreed to the published version of the manuscript.

Acknowledgments: This paper has been prepared in the framework of the MIUR Progetto di Eccellenza.

References

1. Cordain, L.; Miller, J.B.; Eaton, S.B.; Mann, N.; Holt, S.H.A.; Speth, J.D. Plant-animal subsistence ratios and macronutrient energy estimations in worldwide hunter-gatherer diets. *Am. J. Clin. Nutr.* **2000**, *71*, 682–692. [CrossRef] [PubMed]
2. EFSA. Guidance on Safety assessment of botanicals and botanical preparations intended for use as ingredients in food supplements. *EFSA J.* **2009**, *7*, 1249.
3. Food Processing Website. Available online: https://www.foodprocessing.com/articles/2012/defining-botanicals/ (accessed on 2 March 2020).
4. Regulation (EC) No 178/2002 of the European Parliament and of the Council of 28 January 2002 laying down the general principles and requirements of food law, establishing the European Food Safety Authority and laying down procedures in matters of food safety. *Off. J. Eur. Union L* **2002**, *31*, 1–24.
5. Diplock, A.; Aggett, P.J.; Ashwell, M.; Bornet, F.; Fern, E.B.; Roberfroid, M.B. The buckling of a cylindrical shell. *Br. J. Nutr.* **1999**, *81*, S1–S27. [CrossRef]
6. European Council Regulations No. 2015/2283 Regulation (Eu) 2015/2283 on novel foods. *Off. J. Eur. Union* **2015**, *327*, 1–22.
7. Italian Ministry of Health. Available online: http://www.salute.gov.it/portale/temi/p2_5.jsp?lingua=italiano&area=Alimentiparticolarieintegratori&menu=integratori (accessed on 2 March 2020).
8. EFSA Website. Available online: https://www.efsa.europa.eu/en/topics/topic/food-supplements (accessed on 2 March 2020).
9. Trovato, M.; Ballabio, C. Botanical Products: General Aspects. In *Food Supplements Containing Botanicals: Benefits, Side Effects and Regulatory Aspects*; Restani, P., Ed.; Springer: Cham, Switzerland, 2018; pp. 3–26.
10. Coppens, P.; Pettman, S. The regulatory situation in Europe and other continents. In *Food Supplements Containing Botanicals: Benefits, Side Effects and Regulatory Aspects*; Restani, P., Ed.; Springer: Cham, Switzerland, 2018; pp. 27–59.
11. EU Website. Available online: https://ec.europa.eu/food/safety/labelling_nutrition/claims/health_claims_en (accessed on 2 March 2020).
12. EFSA. General scientific guidance for stakeholders on health claim applications. *EFSA J.* **2016**, *14*, 4367.
13. EU Website. Available online: http://ec.europa.eu/food/safety/labelling_nutrition/claims/register/public/?event=search (accessed on 2 March 2020).
14. Slavin, J. Fiber and prebiotics: Mechanisms and health benefits. *Nutrients* **2013**, *5*, 1417–1435. [CrossRef]
15. International Scientific Association for Probiotics and Prebiotics (ISAPP). Available online: https://isappscience.org/for-scientists/resources/prebiotics/ (accessed on 2 March 2020).
16. Pineiro, M.; Asp, N.G.; Reid, G.; Macfarlane, S.; Morelli, L.; Brunser, J.O.; Tuohy, K. FAO Technical Meeting on Prebiotics. *J. Clin. Gastroenterol.* **2008**, *42*, S156–S159. [CrossRef]
17. Niness, K.R. Inulin and oligofructose: What are they? *J. Nutr.* **1999**, *129*, 1402S–1406S. [CrossRef]
18. Torres, D.P.M.; Gonçalves, M.D.P.F.; Teixeira, J.A.; Rodrigues, L.R. Galacto-Oligosaccharides: Production, properties, applications, and significance as prebiotics. *Compr. Rev. Food Sci. Food Saf.* **2010**, *9*, 438–454. [CrossRef]
19. Macfarlane, G.T.; Steed, H.; Macfarlane, S. Bacterial metabolism and health-related effects of galacto-oligosaccharides and other prebiotics. *J. Appl. Microbiol.* **2008**, *104*, 305–344. [CrossRef] [PubMed]
20. Giovannini, M.; Verduci, E.; Gregori, D.; Ballali, S.; Soldi, S.; Ghisleni, D.; Riva, E.; PLAGOS Trial Study Group. Prebiotic Effect of an Infant Formula Supplemented with Galacto-Oligosaccharides: Randomized Multicenter Trial. *J. Am. Coll. Nutr.* **2014**, *33*, 385–389. [CrossRef] [PubMed]
21. Volman, J.J.; Helsper, J.P.F.G.; Wei, S.; Baars, J.J.P.; van Griensven, L.J.L.D.; Sonnenberg, A.S.M.; Mensink, R.P.; Plat, J. Effects of mushroom-derived β-glucan-rich polysaccharide extracts on nitric oxide production by

bone marrow-derived macrophages and nuclear factor-κb transactivation in Caco-2 reporter cells: Can effects be explained by structure? *Mol. Nutr. Food Res.* **2010**, *54*, 268–276. [CrossRef] [PubMed]

22. EFSA. Scientific opinion on the substantiation of health claims related to beta-glucans from oats and barley and maintenance of normal blood LDL-cholesterol concentrations (ID1236, 1299); increase in satiety leading to a reduction in energy intake (ID 851, 852), reduction of post-prandial glycemic responses (ID 821 824), and "digestive function" (ID 850) pursuant to Article 13(1) of Regulation (EC) No 1924/2006. *EFSA J.* **2011**, *9*, 2207.
23. Battilana, P.; Ornstein, K.; Minehira, K.; Schwarz, J.M.; Acheson, K.; Schneiter, P.; Burri, J.; Jéquier, E.; Tappy, L. Mechanisms of action of β-glucan in postprandial glucose metabolism in healthy men. *Eur. J. Clin. Nutr.* **2001**, *55*, 327–333. [CrossRef]
24. EFSA. Scientific opinion on the substantiation of health claims related to beta-glucans and maitenence of normal blood cholesterol concentrations (ID 754, 755, 757, 801, 1465, 2934) and maintenance or achievement of a normal body weight (ID 820, 823) pursuant to Article 13(1) of Regulation (EC) No 1924/2006. *EFSA J.* **2009**, *7*, 1254.
25. Wang, Y.; Harding, S.V.; Thandapilly, S.J.; Tosh, S.M.; Jones, P.J.H.; Ames, N.P. Barley β-glucan reduces blood cholesterol levels via interrupting bile acid metabolism. *Br. J. Nutr.* **2017**, *118*, 822–829. [CrossRef]
26. Cantrill, R. Phytosterols, Phytostanols and Their Esters. Chemical and Technical Assessment. Available online: http://www.fao.org/fileadmin/templates/agns/pdf/jecfa/cta/69/Phytosterols.pdf (accessed on 2 March 2020).
27. Moreau, R.A.; Whitaker, B.D.; Hicks, K.B. Phytosterols, phytostanols, and their conjugates in foods: Structural diversity, quantitative analysis, and health-promoting uses. *Prog. Lipid Res.* **2002**, *41*, 457–500. [CrossRef]
28. EFSA. Plant Sterols and Blood Cholesterol-Scientific substantiation of a health claim related to plant sterols and lower/reduced blood cholesterol and reduced risk of (coronary) heart disease pursuant to Article 14 of Regulation (EC) No 1924/2006-Scientific. *EFSA J.* **2008**, *781*, 1–12.
29. Liu, J.; Zhang, J.; Shi, Y.; Grimsgaard, S.; Alraek, T.; Fønnebø, V. Chinese red yeast rice (Monascus purpureus) for primary hyperlipidemia: A meta-analysis of randomized controlled trials. *Chin. Med.* **2006**, *1*, 4. [CrossRef]
30. EFSA. Scientific Opinion on the substantiation of health claims related to monacolin K from red yeast rice and maintenance of normal blood LDL cholesterol concentrations (ID 1648, 1700) pursuant to Article 13(1) of Regulation (EC) No 1924/2006. *EFSA J.* **2011**, *9*, 2304.
31. Alberts, A.W. Lovastatin and simvastatin–inhibitors of hmg coa reductase and cholesterol biosynthesis. *Cardiology* **1990**, *77*, 14–21. [CrossRef] [PubMed]
32. Di Lorenzo, C.; Ceschi, A.; Kupferschmidt, H.; Lüde, S.; De Souza Nascimento, E.; Dos Santos, A.; Colombo, F.; Frigerio, G.; Nørby, K.; Plumb, J.; et al. Adverse effects of plant food supplements and botanical preparations: A systematic review with critical evaluation of causality. *Br. J. Clin. Pharmacol.* **2015**, *79*, 578–592. [CrossRef] [PubMed]
33. EFSA. Scientific opinion on the safety of monacolins in red yeast rice. *EFSA J.* **2018**, *16*, 5368.

7

Characteristics of Effervescent Tablets of Lactobacilli Supplemented with Chinese Ginseng (*Panax ginseng* C.A. Meyer) and *Polygonatum sibiricum*

Feng Zhao *, Meng Li †, Lingling Meng †, Jinhan Yu and Tiehua Zhang

College of Food Science and Engineering, Jilin University, 5333 Xi'an Road, Changchun 130062, China; lmeng18@mails.jlu.edu.cn (M.L.); mengll19@mails.jlu.edu.cn (L.M.); yjhsqcg@163.com (J.Y.); zhangth@jlu.edu.cn (T.Z.)

* Correspondence: phoenix_zhao@jlu.edu.cn

† The two authors contribute equally to this work.

Featured Application: Chinese ginseng (*Panax ginseng* C.A. Meyer) and *Polygonatum sibiricum* are two medicine food homology herbs widely used in many countries, which have many functional benefits. This study demonstrated that it is possible to develop a formulation of lactobacilli effervescent tablets supplemented with Chinese ginseng and *P. sibiricum*, which provides new ideas for the development of functional probiotic products.

Abstract: Development of probiotic products has always been popular in the food industry. Considering the advantages of effervescent tablets, developing probiotic products in effervescent tablet form was conducted in this study. Besides three *Lactobacillus* species, whole root powders of two medicine food homology herbs, Chinese ginseng (*Panax ginseng* C.A. Meyer) and *Polygonatum sibiricum*, were added to the formulation in equal amounts for multiple health care functions. Using the plate counting method, the viability of lactobacilli was measured. After tabletting, lactobacilli viability in tablets containing the two herbs, L-group (20 mg herbs/tablet), M-group (60 mg herbs/tablet), and H-group (100 mg herbs/tablet) was higher than that in the control (containing no herbs). After tablet disintegration, the survival rate of lactobacilli after gastrointestinal fluids treatment was measured; it was higher for the L-group and the H-group than for the control. After incubation with dissolved tablets for 1 h, the lethal rate of *Staphylococcus aureus* and *Escherichia coli* O157:H7 for tablets containing the herbs was lower than that for the control. In the organoleptic assessment test, the L-group and the control were preferred to the M-group and the H-group. During storage at 25 °C for two months, the viability of lactobacilli in tablets containing the herbs was similar to that in the control. In conclusion, the formulation of the L-group has the best characteristics.

Keywords: lactobacilli effervescent tablets; Chinese ginseng; *Polygonatum sibiricum*; lactobacilli viability; antibacterial activity; organoleptic assessment; storage stability

1. Introduction

Probiotics are defined as "live microorganisms which when administered in adequate amounts confer a health benefit on the host" (FAO/WHO 2002), such as stimulation of the immune system, maintenance of mucosal integrity, production of important digestive enzymes and others [1]. Most probiotics belong to the genera of *Bifidobacterium* and *Lactobacillus* [2]. *Lactobacillus* species are normal inhabitants of the human gastrointestinal tract, and some of them are generally recognized as safe because of a long history of human consumption [3]. Many pieces of research have led to the conviction that certain strains from the genera *Lactobacillus* can promote health in humans and animals. Among them, *Lactobacillus acidophilus* and *Lactobacillus rhamnosus* have been successfully used in restoring the imbalances associated with inflammatory bowel diseases (IBD) [4,5]. Meanwhile, *Lactobacillus plantarum* has the potential to alleviate aluminium toxicity [6] and inhibit pathogenic fungi [7]. Therefore, these lactobacilli might be useful as supporting therapeutic agents. Considering their probiotic properties, some isolates of these lactobacilli, such as *L. acidophilus* LA1, *L. rhamnosus* GG, and *L. plantarum* Lp01 are already widely used as food supplements and produced on an industrial scale [8].

Due to the beneficial health properties, functional foods have been playing an outstanding role in the food market [9]. As one kind of functional foods, probiotic-supplemented food products are more and more popular for their favorable impact on consumer health. Probiotic products available on the market are mainly fermented dairy products, and fruit drinks and powders containing probiotics can be seen in the marketplace in recent years. However, the most popular forms of probiotic products, liquid, semi-solid, and powder, require more space for transportation and storage, which may increase the price of end products. To overcome such problems, compaction of powders containing probiotics in the shape of tablets is a more suitable strategy [10]. In addition to reducing the bulk volume of other forms, products in tablet form are extremely stable, surpassing the stability of liquid form [11]; thus they lead to prolonged shelf life.

At present, the demand for ready-to-eat food and drinks is increasing day by day. Ready-to-drink effervescent tablets can meet consumer demands. Meanwhile, effervescent tablets containing probiotics can be added to any liquid product, which would provide a pleasant taste and facilitate the daily ingestion of probiotics. They are especially suitable for children, the elderly, and people who have difficulty in swallowing pills. Additionally, carbon dioxide gas released during effervescent tablet dissolving could stabilize the gastric mucosa and promote absorption, resulting in benefits to consumer health [12]. Therefore, water-soluble effervescent tablets are a good choice for probiotic-supplemented food products.

To our knowledge, effervescent tablets containing probiotics are usually used for the prevention of vaginal infections [13,14], but little research has been done on the development of effervescent tablets supplemented with probiotics for application in the food industry. Using *L. acidophilus* and *Saccharomyces boulardii* as probiotics supplements, Nagashima, Pansiera, Baracat and Gómez [12] had developed probiotic effervescent tablets for ready-to-drink. Considering the health needs of consumers and the good properties of probiotics, more studies should be conducted to develop a wider variety of effervescent tablet products supplemented with probiotics, especially with multiple health care functions.

Chinese ginseng (*Panax ginseng* C.A. Meyer) is the medicine food homology plant, which has been used for over 2000 years as a medicine in China and is popularly used in more than 35 countries as food, a health supplement, and a natural remedy [15]. Ginseng possesses many beneficial health properties, such as the alleviation of menopause symptoms and some neurological disorders, regulation of cardiovascular disease and hyperglycemia in type 2 diabetes, and improvement of the immune function [16]. *Polygonatum sibiricum* is another traditional herbal medicine and foodstuff widely used in China, Korea, and Japan for hundreds of years [17]. The dried root of *P. sibiricum* shows anti-inflammatory, immunoregulatory, and anti-diabetic activities [18]. Hence, the present work aimed to develop effervescent tablet products containing both probiotic lactobacilli and Chinese ginseng and *P. sibiricum* for more health care functions. Characteristics of the effervescent tablet products were investigated, especially the effect of Chinese ginseng and *P. sibiricum* on the properties of lactobacilli effervescent tablets.

2. Materials and Methods

2.1. Strains

Three lyophilized strains of lactobacilli obtained from Clerici Sacco Co. (Italy) were used in the preparation of effervescent tablets. They were *L. acidophilus* LA3, *L. rhamnosus* IMC501, and *L. plantarum* BG112. These strains are often used in functional foods as probiotic strains and dietary supplements [19–21]. In the antibacterial experiment, *Staphylococcus aureus* NCTC 8325-4 and *Escherichia coli* O157:H7 NCTC 12900 were used. *S. aureus* NCTC 8325-4 belongs to the gram-positive bacterium, which was kindly donated by Professor Baolin Sun working in the University of Science and Technology of China. *E. coli* O157:H7 NCTC 12900, one of the gram-negative bacteria, was obtained from the National Culture Type Collection (Colindale, London, UK).

2.2. Preparation of Effervescent Tablets

In order to maintain high probiotic activity, probiotics used in product production should possess high cell viability. According to the viability of three kinds of *Lactobacillus* in lyophilized powder under the same culture condition as in our preliminary experiment, the proportion of three lactobacilli strains in the mixed lactobacilli powder for effervescent tablet preparation was achieved, which was 5:4:1 for *L. plantarum*: *L. rhamnosus*: *L. acidophilus*. As citric acid and sodium bicarbonate are the common effervescent agents used in pharmaceutical and nutraceutical industries to produce fast dissolving effervescent tablets, the two agents were added to the effervescent tablets in this study. Additionally, the formulation of effervescent tablets contained povidone as a tablet binder and polyethylene glycol 6000 (PEG6000) as a lubricating agent. To determine the effect of Chinese ginseng and *P. sibiricum* on the properties of lactobacilli effervescent tablets, effervescent tablets containing different contents of Chinese ginseng and *P. sibiricum* were prepared. Whole root powders of the two herbs were obtained from Changchun Huacheng Biological Co., Ltd. (Changchun, China). The composition formulas for the lactobacilli effervescent tablets are given in Table 1. Each ingredient for tablet preparation was calibrated through an 80-mesh screen, and then the weighed ingredients were mixed thoroughly according to the formulation. A single punch tabletting machine (Hebi Innovative Instruments Co., Ltd., Henan, China) equipped with a 12-mm flat-faced round punch was used for the preparation of the effervescent tablets.

Table 1. Formulations of lactobacilli effervescent tablets supplemented with different contents of Chinese ginseng and *Polygonatum sibiricum*.

Ingredients	Tablets Formulations (Quantity in mg/Tablet)			
	Control	L-Group	M-Group	H-Group
Lactobacilli mixed powder	150	150	150	150
Citric acid	350	350	350	350
Sodium bicarbonate	350	350	350	350
Povidone	30	30	30	30
PEG6000	20	20	20	20
Chinese ginseng powder	0	10	30	50
Polygonatum sibiricum powder	0	10	30	50

2.3. Measurement of Weight and Thickness of Tablets

For each kind of tablet, ten tablets were individually and randomly weighed on an analytical balance (OHAUS International Trade (Shanghai) Co., Ltd., Shanghai, China) to determine their weight, and their thickness was also measured by a ruler.

2.4. Determination of Disintegration Time

According to the method for measurement of disintegration time of effervescent tablets in Chinese Pharmacopoeia (2015 Edition), the disintegration time of the effervescent tablets prepared in this study was tested. For each kind of effervescent tablet, the disintegration time of six tablets was individually determined in 200 mL of distilled water at 20 ± 5 °C. Disintegration time within 5 min is considered acceptable.

2.5. Change of Viability of Lactobacilli Cells after Tabletting and Tablet Disintegration

In order to determine survival rates of lactobacilli cells after the tablets preparation, the number of viable lactobacilli cells in the mixed lactobacilli powder before tabletting and in the tablets was measured using the pouring plate method. Firstly, the mixed lactobacilli powder or the tablets were dissolved in sterile distilled water. Then, the dissolved sample was ten-fold diluted with a 0.90% NaCl solution, and pour-plated on de Man-Rogosa-Sharpe (MRS) agar (Oxoid Ltd., Basingstoke, Hants, UK). Each dilution sample was measured in triplicate. After incubation at 37 °C for 48 h, the number of colonies was counted. Two independent experiments were performed. The survival rate of lactobacilli cells after tablet preparation equals to the ratio of viable cells in the tablets to those in the mixed lactobacilli powder.

Furthermore, to investigate the viability change of lactobacilli cells after tablet disintegration, the remaining tablet solution after counting was placed at 25 °C for 48 h, then the number of viable lactobacilli cells was measured using the pouring plate method. The survival rate of lactobacilli cells after tablets disintegration was calculated by the ratio of viable cells in tablet solution after disintegration for 48 h to those for 0 h.

2.6. Effect of Gastrointestinal Fluids on the Viability of Lactobacilli Cells

Firstly, one effervescent tablet was dissolved in 15 mL of sterile distilled water. Then, 0.1 mL and 1.0 mL samples from the same solution were added to 9.9 mL and 9.0 mL of sterile simulated gastric fluid (0.045 M HCl, 1% pepsin, pH 1.7), respectively. After incubation at 37 °C for 30 min, 1.0 mL aliquot was removed and added to 9.0 mL of sterile simulated intestinal fluid (0.05 M KH_2PO_4, pH 6.8, added with 0.6% of bile salts), which was further incubated at 37 °C for 150 min. The number of viable lactobacilli cells before and after gastrointestinal fluids treatment was determined using the pouring plate method. Meanwhile, the survival rate after gastric or enteric fluid treatment was calculated respectively, which equals the ratio of viable cells after treatment to those before treatment. Two independent experiments were performed.

2.7. Analysis of the Antibacterial Activity of the Tablets

Antibacterial studies were performed against *S. aureus* and *E. coli* O157:H7. After activation from the stocked strain, cultures of *S. aureus* or *E. coli* O157:H7 were inoculated into sterile distilled water, and the initial cell counts were measured by the pouring plate method using tryptic soy agar (TSA). Each sample was measured in duplicate. Then one effervescent tablet was added to 15 mL of the bacterial solution, and the dissolution time was recorded. After incubation for one hour (including dissolution time) at room temperature, the number of *S. aureus* or *E. coli* O157:H7 was determined by the staph express count plate or *E. coli*/Coliform count plate of 3M Petrifilm™ (3M Center, St. Paul, MN, USA). Each sample was measured in duplicate. The testing slips were incubated at 37 °C for 48 h. Two independent experiments were performed. The antibacterial activity of the tablets was assessed by the following equation:

$$\text{antibacterial ratio} = \left(1 - \frac{\text{Cell counts of bacteria after incubation with tablets for one hour}}{\text{Initial cell counts of bacteria}}\right) \times 100\%$$

Meanwhile, the pH of the solution was measured, including pH before adding tablets, pH at the end of dissolving tablets, and pH after incubation with tablets for one hour. The pH measurement was performed for three independent experiments.

2.8. Organoleptic Assessment

Twenty panelists (10 males and 10 females) aged between 22 and 25 years participated in the organoleptic assessment. The panelists were selected from students at the College of Food Science and Engineering at Jilin University, China. The study was reviewed and approved by the college of Food

Science and Engineering at Jilin University. All participants were familiar with basic organoleptic assessment techniques, and all of them agreed to participate in the test. Before the organoleptic assessment, the panelists participated in briefing sessions to familiarize themselves with the specific vocabulary used to describe the effervescent tablet solution attributes and with the evaluation scales.

Each kind of sample solution was prepared by adding one tablet into 200 mL distilled water at room temperature. After disintegration, the panelists were presented with 20 mL of each sample in see-through polypropylene cups. Different samples were labeled with random numbers and presented to each panelist in random order. Between samples evaluation, panelists were asked to cleanse their palate with water. In addition, panelists were required to have a break before starting the next evaluation [22].

Attributes of appearance, color, aroma, flavor, and overall liking were evaluated in a 9-point hedonic scale ranging from 1 ("dislike extremely") to 9 ("like extremely"). Afterwards, the products were ranked and evaluated by the Friedman test [23] to verify differences between samples.

2.9. *Stability of the Tablets during Storage*

In order to study the stability of tablets during storage, the tablets were stored individually in vacuum packages (Sealed Air Co., Charlotte, NC, USA), which are transparent multi-layer co-extruded cross-linked vacuum shrinkable bags with high oxygen barrier, high sealing strength, and good wear resistance and shrinkage properties, and then incubated at 25 °C for two months. At a certain storage time (0, 15, 30, 45 and 60 days), one tablet of each kind of tablets was dissolved in 15 mL sterile distilled water, and then the number of lactobacilli in the solution was measured in triplicate using MRS agar by the pouring plate method. Two independent experiments were performed.

2.10. *Statistical Analysis*

One-way analysis of variance (ANOVA) and student's test were used to analyze possible statistically significant differences among the samples. The significance level was 0.05. All the analyses were performed using IBM SPSS Statistics 22 (Chicago, IL, USA). The figure was produced by Microcal Origin 9.2 (Northampton, MA, USA).

3. Results and Discussion

3.1. *Physical Properties of the Tablets*

Round, flat disc-shaped tablets were obtained in this study. As powders of Chinese ginseng and *P. sibiricum* are yellow, and other raw materials are white powders, the color of tablets without Chinese ginseng and *P. sibiricum* (Control) was white, while tablets supplemented with the two herbs showed pale yellow. Besides the color, weight and thickness of tablets prepared by different formulations were different. As shown in Table 2, the mean weight of the control was 0.82 g per tablet, which was increased with an increase in the content of the two herbs. Except for the H-group (100 mg herbs/tablet), the thickness of the other three tablets showed similar results (Table 2). After adding the tablets to distilled water, the effervescence was mediated by the presence of citric acid and sodium bicarbonate. The disintegration time of the control was short, at about 3.19 min. Interestingly, this parameter was influenced by the presence of the herbs, showing prolonged disintegration significantly with increasing content of the two herbs ($p < 0.05$). It was 4.48, 6.92, and 9.70 min for the L-group (20 mg herbs/tablet), the M-group (60 mg herbs/tablet), and the H-group, respectively (Table 2). The result indicated that the presence of the two herbs has a slow-releasing effect on the disintegration of effervescent tablets. A disintegration time within 5 min for oral effervescent tablets is considered acceptable in the pharmacopoeia of several countries. The disintegration time depends on the disintegrating solvent, solvent temperature and solvent volume, thus suitable disintegrating conditions should be studied for the M-group and H-group tablets.

Table 2. Weight, thickness and disintegration time of the lactobacilli effervescent tablets supplemented with different contents of Chinese ginseng and *Polygonatum sibiricum*.

Tablets	Weight (g)	Thickness (mm)	Disintegration Time (min)
Control	0.82 ± 0.02 [a]	7.05 ± 0.37 [a]	3.19 ± 0.41 [a]
L-group	0.85 ± 0.03 [b]	6.90 ± 0.39 [a]	4.48 ± 0.31 [b]
M-group	0.88 ± 0.02 [c]	7.40 ± 0.61 [a]	6.92 ± 0.33 [c]
H-group	0.92 ± 0.02 [d]	8.15 ± 0.24 [b]	9.70 ± 0.42 [d]

All data show the means ± SD. Different letters in the same column indicate a significant difference.

3.2. Change of Viability of Lactobacilli after Tabletting and Tablet Disintegration

In order to achieve benefits from probiotics, probiotic products must contain at least 10^6 CFU (Colony Forming Unit)/g or be eaten in sufficient amounts to yield a daily intake of 10^8 CFU [24]. Therefore, the number of viable lactobacilli cells in tablets was investigated. As shown in Table 3, at least 1.55 ± 0.80 billion viable cells per tablet were found after disintegration, which meets the intake requirement for probiotics. However, compared with the mixed lactobacilli powder before tabletting, the number of viable cells in tablets decreased remarkably for four kinds of tablets. Nagashima, Pansiera, Baracat and Gómez [12] had also found that there was up to 2.3 logarithmic cycles reduction in the number of viable *L. acidophilus* in effervescent probiotics tablets after tabletting. Chan and Zhang [25] had observed that cellular viability decrease was related to the applied compression force in tabletting. Under mechanical stress, some cells cannot tolerate such compression, which caused damages to the cell walls and membranes or even loss of viability [12]. But it is worth noting that the survival rate of lactobacilli cells was higher for tablets containing the herbs than that for the control, and the survival rate enhanced significantly with the increase of the herbs content in tablets ($p < 0.05$) (Table 3). This result demonstrated that Chinese ginseng and *P. sibiricum* can protect the viability of lactobacilli cells in the tablets. Perhaps some active ingredients in the herbs, such as polysaccharides, might maintain the viability of the lactobacilli. As we know, prebiotics supply a fermentable carbohydrate for probiotic bacteria in the colon, stimulating the growth and activity [26]. Thus, we further speculated that the two herbs may have similar functions with prebiotics, which would protect or promote the viability of beneficial bacteria after consumption. Therefore, the viability of lactobacilli cells after gastrointestinal juices treatment for four kinds of tablets was investigated, which will be discussed in a later part in this study.

Table 3. Viability of lactobacilli cells in the mixed lactobacilli powder before tabletting and in different kinds of lactobacilli effervescent tablets.

Samples	Number of Viable Cells	The Survival Rate after Tabletting
Mixed lactobacilli powder	(7.14 ± 0.52) × 10^{10} CFU/g powder	
Control tablet	# (1.55 ± 0.80) × 10^9 CFU/Tablet [a]	14.50%
L-group tablet	(5.18 ± 3.71) × 10^9 CFU/Tablet [b]	48.37%
M-group tablet	(7.00 ± 1.14) × 10^9 CFU/Tablet [b,c]	65.36%
H-group tablet	(9.03 ± 1.77) × 10^9 CFU/Tablet [c]	84.31%

All data show the means ± SD. # ANOVA was performed among different kinds of effervescent tablets. Different letters in the same column indicate a significant difference.

What is the change of lactobacilli viability after tablet disintegration? Do the herbs protect viability or stimulate the growth of lactobacilli after tablet disintegration? Surprisingly, after disintegration for 48 h, the number of lactobacilli cells for the control tablet increased more than 2-fold, while the survival rate for tablets containing the herbs decreased by 10.5%–23.75% (Table 4). In fact, besides polysaccharides, saponins are another main active component in ginseng and *P. sibiricum* which have antimicrobial activity [27–29]. Battinelli, Mascellino, Martino, Lu and Mazzanti [29] found that a total extract of ginseng had lower antimicrobial activity than some pure ginsenosides (saponins in ginseng), and ascribed this lack of antimicrobial activity of the whole plant to possible antagonist effects between ginsenosides and other ginseng components. Considering the protective effect of the herbs on the viability of lactobacilli after tabletting, the changes of the viability of lactobacilli after tabletting and tablet disintegration for tablets containing the herbs may be due to possible antagonistic effect between saponins and other components in the herbs.

Table 4. The survival rate of lactobacilli cells after tablet disintegration for 48 h.

Tablets	The Survival Rate after Tablet Disintegration for 48 h
Control	216.61% ± 0.86 [b]
L-group	76.25% ± 0.13 [a]
M-group	89.50% ± 0.21 [a]
H-group	77.62% ± 0.16 [a]

All data show the means ± SD. Different letters in the same column indicate a significant difference.

3.3. *Effect of Gastrointestinal Fluids on the Viability of Lactobacilli Cells*

As shown in Table 5, the survival rate of lactobacilli cells after gastric juice treatment for each kind of tablets was remarkably different with the different initial amounts of tablet solution inoculated into gastric juice. It was increased 23-, 350-, 186- or 482-fold for tablets of control, L-group, M-group, or H-group, respectively, when the initial inoculum increased from 0.1 mL to 1.0 mL. With a 10-fold increment in the initial inoculum, the survival rate of lactobacilli cells after gastric juice treatment increased more than 10-fold for all the kinds of tablets, which demonstrated that more intake of the probiotic product would greatly increase the levels of probiotics reaching the intestine. Meanwhile, it can be seen that the effervescent tablets supplemented with the herbs have a higher survival rate of lactobacilli cells after gastric fluid treatment than the control at 1.0 mL initial inoculum, but this phenomenon cannot be found at 0.1 mL initial inoculum (Table 5). This result indicates that the herbs supplemented in tablets have a protective effect on the viability of lactobacilli during gastric fluid treatment, and this protective effect of the herbs is dose-dependent. This protective effect caused by the herbs should also be a comprehensive effect of antimicrobial activity and probiotic activity derived from components in the herbs. However, in the gastric juice environment, antimicrobial components in the herbs may not play their role effectively, and/or probiotic activity of components may be improved, thus the protective effect is prominent.

Table 5. The survival rate of lactobacilli cells after contact with gastric juice for 30 min followed by exposure to enteric juice for 150 min for different kinds of lactobacilli effervescent tablets.

Tablets	The Initial Amount of Tablet Solution Inoculated into Gastric Juice	Survival Rate (%)		
		Gastric Juice Treatment (N_g/N_0) #	Enteric Juice Treatment (N_e/N_g) #	Enteric Juice Treatment (N_e/N_0) #
Control	0.1 mL	0.0369	0.0000	0.0000
L-group	0.1 mL	0.0063	0.3992	0.0000
M-group	0.1 mL	0.0077	0.0000	0.0000
H-group	0.1 mL	0.0155	0.0000	0.0000
Control	1.0 mL	0.8660	0.1167	0.0009
L-group	1.0 mL	2.2162	0.3444	0.0076
M-group	1.0 mL	1.4232	0.0442	0.0006
H-group	1.0 mL	7.4842	0.3239	0.0294

N_0 is the number of viable lactobacilli cells before gastric fluid treatment (CFU/Tablet). N_g is the number of viable lactobacilli cells after gastric fluid treatment (CFU/Tablet). N_e is the number of viable lactobacilli cells after enteric fluid treatment (CFU/Tablet).

After enteric juice treatment, there were no viable lactobacilli cells at 0.1 mL initial inoculum for three kinds of tablets, while viable cells could be examined in all the kinds of tablets at 1.0 mL initial inoculum (Table 5). This result also confirmed that more intake of the product would significantly increase the levels of probiotics in the intestine. However, compared with the control, the survival rate of lactobacilli cells after intestinal juice treatment only increased 2.95-, 0.13- and 2.77-fold for L-group, M-group, and H-group, respectively. Meanwhile, there was no dose-dependent protective effect of the herbs on the viability of lactobacilli cells after enteric juice treatment when compared to the gastric fluid treatment. Nagashima, Pansiera, Baracat and Gómez [12] had also found that the number of *L. acidophilus* decreased significantly after effervescent probiotics products contact with artificial enteric juice; they ascribed this decline to the sharp change in the pH from 2.0 in the gastric juice to 6.8 in the enteric juice, and the presence of bile salts. Therefore, the presence of bile salts in enteric juice and the pH variation from 1.7 to 6.8 might greatly destroy the viability of lactobacilli and thus weaken the protective effect of the herbs in this study. Additionally, an increase of antimicrobial activity and/or a decrease of probiotic activity of components in the herbs in the enteric juice environment may be another reason for the reduced protective effect of the herbs.

Generally, after gastrointestinal fluids treatment, the survival rates of lactobacilli for the L-group (0.0076%) and the H-group (0.0294%) were both higher than that for the control (0.0009%), while it was similar between the M-group (0.0006%) and the control. It is confirmed that the herbs supplemented in the lactobacilli effervescent tablets have a certain protective effect on the viability of lactobacilli during gastrointestinal fluids treatment, but for the better protective effect the optimal concentration of the herbs in probiotic products should be further investigated.

3.4. Antibacterial Activity of the Tablets

The goal in administering probiotic products is to induce a balanced enteric microbiota, which will have a favorable impact on consumer health. Enteric microbiota include both beneficial and harmful microflora. As mentioned above, the tablets supplemented with Chinese ginseng and *P. sibiricum* have a certain favorable effect on the activity of some lactobacilli. In order to investigate the antibacterial activity of the lactobacilli effervescent tablets, an in vitro bacteriostatic experiment against *S. aureus* and *E. coli* O157:H7, two common pathogens in clinical infection and food contamination, was conducted. After incubation with the control tablet for one hour, about 95.11% and 97.86% of *S. aureus* and *E. coli* O157:H7 were killed, respectively (Table 6). While the antibacterial ratio against both bacteria was decreased significantly with an increase in the content of the two herbs in the tablets ($p < 0.05$), there was still a high antibacterial ratio for these tablets, which was more than 78% for the H-group. Because the treatment time of the antibacterial experiment was relatively short, which was 1 h, we considered that the disintegration progress of tablets may be an important factor affecting the antibacterial activity. As shown in Table 6, the dissolution time of the tablets was prolonged with increasing content of the two herbs ($p < 0.05$), which is opposite to the change trend of antibacterial activity. The effervescence mediated by the citric acid and sodium bicarbonate ensures a rapid and complete distribution of the active ingredients in products to solutions [14], and can rapidly create an anaerobic microenvironment by released CO_2 [30], which can also decrease pH of the solution (Table 6). These features are harmful to bacteria which cannot withstand the environment. As the dissolution time of the tablets was prolonged with increased content of the two herbs (Table 6), this would decrease release rates of active ingredients and CO_2 with an increase in the content of the herbs, which may lower the antibacterial activity of the tablets with increased content of the herbs. Additionally, under the condition of the antibacterial experiment in this study, antagonist effects between antimicrobial and probiotic components of the herbs may lead to weak antibacterial activity of the tablets containing the herbs in a dose-dependent manner. Therefore, the antibacterial activity was highest for the control, which decreased significantly with an increase in the content of the two herbs in tablets under the condition of the antibacterial experiment in this study (Table 6). According to the previous results on the change of viability of lactobacilli after tablet disintegration for 48 h (Table 4), we deduced that the antibacterial activities of the four kinds of tablets against *S. aureus* and *E. coli* O157:H7 would be different when prolonged the treatment time.

Table 6. Antibacterial activity of different kinds of lactobacilli effervescent tablets against *Staphylococcus aureus* and *Escherichia coli* O157:H7 for one-hour incubation.

Tablets	Antibacterial Ratio against *S. aureus*	Antibacterial Ratio against *E. coli* O157:H7	Dissolution Time (min)	pH of Solution		
				Without Tablets	End of Tablets Dissolving	Incubation for 1 h
Control	95.11% ± 0.01 ^{d,A}	97.86% ± 0.01 ^{c,B}	1.99 ± 0.36 ^{a}	6.38 ± 0.09 $^{\beta}$	5.61 ± 0.03 $^{\alpha}$	5.71 ± 0.08 $^{\alpha}$
L-group	90.00% ± 0.01 ^{c,A}	97.39% ± 0.00 ^{c,B}	2.28 ± 0.26 ^{a}	6.42 ± 0.06 $^{\beta}$	5.56 ± 0.08 $^{\alpha}$	5.58 ± 0.08 $^{\alpha}$
M-group	83.16% ± 0.02 ^{b,A}	90.96% ± 0.02 ^{b,B}	3.27 ± 0.28 ^{b}	6.59 ± 0.05 $^{\beta}$	5.57 ± 0.04 $^{\alpha}$	5.60 ± 0.03 $^{\alpha}$
H-group	78.27% ± 0.03 ^{a,A}	83.87% ± 0.04 ^{a,B}	4.45 ± 0.04 ^{c}	6.72 ± 0.11 $^{\beta}$	5.52 ± 0.03 $^{\alpha}$	5.53 ± 0.03 $^{\alpha}$

All data show the means ± SD. Different lowercase English letters in the same column indicate a significant difference; different uppercase English letters or lowercase Greek letters in the same row indicate a significant difference, respectively.

Meanwhile, the antibacterial activity of each kind of tablet was significantly higher against *E. coli* O157:H7 than against *S. aureus* ($p < 0.05$) (Table 6). Xue, Yang, Zhao, Hou, Zhang, Zhang and Ren [28] had found that ginsenosides cause bacterial death by directly destroying the membrane system. As we know, the cell wall of *S. aureus* is thicker than that of *E. coli* O157:H7, which will reduce the speed and content of CO_2 and active ingredients (such as saponins) reaching the cell membrane, causing higher antibacterial activity against *E. coli* O157:H7 than against *S. aureus* for each kind of tablet.

3.5. Organoleptic Assessment

An organoleptic assessment was performed to measure the acceptability of the four kinds of effervescent tablets. As shown in Table 7, except for appearance and overall liking attributes, there was no significant difference among different kinds of tablets. In respect of the appearance of the tablet solution, panelists evaluated the L-group as largely like (7.30 ± 1.17), while the H-group was considered slightly appreciated (5.90 ± 1.86). After disintegration, a small amount of light-yellow foam was floating on the solution of the H-group, resulting in a lower appearance score for it. The overall liking classified the H-group as slightly like (5.30 ± 1.56) and the L-group and the control as moderately like (6.45 ± 1.43 and 6.05 ± 1.39, respectively), while the evaluation for the M-group (5.70 ± 1.45) was between them. Besides the appearance attribute, the flavor was also a main reason for a lower overall liking score for the H-group solution, although there was no significant difference in the flavor attribute between the four kinds of tablets ($p > 0.05$). As can be seen from Table 7, the lowest score of flavor attribute was found for H-group solution (5.70 ± 1.34), as most panelists felt relatively high bitterness in the H-group solution. Panelists participated in the organoleptic assessment aged between 22 and 25 years, do not like consuming bitter foods. Perhaps these effervescent tablets may be evaluated differently if older people participate in the organoleptic assessment. According to the preference ranking test results (Table 8), the L-group received the highest value in the sum of the orders (59), but its preference did not present statistical difference ($p > 0.05$) for the control and the M-group. The H-group was the less preferred along with the M-group, reinforcing the results obtained in the organoleptic assessment.

Table 7. Organoleptic assessment of the lactobacilli effervescent tablets supplemented with different contents of Chinese ginseng and *Polygonatum sibiricum*.

Tablets	Appearance	Color	Aroma	Flavor	Overall Liking
Control	7.10 ± 1.41 ^{a,b}	7.25 ± 0.97 ^{a}	6.15 ± 1.31 ^{a}	6.30 ± 1.49 ^{a}	6.05 ± 1.39 ^{a}
L-group	7.30 ± 1.17 ^{b}	7.20 ± 0.95 ^{a}	6.40 ± 1.39 ^{a}	6.40 ± 1.43 ^{a}	6.45 ± 1.43 ^{a,b}
M-group	6.20 ± 1.58 ^{a,b}	6.75 ± 1.37 ^{a}	6.35 ± 1.22 ^{a}	6.10 ± 1.71 ^{a}	5.70 ± 1.45 ^{a}
H-group	5.90 ± 1.86 ^{a}	6.55 ± 1.54 ^{a}	6.40 ± 1.23 ^{a}	5.70 ± 1.34 ^{a}	5.30 ± 1.56 ^{a}

All data show the means ± SD. Different letters in the same column indicate a significant difference.

Table 8. Results of the preference ranking test of the lactobacilli effervescent tablets supplemented with different contents of Chinese ginseng and *Polygonatum sibiricum*.

Tablets	Control	L-Group	M-Group	H-Group
Control	-	1 ns	10 ns	23 *
L-group		-	11 ns	24 *
M-group			-	13 ns
H-group				-

* Significant critical difference (5%) minimum of 21, for four samples and 20 panelists, according to the Friedman test. ns non-significant.

3.6. Stability of the Tablets during Storage

Figure 1 shows the survival of lactobacilli in different kinds of lactobacilli effervescent tablets after storage at 25 °C for 60 days. After storage for 15 days, the number of lactobacilli cells was reduced by 1.20, 1.79, 2.08, and 2.35 logarithmic cycles for the control, L-group, M-group, and H-group, respectively. This result demonstrated that the viability of lactobacilli decreased significantly with the increase of the content of the herbs in tablets in the early stage of storage (0–15 days). Nevertheless, in the later stage of storage (15–60 days), the viability of lactobacilli in the tablets supplemented with the herbs was similar to that in the control (Figure 1). Considering the diversity of drug-resistance ability of microorganism cells to antimicrobial substances, we speculated that some sensitive cells in the tablets may be inactivated by the herbs in a dose-dependent manner in the early stage of storage, while the cells that can tolerate the herbs could maintain their viability throughout the storage period. Nagashima, Pansiera, Baracat and Gómez [12] had also reported that the number of *L. acidophilus* in effervescent probiotics tablets decreased from 5.18 to 2.91 logarithmic cycles after storage for 60 days at 25 °C. In this study, the number of viable lactobacilli cells was about 5.80 logarithmic cycles in all kinds of tablets at the end of storage (Figure 1). In order to obtain more probiotic properties, it should be considered to add protectants for lactobacilli viability to the formula.

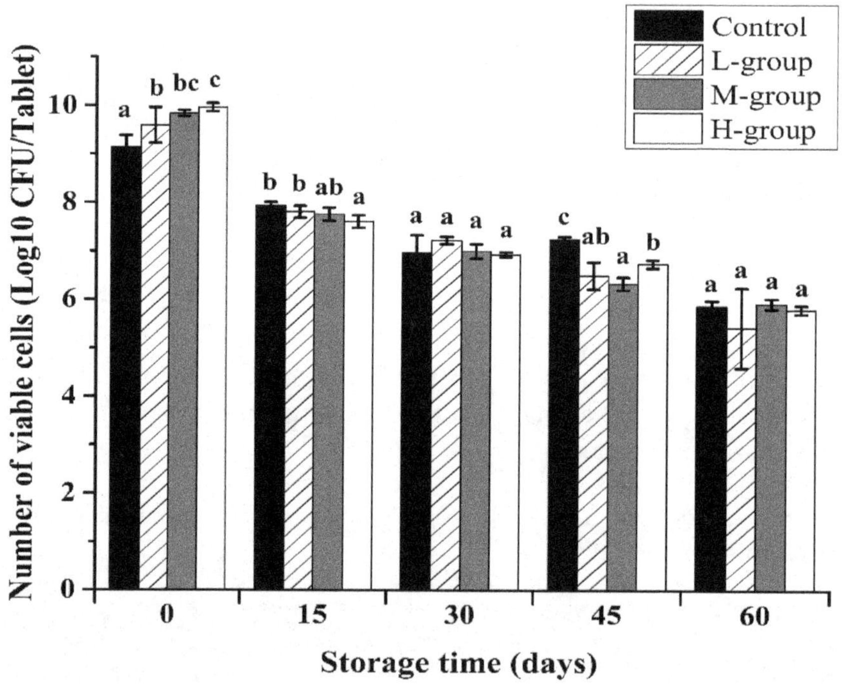

Figure 1. Viability of lactobacilli in different kinds of lactobacilli effervescent tablets stored for 0, 15, 30, 45 and 60 days at 25 °C. All data show the means ± SD. At the same storage period, different letters indicate a significant difference.

4. Conclusions

Our findings demonstrate that it is possible to develop an optimal formulation of lactobacilli effervescent tablets supplemented with Chinese ginseng and *P. sibiricum*, combining functional benefits of lactobacilli and both herbs. In terms of form, the effervescent tablet product exceeds the stability of the liquid form, thereby prolonging the shelf life. Compared with the capsule product, the effervescent tablet has the advantages of simple processing, rapid disintegration, dissolving in water, and easy to take. The effervescent tablet is more suitable for children, the elderly, and people who have difficulty in swallowing pills. According to the results in this study, the formulation of the L-group (60 mg herbs/tablet) would be the best choice for industrial production, which can effectively protect the viability of lactobacilli after tabletting and gastrointestinal juices treatment, together with the high antibacterial ability and the preferred organoleptic characteristics. Meanwhile, the L-group was relatively stable during storage. For a better probiotic effect of the L-group, consumers should drink it in time after disintegration, which would be conducive to retaining higher viability of lactobacilli reaching the intestine and help to create better antibacterial activity in the intestine, leading to a more beneficial enteric microbiota. The main purpose of this study was to investigate the effect of Chinese ginseng and *P. sibiricum* on the properties of effervescent tablets, thus no sweetener was added to the formulations of the lactobacilli effervescent tablets. Considering the younger consumer perspective, manufacturers can add some beneficial sweeteners, such as the prebiotic fiber inulin, to the formula. Additionally, an in vivo experiment should be studied for understanding more health care functions of the lactobacilli effervescent tablets supplemented with Chinese ginseng and *P. sibiricum*.

Author Contributions: Conceptualization, F.Z. and T.Z.; methodology, F.Z., M.L., L.M. and J.Y.; validation, M.L. and L.M.; formal analysis, F.Z.; investigation, M.L., L.M. and J.Y.; resources, F.Z.; data curation, F.Z.; writing—original draft preparation, F.Z.; writing—review and editing, M.L. and L.M.; visualization, F.Z.; supervision, F.Z.; project administration, F.Z.; funding acquisition, F.Z. All authors have read and agreed to the published version of the manuscript.

Acknowledgments: We would like to acknowledge technician Yan Chen for equipment maintenance, and thank Shuning Zhong for assistance in provision of some necessary literature.

References

1. Holzapfel, W.H.; Schillinger, U. Introduction to pre- and probiotics. *Food Res. Int.* **2002**, *35*, 109–116. [CrossRef]
2. Bove, P.; Gallone, A.; Russo, P.; Capozzi, V.; Albenzio, M.; Spano, G. Probiotic features of *Lactobacillus plantarum* mutant strains. *Appl. Microbiol. Biotechnol.* **2012**, *96*, 431–441. [CrossRef]
3. Ouwehand, A.C.; Salminen, S.; Isolauri, E. Probiotics: An overview of beneficial effects. *Antonie Van Leeuwenhoek* **2002**, *82*, 279–289. [CrossRef]
4. Claes, I.J.J.; Lebeer, S.; Shen, C.; Verhoeven, T.L.A.; Dilissen, E.; De Hertogh, G.; Bullens, D.M.A.; Ceuppens, J.L.; Van Assche, G.; Vermeire, S.; et al. Impact of lipoteichoic acid modification on the performance of the probiotic *Lactobacillus rhamnosus* GG in experimental colitis. *Clin. Exp. Immunol.* **2010**, *162*, 306–314. [CrossRef]
5. Mohamadzadeh, M.; Pfeiler, E.A.; Brown, J.B.; Zadeh, M.; Gramarossa, M.; Managlia, E.; Bere, P.; Sarraj, B.; Khan, M.W.; Pakanati, K.C.; et al. Regulation of induced colonic inflammation by *Lactobacillus acidophilus* deficient in lipoteichoic acid. *Proc. Natl. Acad. Sci. USA* **2011**, *108*, 4623–4630. [CrossRef]
6. Yu, L.; Zhai, Q.; Liu, X.; Wang, G.; Zhang, Q.; Zhao, J.; Narbad, A.; Zhang, H.; Tian, F.; Chen, W. *Lactobacillus plantarum* CCFM639 alleviates aluminium toxicity. *Appl. Microbiol. Biotechnol.* **2016**, *100*, 1891–1900. [CrossRef] [PubMed]
7. Wang, H.; Yan, Y.; Wang, J.; Zhang, H.; Qi, W. Production and characterization of antifungal compounds produced by *Lactobacillus plantarum* IMAU10014. *PLoS ONE* **2012**, *7*, e29452. [CrossRef] [PubMed]

8. Giraffa, G.; Chanishvili, N.; Widyastuti, Y. Importance of lactobacilli in food and feed biotechnology. *Res. Microbiol.* **2010**, *161*, 480–487. [CrossRef] [PubMed]
9. Tripathi, M.K.; Giri, S.K. Probiotic functional foods: Survival of probiotics during processing and storage. *J. Funct. Foods* **2014**, *9*, 225–241. [CrossRef]
10. Zea, L.P.; Yusof, Y.A.; Aziz, M.G.; Ling, C.N.; Amin, N.A.M. Compressibility and dissolution characteristics of mixed fruit tablets made from guava and pitaya fruit powders. *Powder Technol.* **2013**, *247*, 112–119. [CrossRef]
11. Maximiano, F.P.; Costa, G.H.Y.; de Sá Barreto, L.C.L.; Bahia, M.T.; Cunha-Filho, M.S.S. Development of effervescent tablets containing benznidazole complexed with cyclodextrin. *J. Pharm. Pharmacol.* **2011**, *63*, 786–793. [CrossRef] [PubMed]
12. Nagashima, A.I.; Pansiera, P.E.; Baracat, M.M.; Gómez, R.J.H.C. Development of effervescent products, in powder and tablet form, supplemented with probiotics *Lactobacillus acidophilus* and *Saccharomyces boulardii*. *Food Sci. Technol.* **2013**, *33*, 605–611. [CrossRef]
13. Alam, M.A.; Ahmad, F.J.; Khan, Z.I.; Khar, R.K.; Ali, M. Development and evaluation of acid-buffering bioadhesive vaginal tablet for mixed vaginal infections. *AAPS PharmSciTech* **2007**, *8*, 229–236. [CrossRef]
14. Maggi, L.; Mastromarino, P.; Macchia, S.; Brigidi, P.; Pirovano, F.; Matteuzzi, D.; Conte, U. Technological and biological evaluation of tablets containing different strains of lactobacilli for vaginal administration. *Eur. J. Pharm. Biopharm.* **2000**, *50*, 389–395. [CrossRef]
15. Baeg, I.-H.; So, S.-H. The world ginseng market and the ginseng (Korea). *J. Ginseng. Res.* **2013**, *37*, 1–7. [CrossRef] [PubMed]
16. Li, X.; Luo, J.; Anandh Babu, P.V.; Zhang, W.; Gilbert, E.; Cline, M.; McMillan, R.; Hulver, M.; Alkhalidy, H.; Zhen, W.; et al. Dietary supplementation of Chinese ginseng prevents obesity and metabolic syndrome in high-fat diet-fed mice. *J. Med. Food* **2014**, *17*, 1287–1297. [CrossRef]
17. Zhang, H.; Cai, X.T.; Tian, Q.H.; Xiao, L.X.; Zeng, Z.; Cai, X.T.; Yan, J.Z.; Li, Q.Y. Microwave-assisted degradation of polysaccharide from *Polygonatum sibiricum* and antioxidant activity. *J. Food Sci.* **2019**, *84*, 754–761. [CrossRef]
18. Tang, C.; Yu, Y.; Guo, P.; Huo, J.; Tang, S. Chemical constituents of *Polygonatum sibiricum*. *Chem. Nat. Compd.* **2019**, *55*, 331–333. [CrossRef]
19. Moraes Filho, M.L.; Busanello, M.; Prudencio, S.H.; Garcia, S. Soymilk with okara flour fermented by *Lactobacillus acidophilus*: Simplex-centroid mixture design applied in the elaboration of probiotic creamy sauce and storage stability. *LWT-Food Sci. Technol.* **2018**, *93*, 339–345. [CrossRef]
20. Moraes, M.L.; Busanello, M.; Garcia, S. Probiotic creamy soy sauce with *Lactobacillus plantarum* BG 112. *Br. Food J.* **2019**, *121*, 2746–2758. [CrossRef]
21. Coman, M.M.; Cecchini, C.; Verdenelli, M.C.; Silvi, S.; Orpianesi, C.; Cresci, A. Functional foods as carriers for SYNBIO®, a probiotic bacteria combination. *Int. J. Food Microbiol.* **2012**, *157*, 346–352. [CrossRef] [PubMed]
22. Phat, C.; Moon, B.; Lee, C. Evaluation of umami taste in mushroom extracts by chemical analysis, sensory evaluation, and an electronic tongue system. *Food Chem.* **2016**, *192*, 1068–1077. [CrossRef] [PubMed]
23. Newell, G.J.; MacFarlane, J.D. Expanded tables for multiple comparison procedures in the analysis of ranked data. *J. Food Sci.* **1987**, *52*, 1721–1725. [CrossRef]
24. Chávarri, M.; Marañón, I.; Ares, R.; Ibáñez, F.C.; Marzo, F.; Villarán, M.D.C. Microencapsulation of a probiotic and prebiotic in alginate-chitosan capsules improves survival in simulated gastro-intestinal conditions. *Int. J. Food Microbiol.* **2010**, *142*, 185–189. [CrossRef] [PubMed]
25. Chan, E.S.; Zhang, Z. Encapsulation of probiotic bacteria *Lactobacillus acidophilus* by direct compression. *Food Bioprod. Process.* **2002**, *80*, 78–82. [CrossRef]
26. Gibson, G.R.; Probert, H.M.; Loo, J.V.; Rastall, R.A.; Roberfroid, M.B. Dietary modulation of the human colonic microbiota: Updating the concept of prebiotics. *Nutr. Res. Rev.* **2004**, *17*, 259–275. [CrossRef]
27. Cui, X.; Wang, S.; Cao, H.; Guo, H.; Li, Y.; Xu, F.; Zheng, M.; Xi, X.; Han, C. A Review: The bioactivities and pharmacological applications of *Polygonatum sibiricum* polysaccharides. *Molecules* **2018**, *23*, 1170. [CrossRef]
28. Xue, P.; Yang, X.; Zhao, L.; Hou, Z.; Zhang, R.; Zhang, F.; Ren, G. Relationship between antimicrobial activity and amphipathic structure of ginsenosides. *Ind. Crops Prod.* **2020**, *143*, 111929. [CrossRef]
29. Battinelli, L.; Mascellino, M.T.; Martino, M.C.; Lu, M.; Mazzanti, G. Antimicrobial activity of ginsenosides. *Pharm. Pharmacol. Commun.* **1998**, *4*, 411–413. [CrossRef]

30. Murina, F.; Graziottin, A.; Vicariotto, F.; De Seta, F. Can *Lactobacillus fermentum* LF10 and *Lactobacillus acidophilus* LA02 in a slow-release vaginal product be useful for prevention of recurrent vulvovaginal candidiasis?: A clinical study. *J. Clin. Gastroenterol.* **2014**, *48*, S102–S105. [CrossRef]

8

Agaricus bisporus By-Products as a Source of Chitin-Glucan Complex Enriched Dietary Fibre with Potential Bioactivity

Sara M. Fraga and Fernando M. Nunes *

CQ-VR, Chemistry Research Centre—Vila Real, Food and Wine Chemistry Lab, Chemistry Department, Universidade de Trás-os-Montes e Alto Douro, Apartado 1013, 5000-801 Vila Real, Portugal; sarafraga_@hotmail.com

* Correspondence: fnunes@utad.pt

Featured Application: A novel, simple and environmentally friendly method was developed and optimize to produce a dietary fiber ingredient from *Agaricus bisporus* by-products, with suitable characteristics for food application and potential biological activity, as a mean for upgrading mushroom industry wastes.

Abstract: Mushroom production generates large amounts of by-products whose disposal creates environmental problems. The high abundance of biological active non-starch polysaccharides in mushroom cell walls makes these by-products attractive for dietary fiber-based ingredient (DFI) production. Traditional methods of dietary fiber preparation didn't allow to obtain a DFI with suitable chemical and functional properties. In this work a simple and environmentally friendly method was developed and optimized for DFI production using a central composite design with treatment time, hydrogen peroxide and sodium hydroxide concentration as factors and chemical composition, chromatic and functional properties as dependent variables. The chemical composition of the DFI was strongly influenced by the process parameters and its functional and color properties were dependent on its fiber and protein content, respectively. The method developed is simple, uses food grade and low-cost reagents and procedures yielding a DFI with white color, no odor and a high concentration of dietary fiber (>60%) with an identical sugar composition to the original mushroom fiber. Due to the high water and oil retention capacity, this DFI may be used not only for dietary fiber enrichment and reduction of the food energy value but also as a functional ingredient with potential bioactivity.

Keywords: dietary fiber; mushroom; *Agaricus bisporus*; dietary fiber ingredient; chemical composition; functional properties; optimization; central composite design

---

1. Introduction

Mushrooms consumption and production over the last decades has shown a phenomenal growth with several times increase in tonnage [1]. Some of the more common cultivated mushroom species are the button mushroom (*Agaricus bisporus*) which is widely cultivated in Europe and comprising about 32% of the world mushroom production, the Shiitake mushroom (*Lentinus edodes*) which is grown for centuries in China and other oriental countries and the oyster mushroom (*Pleurotus ostreatus*) cultivated in several countries around the world [2]. This increase is related to the increasing awareness of consumers for the importance of a healthy diet [3,4]. Indeed, a variety of substances present in mushrooms have been shown to present beneficial biological effects, from these, polysaccharides comprising the β-D-glucans and heteroglucans are the best known and most potent mushroom-derived substances with antitumor and immunomodulating properties [5–8]. The fungal cell walls are composed by an alkali-insoluble structural skeleton mainly composed of β-(1→3)-glucan covalently linked to chitin [9,10], forming a chitin-glucan complex (CGC). Chitin and CGC have been shown to have very interesting biological activities [11–15]. In addition, several studies have shown that polysaccharides from a variety of mushrooms, including those of *A. bisporus*, have been successfully used as prebiotics [16–22].

Nevertheless, mushroom production generates a large amount of by-products including waste and off-grade mushrooms with no suitable commercial use that ranges between 5% and 20% of production volume [23]. Mushrooms and mushroom by-products, especially those from *A. bisporus*, are rapidly perishable products [24], and they suffer rapid and deleterious transformations resulting in darker products due to the tyrosinase activity and synthesis of melanins [25] and with an unpleasant smell, creating environmental problems for their disposal. The European regulation of waste management, Directive 2008/98/ EC ('Waste Framework Directive'), focused on the reduction of waste generation by 30% in 2025, requires that waste should be managed without endangering human health and harming the environment, in particular without risk to water, air, soil, plants or animals, and without causing a nuisance through noise or odors [26]. To reduce the environmental impact of the agro-food industries and the dependence on raw materials, the implementation of valorization procedures for these materials is stimulated. Some strategies have already been evaluated, for example, the use of *A. bisporus* by-products for non-animal chitin and chitosan production [27]. Nevertheless, most of the methods employed for the extraction of fungal cell wall polysaccharides are tedious and time-consuming involving the use of high temperatures and high concentrated alkaline and acid solutions or using specific enzymatic treatment in combination with synthetic detergents [28–31]. In addition, the use of concentrated reagents can deteriorate the native properties of the obtained products [32]. The production of dietary fiber ingredients (DFI) has been successfully used to upgrade agricultural products and by-products of cereals, fruits, and vegetables [33,34], therefore, the production of a high added value food ingredient based on mushroom dietary fiber from by-products and off-grade mushrooms can be an economical alternative to the simple waste disposal. Nevertheless for the food industry, beyond their nutritional and health benefits, dietary fibers also have technological properties that can be used in food formulations, resulting in texture modification and enhancement of food stability during production and storage, and more importantly, added fibers cannot alter the sensorial properties of foods where they are used. Altogether, these factors will determine their successful use in foods.

The purpose of this work was to develop and optimize a simple and green method for the production of mushroom CGC enriched dietary fiber from *A. bisporus* off-grade mushrooms and in situation of excessive mushroom production, using a response surface methodology based on a central composite design to evaluate the influence of the process variables in the chemical composition, nutritional and functional properties to evaluate its suitability for use as a DFI in food formulations.

2. Materials and Methods

2.1. Materials

As the method developed in this work is intended to be used for the valorization of off-grade mushrooms with no commercial value and the excesses of mushroom production, for reasons of simplicity and easier management, the *A. bisporus* mushrooms were bought on the local market for obtaining the DFI. Samples were stored in dark conditions at 4 °C until experiments began for a maximum of one day. All reagents used were of analytical grade. All reported values, unless otherwise stated, are expressed on a dry weight basis and are the average values of the analysis of at least two different replicates.

2.2. Method for Preparation of Mushroom DFI

Preliminary experiments in our lab allow concluding (detailed later) that to obtain a food ingredient based on dietary fiber from mushrooms with good technological properties, i.e., with a white color and no aroma, an alkaline oxidative treatment using sodium hydroxide and hydrogen peroxide was the most appropriate, and this method was further optimized concerning the treatment time, sodium hydroxide concentration and hydrogen peroxide concentration (Table 1). For obtaining mushroom DFI, mushrooms (300 g) were sliced and ground in a Waring blender (3 min) and transferred to the treatment solution (1 L) whose composition was varied according to Table 1. The material was stirred at 300 rpm at room temperature (20–22 °C) during the time for each specific treatment. After the treatment, the solution pH was neutralized with concentrated sulfuric acid to pH 6–7, and hydrogen peroxide was destroyed by adding $NaHSO_3$. The material was filtrated, re-suspended in water and filtered again. The material was freeze-dried and the solid was ground and weighted. The yield, chemical and functional properties of the prepared mushroom DFI were determined to evaluate the impact of the studied process parameters.

2.3. Dietary Fiber, Protein, Moisture, Lipids, Ash and Caloric Value Content of the DFI

Due to the expected presence of chitin in the DFI, the content and sugar composition of dietary fiber of the mushroom DFI was determined as non-starch polysaccharides (NSP) by the method of Englyst et al. [35,36], being determined by the sum of sugars released after acid hydrolysis, and quantified by anion-exchange chromatography with pulsed amperometric detection (HPAEC-PAD) [37]. Protein content was determined by quantification of the nitrogen content of the mushroom DFI after correction for the nitrogen from glucosamine present and multiplication by 6.25. The total nitrogen content of the DFI was determined by the Dumas method. Moisture, lipids and ash content of the mushroom DFI were determined according to AOAC [38]. Total carbohydrates were calculated by difference. Caloric values, on a dry basis, were computed using the Attwater coefficients [39], corrected for 2% of ash.

2.4. FTIR Analysis

A Unicam Research Series FTIR spectrometer was used. The spectra were recorded in the range of wavenumbers 4000–450 cm^{-1} with 50 scans being taken at 2 cm^{-1} resolution. Pellets were prepared by thoroughly mixing DFI sample or reference polysaccharides (chitin, chitosan, and curdlan) and KBr at a 1:200 sample/KBr weight ratio in a small size agate mortar. The resulting mixture was placed in a Perkin–Elmer manual hydraulic press, and a force of 15 tons was applied for 10 min. The spectra obtained were background corrected and smoothed using the Savitzky–Golay algorithm using PeakFit v4 (AISN Software Inc., Oregon, United States, 1995). Chitin from crab shells (Sigma), Chitosan 66% deacetylation degree (Sigma) and curdlan (Sigma) were used as reference polysaccharides.

2.5. DFI Chromatic Characteristics

The chromatic characteristics of the DFI were evaluated with a Chroma Meter CR-300 Minolta (Osaka, Japan). CIE Lab coordinates were obtained using D65 illuminant a 10 observer as a reference system. L*, a*, and b* parameters were calculated from the average of five color measurements. The equipment was calibrated with a white standard (L* = 97.71; a* = −0.59 and b* = 2.31).

2.6. Water Retention Capacity and Oil Retention Capacity

Water retention capacity (WRC) of the mushroom DFI obtained under the different experimental conditions was determined under external centrifugal force using the method described by Robertson et al. [40]. Fiber (~1 g) was hydrated in water (30 mL) for 18 h, centrifuged (3000× *g*; 20 min), drained, and dried. WRC was calculated as the amount of water retained per g of dry fiber residue.

For determination of the oil retention capacity (ORC) of the mushroom DFI, the same procedure described previously was used, but instead of water 30 mL of corn oil were used.

2.7. Experimental Design

A rotatable central composite design of the experiments was performed with k = 3—treatment time, hydrogen peroxide and sodium hydroxide concentrations as independent variables. Central composite experiments consisted of three sets of experimental points [41]: (1) a factorial design with 2k points, k is the number of x_i variables (factors) with coded levels +1 and −1 for each; (2) a star for 2k points, coded as $+\alpha$ and $-\alpha$ on the axis of the system at a distance of 2k/4 from the origin, that accounts for non-linearity; (3) central points, which are replicated to provide an estimate of the lack of fit of the linear statistical model obtained as well as the pure error of the experiments (due to unreliability in the measurement of the dependent variable) [42]. The main advantage of this methodology is to decrease the number of experimental trials needed to evaluate multiple parameters and their interactions. The established ranges were: sodium hydroxide concentration (C_{NaOH}) 0.1–0.5 M, hydrogen peroxide concentration ($C_{H_2O_2}$)—1.5–4.5%, treatment time (T)—2–6 h. Table 1 shows the coded and uncoded experimental design.

2.8. Statistical Analysis

Data was fit to second-order polynomial Equation (1) for each dependent Y variable, through multiple regression analysis using Statistic® vs. 10 software.

$$Y=\beta_0 + \beta_1X_1 + \beta_2X_2 + \beta_3X_3 + \beta_4{X_1}^2 + \beta_5{X_2}^2 + \beta_5{X_3}^2 + \beta_7X_1X_2 + \beta_8X_1X_3 + \beta_9X_2X_3, \quad (1)$$

β_n are regression equation coefficients and X_n the independent variables. Based on the predicted model equations surface plots were generated. The analysis of the variance was performed to determine the lack of fit and the significance of the effects of each of the three independent factors, using the mean square pure error as the error term. This provides a more sensitive test of model fit because the effects of the additional higher-order terms are removed from the error.

2.9. Principal Component Analysis (PCA)

PCA is one of the most often used chemometric methods for data reduction and exploratory analysis of high-dimensional data sets [43]. PCA decomposes the original matrix into multiplication of loading (chemical composition, color, and functional properties) and score (dietary fiber samples) matrices. The principal components are linear combinations of the original variables. The principal components are uncorrelated and account for the total variance of the original variables. PCA is an unsupervised method of pattern recognition in the sense that no grouping of the data has to be known before the analysis. The new sub-space defined by the principal components leads to a model that is easier to interpret than the original data set. From these results, it should be possible to highlight several characteristics and correlate them to the chemical composition of the different DFI produced.

3. Results

3.1. Development and Optimization of a Method for Obtaining Mushroom DFI

Preliminary experiments using methods previously described for the production of DFIs from other sources, including the simple hot water extraction [44], ethanol extraction of the low molecular weight material [45] and enzymatic removal of protein [46], rendered a deep yellow-brown material with an unpleasant smell (results not shown). This prompts us to develop an efficient method for the production of mushroom DFI that could render a food ingredient with desirable characteristics for their application in foods. This could be accomplished by using a chemical treatment with an alkaline solution containing hydrogen peroxide at room temperature. Under these conditions, the product obtained presented a white color and with no perceived odor. The method developed for the production of mushroom dietary fiber was optimized considering three process variables: treatment time (T), hydrogen peroxide concentration ($C_{H_2O_2}$) and sodium hydroxide concentration (C_{NaOH}). A rotatable central composite design with $\alpha = 1.68$ was used for the optimization of the parameters for the production of mushroom DFI as well as optimization of the DFI physico-chemical, nutritional and functional properties. Table 1 shows the design matrix of factors for the rotatable central composite design. DFI yield, chemical and nutritional composition, color, and functional properties were measured as the output variables.

3.2. *Yield of the Mushroom DFI*

The yield of mushroom DFI obtained varied between a minimum of 15% to a maximum of 53% of the mushroom dry weight (0.77% to 2.8% of the fresh mushroom weight for a mushroom water content of 94.7%) (Table 1). Based on the central composite design, each of the three factors (T, $C_{H_2O_2}$, and C_{NaOH}) had a significant effect on the mushroom DFI yield (Table 2). There was also observed a significant interaction between T and C_{NaOH}. Using multiple regression analysis, a second-order polynomial equation model based on codded levels was used to fit the experimental results. This model which consists of the factors found to be significant is shown in Table A1. The ANOVA results of the model obtained indicated an adequate performance with $R^2 = 0.64$, implying that 64% of the variations observed for the mushroom DFI yield are explained by the factors considered. It was therefore considered that the model provided a good description of the experimental data. Nevertheless, the F-test for the lack of fit was also significant ($p < 0.05$) therefore a more complicated model or additional factors (for example variability of the mushrooms used in each experiment) are required to a higher fit of the experimental data [41]. Figure 1 shows the three-dimension response surface curves of mushroom DFI yield for each pair of factors by keeping the third factor constant at the level where it presented the maximum value. The factor T presented the highest positive effect (Table 2, Figure 1a) on the mushroom DFI yield (maximum for the +1.682 level), followed by the factor $C_{H_2O_2}$ were it was observed a positive effect (Table 2; Figure 1b) for the linear effect and a negative effect for the quadratic effect (maximum value for the $C_{H_2O_2} > 0$ level). The interaction between the factor T and C_{NaOH} and the linear effect of the factor C_{NaOH} both had a positive effect on the DFI yield (Table 2, Figure 1a).

Table 1. Coded and actual variables for the experimental design for the optimization of mushroom dietary fiber isolation, yield (in relation to the initial mushroom fresh weight) and chemical composition concerning the fiber, protein, fat and ash of the dietary fiber ingredient (DFI) obtained in each experiment.

Coded			Actual								
C_{NaOH} (M)	$C_{H_2O_2}$ (%)	Time (h)	C_{NaOH} (M)	$C_{H_2O_2}$ (%)	Time (h)	Run Number	Yield (g/100 g)	Fiber (g/100 g)	Protein [1] (g/100 g)	Fat (g/100 g)	Ash (g/100 g)
−1	−1	−1	0.181	2.1	2.81	12	1.21	64.9	17.1	2.2	5.0
+1	−1	−1	0.419	2.1	2.81	10	0.77	64.8	10.6	2.1	2.4
−1	+1	−1	0.181	3.9	2.81	5	0.92	60.1	21.1	1.9	2.2
+1	+1	−1	0.419	3.9	2.81	3	1.22	63.7	12.0	2.1	3.9
−1	−1	+1	0.181	2.1	5.19	2	1.44	56.9	20.0	1.7	5.5
+1	−1	+1	0.419	2.1	5.19	8	2.78	37.9	30.8	2.5	18.1
−1	+1	+1	0.181	3.9	5.19	14	2.34	42.6	32.7	1.8	10.3
+1	+1	+1	0.419	3.9	5.19	13	2.22	49.2	24.7	2.1	9.5
−α	0	0	0.1	3	4	11	1.73	42.4	28.9	2.0	6.8
+α	0	0	0.5	3	4	16	2.14	42.7	28.5	2.1	11.5
0	−α	0	0.3	1.5	4	9	1.15	48.9	27.6	1.9	5.0
0	+α	0	0.3	4.5	4	6	2.20	45.1	28.7	1.7	6.3
0	0	−α	0.3	3	2	7	1.57	51.8	27.9	2.2	2.6
0	0	+α	0.3	3	6	20	1.84	44.8	34.5	1.9	5.0
0	0	0	0.3	3	4	19	2.02	42.4	39.2	2.0	5.4
0	0	0	0.3	3	4	17	1.94	49.8	23.1	1.7	8.3
0	0	0	0.3	3	4	18	1.90	46.6	40.1	2.1	5.1
0	0	0	0.3	3	4	4	2.09	53.8	23.8	2.2	6.5
0	0	0	0.3	3	4	15	2.13	55.8	23.0	1.7	6.1
0	0	0	0.3	3	4	1	1.72	47.1	31.8	2.0	3.2
Original								30.3	22.7	5.2	9.2

[1] Protein content calculated from the difference from total nitrogen minus glucosamine nitrogen.

Table 2. Analysis of Variance Results for the physico-chemical and functional response variables of mushroom dietary fiber ingredient (DFI).

		Factor											
		Time (L)	Time (Q)	$C_{H_2O_2}$ (L)	$C_{H_2O_2}$ (Q)	C_{NaOH} (L)	C_{NaOH} (Q)	Time X $C_{H_2O_2}$	Time X C_{NaOH}	$C_{H_2O_2}$ X C_{NaOH}	Lack of Fit	Pure Error	Total SS
DFI Yield	SS	2.096	0.024	0.373	0.260	0.173	0.221	0.004	0.231	0.064	1.591	0.111	5.090
	Df	1	1	1	1	1	1	1	1	1	5	5	19
	F	94.65	1.12	16.86	11.76	7.80	9.98	0.183	10.44	2.92	14.37		
	$p<$	0.0002	0.338	0.009	0.018	0.038	0.025	0.687	0.023	0.147	0.0055		
Protein Yield	SS	0.427	0.0124	0.0389	0.0680	0.0335	0.0350	0.0005	0.0561	0.102	0.382	0.118	1.257
	Df	1	1	1	1	1	1	1	1	1	5	5	19
	F	18.088	0.567	1.648	2.881	1.422	1.483	0.0227	2.379	4.304	3.237		
	$p<$	0.008	0.500	0.255	0.150	0.287	0.278	0.886	0.184	0.093	0.112		
Fat Yield	SS	0.000589	0.000002	0.000044	0.00016	0.000094	0.000026	0	0.00200	0.000019	0.00059	0.000102	0.00181
	Df	1	1	1	1	1	1	1	1	1	5	5	19
	F	29.01	0.111	2.148	7.657	4.628	1.286	0.0012	9.860	0.941	5.818		
	$p<$	0.003	0.752	0.203	0.039	0.084	0.308	0.973	0.026	0.377	0.038		
L*	SS	11.659	15.892	29.191	105.050	14.185	8.990	2.040	41.284	6.820	125.06	6.875	369.27
	Df	1	1	1	1	1	1	1	1	1	5	5	19
	F	8.479	11.558	21.230	76.399	10.316	6.538	1.484	30.024	4.960	18.191		
	$p<$	0.033	0.019	0.006	0.0003	0.024	0.051	0.278	0.003	0.076	0.003		
a*	SS	0.587	3.785	2.291	7.757	2.304	2.030	0.648	1.641	0.546	5.914	0.144	28.075
	Df	1	1	1	1	1	1	1	1	1	5	5	19
	F	20.369	131.36	79.533	269.25	79.978	70.457	22.488	56.959	18.951	41.054		
	$p<$	0.006	0.00009	0.0003	0.00002	0.0003	0.0004	0.005	0.0006	0.007	0.0005		
b*	SS	7.670	38.664	1.310	29.751	13.560	66.903	8.757	1.020	5.254	98.375	1.422	252.40
	Df	1	1	1	1	1	1	1	1	1	5	5	19
	F	26.969	135.96	4.607	104.61	47.681	235.25	30.793	3.587	18.475	69.183		
	$p<$	0.003	0.00008	0.085	0.0002	0.001	0.00002	0.003	0.117	0.008	0.0001		
WRC	SS	67.870	93.966	0.337	88.368	2.126	82.042	12.880	31.859	3.521	93.974	12.770	448.08
	Df	1	1	1	1	1	1	1	1	1	5	5	19
	F	26.575	39.793	0.132	34.601	0.832	32.124	5.043	12.475	1.379	7.359		
	$p<$	0.004	0.002	0.731	0.002	0.403	0.002	0.075	0.017	0.293	0.023		
ORC	SS	18.817	56.560	1.049	30.534	0.569	5.400	19.965	49.581	15.207	20.792	3.527	210.94
	Df	1	1	1	1	1	1	1	1	1	5	5	19
	F	26.679	80.191	1.487	43.291	0.806	7.656	28.306	70.297	21.560	5.896		
	$p<$	0.004	0.0003	0.277	0.001	0.410	0.039	0.003	0.0004	0.006	0.037		

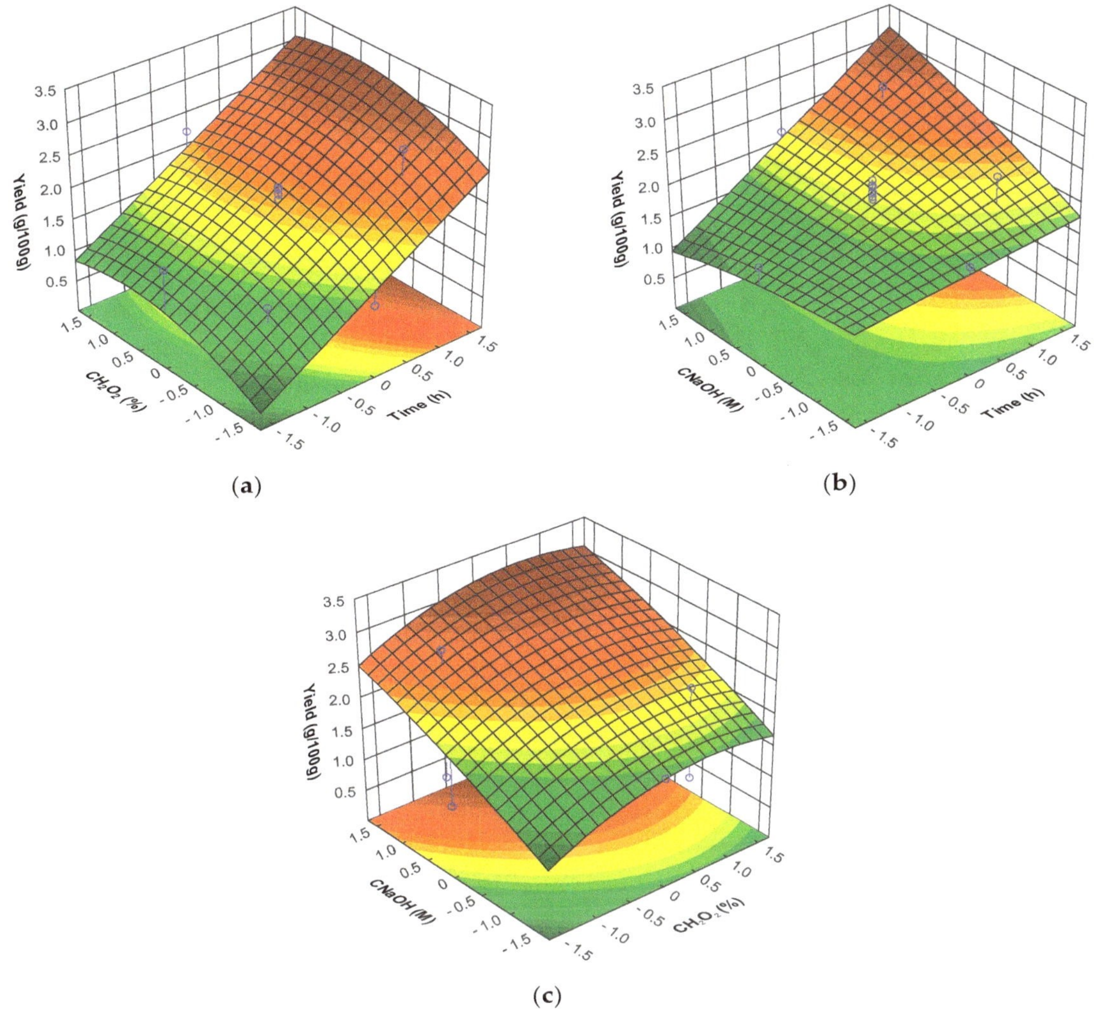

Figure 1. Response surfaces for mushroom DFI yield as a function of: (**a**) time and hydrogen peroxide concentration (at sodium hydroxide concentration level of 1.682); (**b**) time and sodium hydroxide concentration (at hydrogen peroxide concentration level of 1); (**c**) hydrogen peroxide concentration and sodium hydroxide concentration (at time level of 1.682).

These results show that during the treatment of the mushroom material with the alkaline solution containing hydrogen peroxide there was observed an insolubilization of material with treatment time, this insolubilization being promoted by higher NaOH concentrations. According to the response surface analysis, the predicted maximum mushroom DFI yield in the range studied is 2.9% of the mushroom fresh weight (95% prediction interval: 2.1–3.6%) when the factor T is +1.682, the factor $C_{H_2O_2}$ is +0 and the factor C_{NaOH} is +1.682, corresponding to 55% of the mushroom solids. To understand what is being insolubilized during the treatment of the mushroom material, and as the composition of DFIs are important from a legal perspective [47] but also for its nutritional and functional properties, the fiber, protein, lipid and ash contents of the DFI were determined.

3.3. Fibre Content and Composition

As can be observed in Table 1, fiber was the main component of the mushroom DFI for all the conditions employed and ranged from 45.9% to 70.4%. Only the factor T had a significant negative effect on the DFI fiber content (Table 2), therefore although higher treatment times resulted in higher DFI yields, there was also observed a decrease in the relative abundance of dietary fiber in the DFI. The previously described increase in the DFI yield with T is not related to an increase in fiber retention during the treatment as there was not observed a correlation between fiber yield and treatment time (R^2

= 0.2092). For obtaining a mushroom DFI with higher fiber contents the lower processing times assure this value (Table 1). The yield of dietary fiber obtained ranged between 0.50% of the mushroom's fresh weight to 1.3%, corresponding to a yield of fiber between 31% and 81% of original mushroom fiber content (on average 54%). This yield is explained by the fact that some of the *A. bisporus* polysaccharides are water and alkali-soluble [48].

In Table 3 it is shown the sugar composition of the mushroom DFI obtained for the different experimental conditions tested. In addition, the sugar composition of the fiber of the freeze-dried mushrooms is shown. The method applied resulted in a relative increase of the fiber in the DFI from 1.9 to 2.9 times in comparison with the original mushroom, showing the efficiency of the method employed for enriching the DFI with the original mushroom fiber. As can be observed, the main sugars present in the mushroom DFI were glucose followed by glucosamine and xylose that together account for more than 91% of the total sugars present. Smaller amounts of mannose, glucuronic acid, fucose, and galacturonic acid were also present. This sugar composition is similar to that described in previous works that have shown that *A. bisporus* cell walls are composed predominantly by β(1→3)-linked glucan containing some β(1→6) linkages containing also chitin [27,48,49]. FTIR analysis of the DFI confirms the presence of chitin (Figure 2). The spectra had characteristic bands at 3400–3480 cm^{-1} that responded to OH-3 and CH_2OH-6 intra- and intermolecular hydrogen bonds, bands at 1650 cm^{-1} for amide I, and 1557 cm^{-1} for amide II vibrational mode. The chitin present in the mushroom DFI is in an antiparallel α-conformation [50] as there is observed a split of the amide I vibration band at 1655 cm^{-1}, identical to the reference crustacean chitin (Figure 2). These results confirmed that the glycosaminoglycans of DFI from *A. bisporus* were in highly acetylated form. The ratio of intensities of the bands at ~1379 and ~2920 cm^{-1} has been suggested as the crystallinity index for chitin and chitosan [51]. The crystallinity index of the DFI chitin was similar to that of the reference chitin (1.07 vs. 1.12, respectively) and higher than that observed for the reference chitosan (0.78). The crystallinity index obtained mushroom DFI was higher than that obtained by Wu et al. [27], this being probably due to the preparation method used by these authors (1M NaOH at 95 °C during 30 min followed by 2% acetic acid at 95 °C during 6 h). A clear spectrum of the glucan in DFI could not be observed, due to the overlapping of chitin bands and the lack of unique bands in β-glucans when compared to chitin (Figure 3). This composition of dietary fiber is similar to that previously described [52], although in our work the amount of glucosamine was lower, and this can be related with different times after harvesting of the mushrooms [53] or to different *A. bisporus* strains used [54], nevertheless the chitin content of the *A. bisporus* obtained in this work is in agreement with previous works [27,48,49,55]. Although the relative abundance of the different sugars in the mushroom DFI is similar to that observed for the original mushroom there was a decrease in the relative abundance of fucose (−60%), galactose (−70%), and glucuronic acid (−60%). The other sugars present increased their relative abundance by 10% for glucose, 70% for xylose and 30% for mannose. Galacturonic acid was not detected in the original mushrooms but was present in most of the DFI obtained, and the relative abundance of glucosamine was on average the same as that found in the original mushroom dietary fiber.

Table 3. Sugar composition of starting material (g/100 g) and mushroom dietary fiber ingredient (g/100 g ashless basis).

	Fuc	GlcNH2	Gal	Glc	Xyl	Man	GalA	GlcA	Total
Original	0.2 (0.0) ^{a}	7.1 (0.1) ^{j}	1.5 (0.1) ^{a,b}	18.4 (0.4) ^{j}	1.1 (0.1) ^{h}	0.5 (0.1) ^{c}	n.d. ^{a}	1.4 (0.3) ^{a,b,c}	30.3 (0.7) ^{j}
1	0.1 (0.0) ^{a}	21.1 (0.7) ^{a}	0.5 (0.1) ^{g}	38.1 (2.3) ^{a,b}	5.2 (0.2) ^{a}	1.6 (0.1) ^{a,b}	0.1 (0.1) ^{a}	1.6 (0.5) ^{a,b,c}	68.4 (2.9) ^{a}
2	0.1 (0.0) ^{a}	20.3 (0.6) ^{a,b}	0.7 (0.0) ^{e,f,g}	36.9 (1.5) ^{a,b,c}	5.1 (0.3) ^{a}	1.8 (0.0) ^{a}	0.2 (0.1) ^{a}	1.2 (0.3) ^{a,b,c}	66.4 (0.9) ^{a,b}
3	0.1 (0.0) ^{a}	20.8 (0.3) ^{a}	0.7 (0.0) ^{e,f,g}	31.7 (2.0) ^{d,e,f}	4.9 (0.4) ^{a,b,c}	1.6 (0.1) ^{a,b}	0.3 (0.0) ^{a}	1.2 (0.2) ^{a,b,c}	61.5 (2.6) ^{b,c}
4	0.1 (0.0) ^{a}	17.4 (0.6) ^{c,d}	0.6 (0.0) ^{f,g}	40.0 (2.7) ^{a}	4.5 (0.0) ^{a,b,c,d}	1.5 (0.1) ^{a,b}	0.2 (0.2) ^{a}	1.9 (0.5) ^{a,b}	66.2 (2.5) ^{a,b}
5	0.2 (0.0) ^{a}	16.5 (0.2) ^{d,e}	0.7 (0.1) ^{e,f,g}	34.8 (0.9) ^{b,c,d,e}	4.3 (0.3) ^{b,c,d,e}	1.5 (0.1) ^{a,b}	0.1 (0.2) ^{a}	2.1 (0.4) ^{a}	60.2 (0.5) ^{c}
6	0.2 (0.0) ^{a}	12.6 (1.3) ^{h,i}	1.3 (0.0) ^{a,b,c,d}	26.1 (1.1) ^{g,h,i}	3.3 (0.0) ^{g}	1.4 (0.0) ^{a,b}	0.1 (0.1) ^{a}	1.4 (0.3) ^{a,b,c}	46.3 (0.9) ^{h,i}
7	0.2 (0.0) ^{a}	12.3 (0.2) ^{h,i}	1.0 (0.0) ^{c,d,e,f}	27.7 (1.4) ^{f,g,h}	3.2 (0.3) ^{g}	1.3 (0.1) ^{b}	0.2 (0.1) ^{a}	1.5 (0.2) ^{a,b,c}	47.5 (1.9) ^{h,i}
8	0.2 (0.0) ^{a}	13.9 (0.2) ^{f,g,h}	1.1 (0.1) ^{b,c,d,e}	32.1 (1.4) ^{c,d,e,f}	3.9 (0.3) ^{d,e,f,g}	1.2 (0.1) ^{b}	0.1 (0.2) ^{a}	1.9 (0.4) ^{b}	54.4 (1.6) ^{d,e,f}
9	0.2 (0.0) ^{a}	15.0 (0.4) ^{e,f,g}	0.9 (0.0) ^{d,e,f,g}	22.6 (0.6) ^{i,j}	4.2 (0.1) ^{c,d,e,f}	1.6 (0.0) ^{a,b}	0.2 (0.0) ^{a}	0.7 (0.2) ^{a,b,c}	45.5 (0.7) ^{i}
10	0.2 (0.0) ^{a}	13.6 (0.2) ^{f,g,h}	1.1 (0.0) ^{b,c,d,e}	27.3 (1.0) ^{f,g,h,i}	3.6 (0.2) ^{e,f,g}	1.4 (0.1) ^{a,b}	0.2 (0.0) ^{a}	0.9 (0.1) ^{a,b,c}	48.3 (1.4) ^{g,h,i}
11	0.2 (0.0) ^{a}	15.3 (0.4) ^{e,f}	1.0 (0.1) ^{c,d,e,f}	27.5 (0.9) ^{f,g,h,i}	4.2 (0.1) ^{c,d,e,f}	1.8 (0.1) ^{a}	0.2 (0.0) ^{a}	1.1 (0.2) ^{a,b,c}	51.5 (1.2) ^{f,g,h}
12	0.2 (0.0) ^{a}	11.5 (0.1) ^{i}	1.6 (0.1) ^{a}	28.8 (0.8) ^{f,g,h}	3.2 (0.1) ^{g}	1.5 (0.1) ^{a,b}	0.0 (0.0) ^{a}	1.2 (0.2) ^{a,b,c}	48.1 (0.7) ^{g,h,i}
13	0.2 (0.0) ^{a}	15.1 (0.1) ^{e,f,g}	1.0 (0.1) ^{c,d,e,f}	29.9 (0.5) ^{e,f,g}	4.2 (0.0) ^{c,d,e,f}	1.5 (0.0) ^{a,b}	0.2 (0.0) ^{a}	1.1 (0.2) ^{a,b,c}	53.2 (0.1) ^{e,f,g}
14	0.2 (0.0) ^{a}	13.4 (0.5) ^{g,h}	1.3 (0.0) ^{a,b,c,d}	26.1 (0.1) ^{g,h,i}	3.6 (0.1) ^{e,f,g}	1.4 (0.0) ^{a,b}	0.2 (0.0) ^{a}	1.0 (0.2) ^{a,b,c}	47.2 (0.4) ^{h,i}
15	0.2 (0.0) ^{a}	13.3 (0.6) ^{g,h}	1.3 (0.0) ^{a,b,c,d}	24.2 (0.0) ^{h,i}	3.6 (0.1) ^{e,f,g}	1.2 (0.1) ^{b}	n. d. ^{a}	1.0 (0.2) ^{a,b,c}	44.8 (0.6) ^{i}
16	0.2 (0.0) ^{a}	18.8 (0.3) ^{b,c}	1.0 (0.0) ^{c,d,e,f}	26.6 (0.7) ^{g,h,i}	5.0 (0.1) ^{a,b}	1.6 (0.0) ^{a,b}	0.3 (0.0) ^{a}	0.8 (0.2) ^{b,c}	54.3 (0.4) ^{d,e,f}
17	0.2 (0.0) ^{a}	12.8 (0.3) ^{h,i}	1.3 (0.1) ^{a,b,c,d}	28.9 (0.3) ^{f,g,h}	3.5 (0.0) ^{f,g}	1.2 (0.1) ^{b}	n. d. ^{a}	1.2 (0.3) ^{a,b,c}	49.1 (0.4) ^{f,g,h,i}
18	0.1 (0.0) ^{a}	15.3 (0.0) ^{e,f}	0.8 (0.1) ^{e,f,g}	34.0 (2.0) ^{b,c,d,e}	4.1 (0.1) ^{d,e,f}	1.4 (0.0) ^{a,b}	0.1 (0.2) ^{a}	1.7 (0.3) ^{a,b,c}	57.5 (1.6) ^{c,d,e}
19	0.1 (0.0) ^{a}	15.3 (0.2) ^{e,f}	0.8 (0.1) ^{e,f,g}	35.7 (0.5) ^{a,b,c,d}	4.2 (0.1) ^{c,d,e,f}	1.3 (0.1) ^{b}	0.1 (0.2) ^{a}	1.8 (0.4) ^{a,b,c}	59.4 (0.1) ^{c,d}
20	0.2 (0.0) ^{a}	15.4 (0.6) ^{e,f}	1.4 (0.1) ^{a,b,c}	25.0 (0.1) ^{g,h,i}	4.1 (0.0) ^{d,e,f}	1.4 (0.1) ^{a,b}	0.2 (0.1) ^{a}	0.9 (0.2) ^{a,b,c}	48.6 (0.9) ^{g,h,i}

Values are presented as mean and standard deviation is inside brackets ($n = 2$); within the same column, values with the same superscript letter are not significantly different ($p < 0.05$, ANOVA and Tukey post-hoc test).

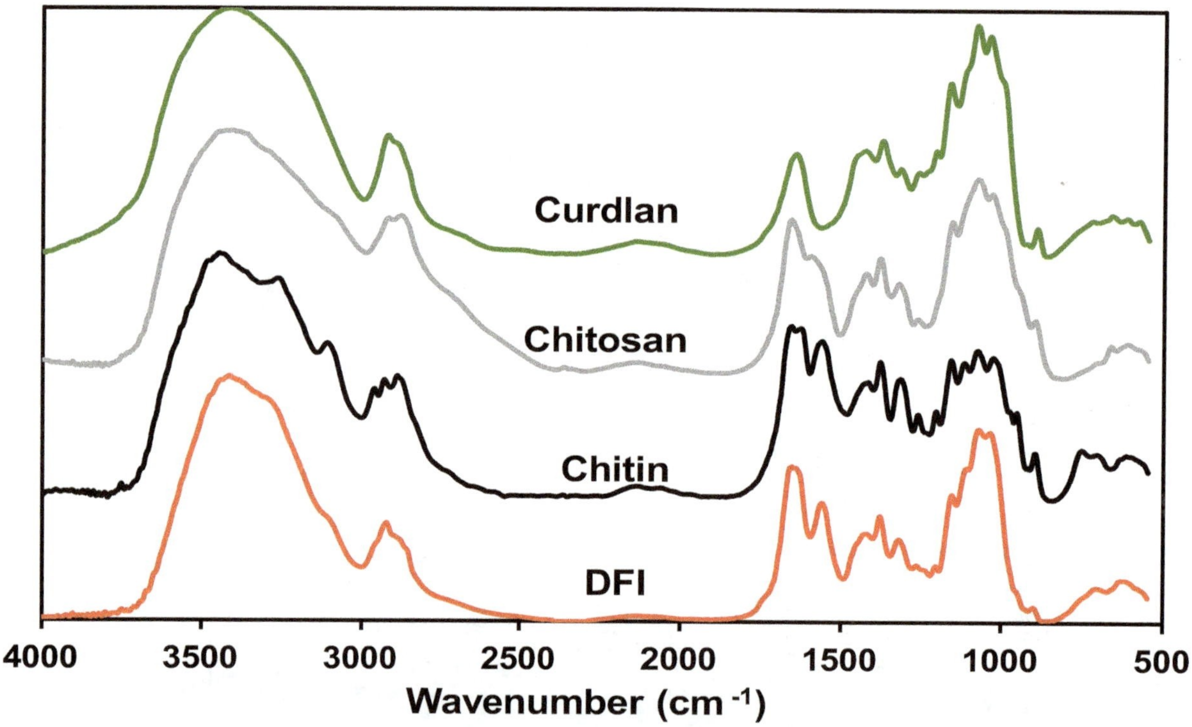

Figure 2. FTIR spectra of the DFI obtained in treatment n° 4 and of the reference polysaccharides chitin, chitosan and curdlan.

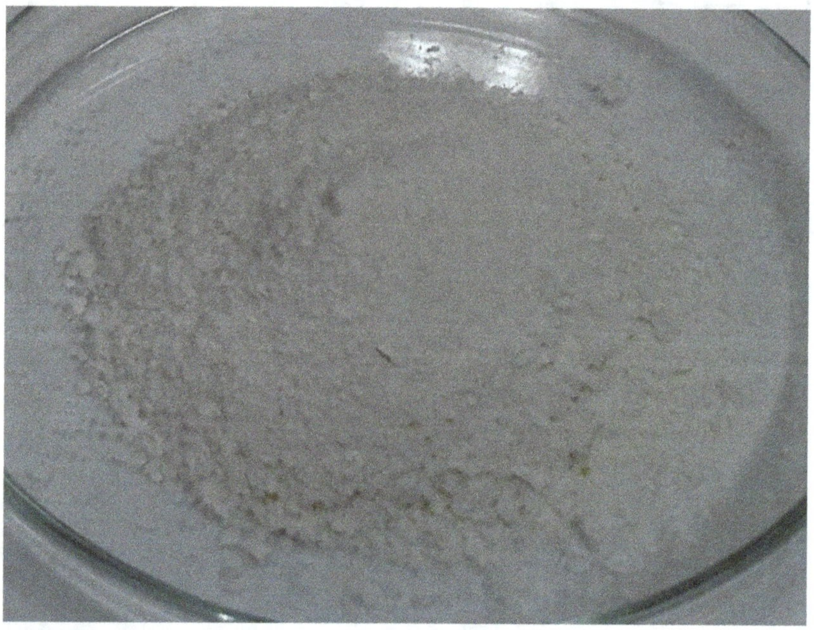

Figure 3. Dietary fiber ingredient obtained for the treatment n° 4. $C_{NaOH} = 0.419$ M; $C_{H_2O_2} = 3.9\%$ and $T = 2.81$ h.

3.4. *Protein, Fat, Ash Content and Energy*

Protein was the second most abundant component of the mushroom DFI, ranging from 11 to 40% (Table 1). The yield of protein obtained varied between a minimum of 0.081% of the mushroom fresh weight to 0.88%, representing between 6.7% and 73% of the original mushroom protein content. Only T had a significant effect on the yield of protein from the mushroom. There was observed an increase in the amount of protein recovered in the DFI with increasing T, nevertheless, the model (Table 3) is not enough to explain the variations observed in the amount of protein recovered in the DFI ($R^2 = 0.33$) during the chemical treatment of the mushroom material. Lower *T* assure lower amounts of protein in the DFI. This higher recovery of protein in the ingredient with increasing *T* was probably due to the denaturation of protein during the treatment in alkaline solution [56], to the crosslinking of protein due to the hydrogen peroxide treatment [57] or due to the alkaline conditions employed leading to the formation of lysinoalanine crosslinks [58].

The fat recovered in the mushroom DFI varied between a minimum of 0.016% of the mushroom fresh weight, to 0.057%, representing between 4.9% and 17.4% of the original mushroom fat content. There is observed an increase in the amount of fat recovered in the DFI with the increasing *T* and increasing C_{NaOH} being observed a significant interaction between these two factors. This higher recovery of fat in the final product was probably due to the precipitation or adsorption of fatty acids released from triglycerides during the alkaline treatment, as also higher C_{NaOH} and increasing *T* resulted in higher amounts of fat recovered.

The caloric values were calculated for each mushroom DFI produced under the different conditions employed and ranged from 261 to 316 kcal on a dry basis (Table 1). As can be observed, and as expected, the DFI with a higher amount of dietary fiber presented the lower caloric values.

3.5. Colour of Mushroom DFI

The mushroom DFI presented a white/yellowish color depending on the treatment conditions (Table 4).

Table 4. Yield, water and oil retention capacity and color parameters [a] obtained for the different runs used for the optimization process.

Run	L*	a*	b*	Water Retention Capacity	Oil Retention Capacity
1	91.0	−0.113	11.39	15.2	11.3
2	89.3	0.320	15.71	18.5	12.0
3	82.1	1.100	17.68	18.5	11.3
4	90.6	−0.470	13.41	21.3	18.9
5	87.4	0.337	18.49	16.3	15.7
6	90.5	−0.467	18.88	8.5	7.8
7	90.3	−0.360	15.24	11.3	10.8
8	75.8	2.930	17.75	9.3	7.0
9	86.9	0.787	21.52	11.4	12.6
10	84.7	1.517	20.37	9.9	10.4
11	81.3	1.037	20.18	11.5	11.5
12	81.0	2.507	22.95	9.2	8.4
13	93.8	−2.623	16.37	10.6	7.4
14	88.2	−0.080	22.72	9.6	7.8
15	89.4	−0.497	22.94	5.9	7.7
16	88.9	−0.677	23.61	4.2	7.7
17	91.9	−0.224	22.34	5.7	7.9
18	89.5	−0.304	22.61	4.7	6.0
19	88.8	−0.273	22.52	6.2	6.9
20	89.1	−0.443	23.51	8.8	6.1

[a] L* defines lightness, a* denotes the red (+)/green (−) value and b* the yellow (+)/blue (−) value.

In theory, the perfect colorless white (white point) has the values L* = 100, a* = 0, b* = 0, therefore, processing conditions rendering DFI with values close to these theoretical values will allow to obtain DFI with a white color. Lightness (L*) was significantly affected by the three factors, being also observed a significant interaction between *T* and $C_{H_2O_2}$ and between $C_{H_2O_2}$ and C_{NaOH} (Table 2). Taking all these effects into account, for obtaining a DFI with a high L* value, the optimum $C_{H_2O_2}$. level is 0 and aiming having a DFI with higher fiber values (Section 3.2), the C_{NaOH} level should be 1.682 and the level for the treatment time factor should be −1 (predicted L* = 103.79; 88.90 to 118.18). For the a* value (red-green coordinate of the color space), all factors, either linear or quadratic effects were significant. In addition, there was observed a significant interaction between all factors (Table 2). There are several combinations of independent variables (T, $C_{H_2O_2}$, C_{NaOH}) that allow to obtain the desired value of a* = 0 as there is observed a significant interaction between all factors (Table 2). Optimum values for a* for factor $T - 1$, important for obtaining high fiber percentage in the DFI, can be obtained with the following combination: levels of $C_{H_2O_2}$ of 1 and of C_{NaOH} of 1 (predicted a* value of 0.785 and prediction interval of −5.760 to 7.330). For the b* value (yellow-blue coordinate of the color space), the linear terms of T and C_{NaOH} and all quadratic terms of the factors had a significant effect (Table 2). Additionally, there was observed a significant interaction between T and $C_{H_2O_2}$ and $C_{H_2O_2}$ and C_{NaOH} (Table 2). For the desired value of b*, all factors should remain at the lower level yielding a b* value of 0.131 (95% prediction interval of −2.814 to 3.076). These results show that the method developed allowed us to obtain a DFI with desirable neutral color values for their application as a food ingredient (Figure 3).

3.6. Mushroom DFI Water and Oil Retention Capacity

The water retention capacity (WRC) of mushroom DFI is shown in Table 4. WRC ranged from a minimum of 4.2 g water/g of DFI to a maximum of 21.3 g water/g of DFI. The highest WRC values obtained for the mushroom DFI are higher than that obtained for dietary fiber concentrates obtained from orange, peach, artichoke and asparagus, mango peel, sugar beet (10–14 g/g), apple and pear (6–7 g/g) and much higher than that observed for wheat and oat bran, carrot, and pea dietary fiber concentrates (3–4 g/g) [59–61] and in the range of that observed for potato fiber (23–25 g/g) [62]. As can be observed in Figure 4a, the WRC of the mushroom DFI was strongly dependent on T, being observed a decrease in the WRC with increasing T, whatever the $C_{H_2O_2}$.

For the $C_{H_2O_2}$ there was observed a minimum for the WRC at the central value of this factor, with lower and higher levels showing a positive effect in the WRC of the DFI. For the C_{NaOH} there were observed to different situations (Figure 4b), for lower treatment times there was observed an increase in the WRC with increasing C_{NaOH}, the reverse was true for higher treatment times. Keeping the level of factor T at the minimum, the effect of C_{NaOH} on the WRC of DFI was much more important than the $C_{H_2O_2}$ (Figure 4c). Whatever the $C_{H_2O_2}$ the higher WRC was observed for the higher C_{NaOH}. For a higher WRC of the DFI the optimum $C_{H_2O_2}$ level was 1.682, the C_{NaOH} level should be 1.682 and the level for factor T should be −1.682 (predicted WRC of 36.0 g/g of DFI with a 95% prediction interval of 29.6 to 42.4 g/g).

The oil retention capacity (ORC) of mushroom DFI is shown in Table 4. ORC varied from a minimum of 6.0 g oil/g of DFI to a maximum of 18.9 g oil/g of DFI. The ORC values obtained for the mushroom DFI were higher than that obtained for dietary fiber concentrates obtained from apple, pea, wheat, carrot (1–2.3 g/g) and sugar beet (5 g/g) [59], apple pomace and citrus by-products (0.6–1.8 mL oil/g) [63], unripe banana flour (~2 mL oil/g) [64]; carrot pulp dried at 50 °C (~6 mL oil/g) [65] and asparagus by-products (5.5–8.5 mL oil/g) [66]. As can be observed in Figure 5a, the ORC of the mushroom DFI was strongly dependent on the $C_{H_2O_2}$ and T, being observed the higher value of ORC for lower T and higher $C_{H_2O_2}$.

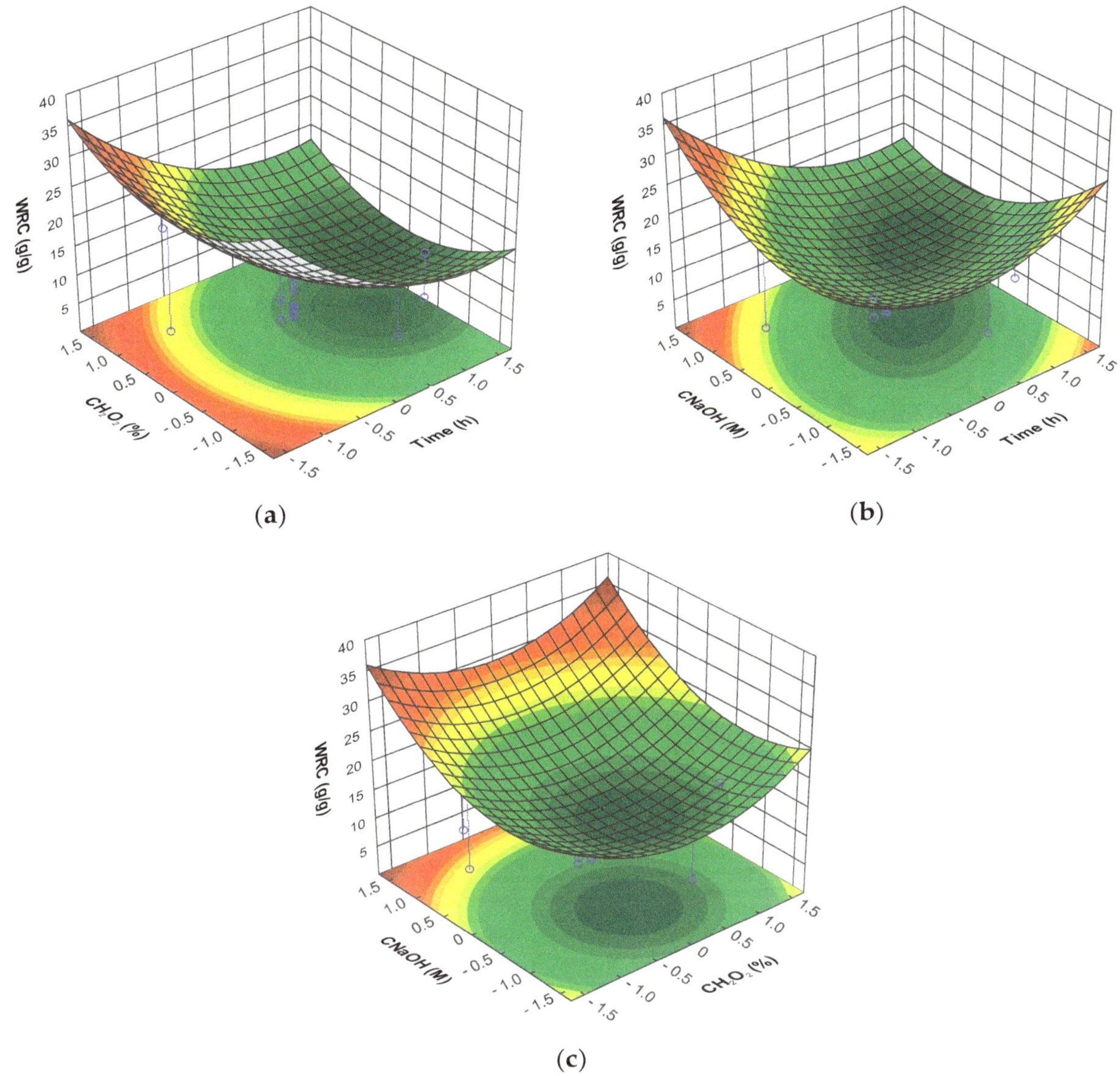

Figure 4. Response surfaces for mushroom DFI water retention capacity (WRC) as a function of: (**a**) time and hydrogen peroxide concentration (at sodium hydroxide concentration level of 1.682); (**b**) time and sodium hydroxide concentration (at hydrogen peroxide concentration level of 1.682); (**c**) hydrogen peroxide concentration and sodium hydroxide concentration (at time level of −1.682).

The same effect was observed for factor C_{NaOH}, for lower T there was observed an increase in the ORC with increasing C_{NaOH}, the reverse was true for high T (Figure 5b). When the effect of the factors C_{NaOH} and $C_{H_2O_2}$ are represented, there was observed that the maximum ORC was obtained or for high C_{NaOH} and $C_{H_2O_2}$ when the treatment time was at the lower level (Figure 5c) the reversed being observed for longer treatment times (result not showed). Using the factor levels where the maximum value is observed ($T = -1.682$; $C_{H_2O_2}$ and $C_{NaOH} = 1.682$) the predicted value of ORC of the DFI is 35.8 g/g of DFI (95% prediction interval between 30.8 to 40.8 g/g).

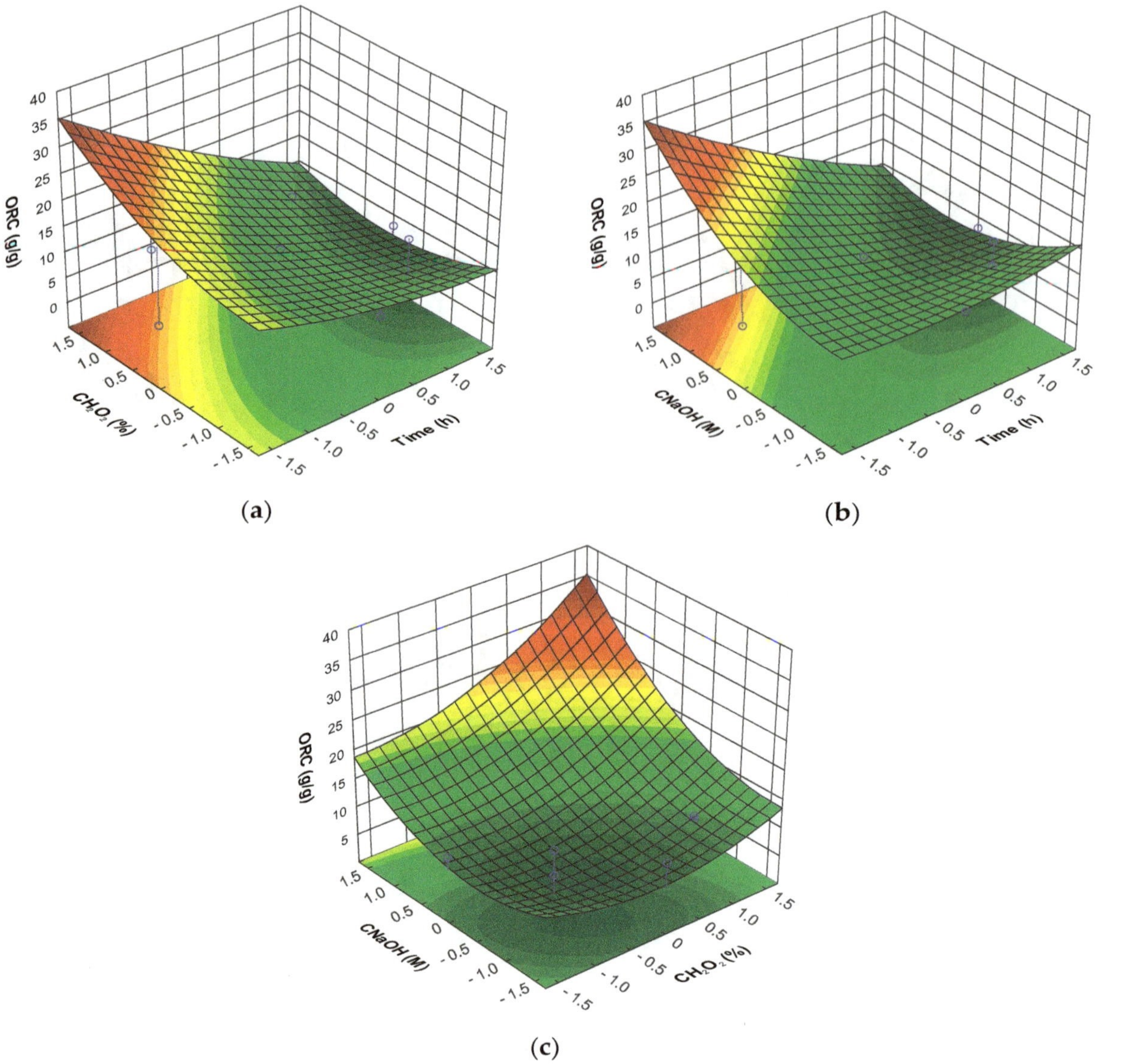

Figure 5. Response surfaces for mushroom DFI oil retention capacity (ORC) as a function of: (**a**) time and hydrogen peroxide concentration (at sodium hydroxide concentration level of 1.682); (**b**) time and sodium hydroxide concentration (at hydrogen peroxide concentration level of 1.682); (**c**) hydrogen peroxide concentration and sodium hydroxide concentration (at time level of −1.682).

3.7. *Effect of Mushroom DFI Chemical Composition on the Colour and Functional Properties*

To understand the effect of the chemical composition of the mushroom DFI obtained under the different processing conditions on the color and functional properties of mushroom DFI, the data obtained was analyzed by principal component analysis (PCA). The first three principal components obtained explained >70% of the total variance in the original data set. The loadings express how well the new PCs correlate with the original variables (Figure 6a and Table 2). The first PC, which explains 44.4% of the total variance, correlates positively with total fiber, glucosamine, glucose, xylose, WRC and ORC and negatively with protein and the b* value. The second PC, which explains 14.6% of the total variance, correlates positively with galacturonic acid content and negatively with glucuronic acid content, and PC3, which explains 13.5% of the total variance correlates positively with the a* value and negatively with lightness (L*). These results show that the WRC and ORC of the DFI are correlated with the total sugar content of the DFI (Figure 6a) and the b* value, related to the yellowness of the DFI is correlated with its protein content.

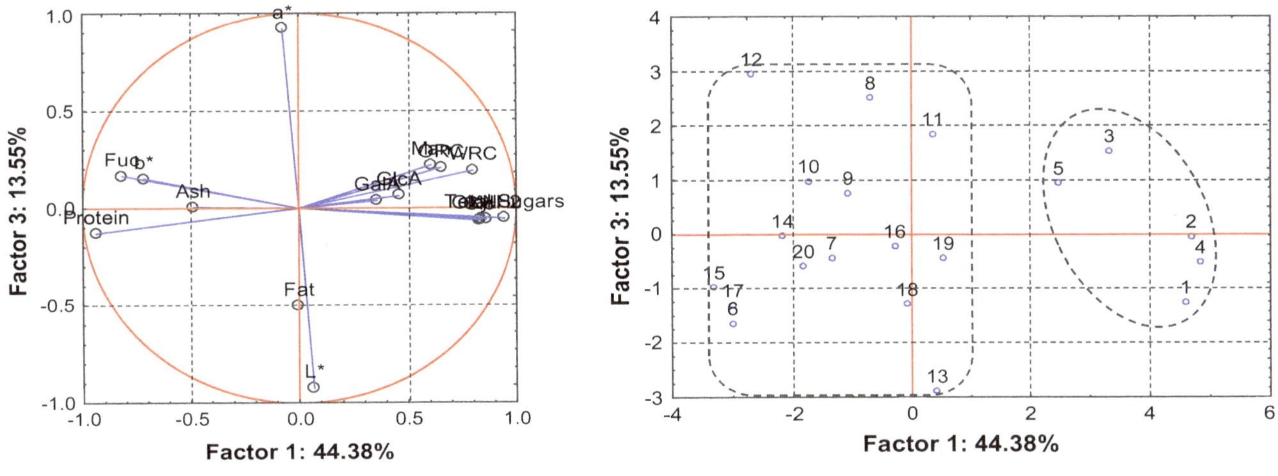

(a) (b)

Figure 6. (**a**) Factor loading plot based on correlations of the mushroom DFI chemical composition, color characteristics and functional properties projected on the space of PC1 vs. PC3; (**b**) scores plot of the mushroom DFI samples projected on the space of PC1 vs. PC3.

The scatter plot of the sample scores on the PC1 and PC3 scores (Figure 6b) shows the formation of two distinct clusters along the PC1. Samples with positive PC1 scores have a high relative content of total sugars and also a high WRC and low protein content and were less yellow, the opposite being true for the samples with negative PC1 scores. The WRC of dietary fibers is dependent on its structure [62,67] and chemical composition [68,69]. The water retained by dietary fiber material generally comprise three types of water, retained by three mechanisms: water bound by the hydrophilic polysaccharides of the fiber, dependent on the chemical composition of the fiber; water held by the fiber in the fiber matrix, mainly dependent on the pore size distribution of the fiber matrix; and water associated with fiber other than bound or matrix water, trapped within the cell wall lumen, dependent on the fiber source, method of preparation and method of measurement. Contrarily the ORC is in part related to its chemical composition but is more largely a function of the porosity of the fiber structure rather than the affinity of the fiber molecule for oil [70].

Samples with high scores on PC3 contain a relatively high a* value and lower L* value. As can be observed in Figure 6b, the group composed by the samples with a high PC1 score, corresponding to the DFI resulting from the 5 first treatments applied, are subdivided according to PC3 forming two groups, samples 3 and 5 contain a higher a* and lower L* values when compared to samples 1, 2 and 4.

4. Discussion

The production of a DFI from *A. bisporus* by-products, besides being a good strategy to reduce wastes generated in the mushroom agro-industry, can yield a DFI that besides having prebiotic activity [19,21,22] can also present a range of other very interesting biological activities. Several studies have shown that *A. bisporus* polysaccharides show immunostimulatory [71–74], antioxidant [74,75], antitumor [76–78], anti-inflammatory [7,79] and anti-sepsis activities [80], as well as antinociceptive inhibition [7,80]. The method developed allowed to concentrate the *A. bisporus* fiber polysaccharides up to 2.9 times, with a chemical composition similar to the initial cell wall, and so the biological activities of these polysaccharides are expected to be enhanced due to the concentration observed during the production process. In addition, it is expected that the original CGC present in *A. bisporus* cell walls is maintained [27,48,49]. CGC has been shown beneficial effects concerning the development of obesity and associated metabolic diabetes and hepatic steatosis, through a mechanism related to the restoration of the composition and/or the activity of gut bacteria, namely, bacteria from clostridial cluster XIVa [81]. Furthermore, CGC has potential beneficial effects concerning the development of atherosclerosis, mainly related to improving the antioxidant status [11,12]. On the other hand, chitin consumption can reduce triglyceride and cholesterol levels in liver and increase excretion of triglycerides in feces [13] and reduce cholesterol levels [14], and linear β-(1$\rightarrow$3)-glucans have shown hypoglycemic activity accompanied by promotion of metabolism and inhibition of inflammation, through suppressing SGLT-1 expression and possibly associated with alteration of gut microbiota [15]. Nevertheless, to be acceptable, a DFI added to a food product must perform in a satisfactorily as a food ingredient [82], namely be bland in taste, color, and odor. Besides the well-established nutritional benefits of adding dietary fiber ingredients to food products, the use of DFI can also have important technological advantages [59]. Of the various technological benefits, the increases in the water retention capacity (WRC) and oil retention capacity (ORC) of foods are one of the main advantages of using DFIs [59,83]. Both WRC and ORC can increase the technological yield of food. WRC of DFIs can be advantageous in sauces and soups, but also for their textural properties, enhancing the flow properties and avoiding lump formation in powdered mixes (e.g., ready-to-eat sauces, mixes of spices, flavoring agents). ORC can be exploited in foods (cooked meat products) to enhance their retention of fat that is normally lost during cooking, being also beneficial for flavor retention [59]. The WRC can have a nutritional interest as well, as increase in water retention has been related to an increase in orocaecal transit time. The water-holding capacity of dietary fiber has been proposed to be valuable in the diet to alter stool bulking [84]. Increased stool weight can cause shorter gut transit times limiting the exposure of the gut to secondary bile acids and other toxins [85,86].

The use of a sodium hydroxide concentration of 0.419 mol/L and hydrogen peroxide of 3.9% during 2.81 h, at room temperature, allow to obtain the highest yield of DFI (1.22% in relation to the fresh weight) with one of the highest dietary fiber (63.7 g/100 g) and lower protein (12.0 g/100 g) contents and highest WRC (21.3 g/g of DFI) and ORC (18.9 g/f of DFI). In addition, the chromatic characteristics of the DFI obtained show that it has a good lightness ($L^* = 90.6$) and neutral (white) color ($a^* = -0.470$ and $b^* = 13.71$).

The by-products of *A. bisporus* production can be successfully used for the production of a DFI using a simple method at room temperature and using food-grade materials, being a good strategy to reduce wastes in the mushroom agro-industry. Due to the simplicity and the efficiency shown in the production of *A. bisporus* DFI, there are no anticipated problems in applying this technology to other abundant mushrooms wastes as those derived from the production of *Lentinus edodes* and the oyster mushroom (*Pleurotus ostreatus*).

Author Contributions: Conceptualization, F.M.N.; investigation, S.M.F.; resources, F.M.N.; writing—original draft preparation, F.M.N.; writing—review and editing, F.M.N. and S.M.F.; supervision, F.M.N.; project administration, F.M.N.; funding acquisition, F.M.N. All authors have read and agreed to the published version of the manuscript.

Acknowledgments: The authors would like to acknowledge to João Coutinho for the nitrogen analysis.

Appendix A

Table A1. Regression equation coefficients for response parameters of mushrooms DFI.

Dependent Variable	Equation [1]	R^2	R^2Adj
DFI Yield	$Y = -1.937 + 0.391X_1 + 0.166X_2 - 0.130X_2^2 + 0.112X_3 - 0.119X_3^2 + 0.170X_1X_3$	0.647	0.483
Protein Yield	$Y = -0.528 + 0.177X_1$	0.339	0.303
Fat Yield	$Y = -0.035 - 0.0066X_1 - 0.0031X_2^2 - 0.005X_1X_3$	0.515	0.424
L*	$Y = 90.20 - 0.92X_1 - 1.13X_1^2 - 1.46X_2 - 2.78X_2^2 - 1.02X_3 - 2.27X_1X_3$	0.596	0.409
a*	$Y = -0.397 + 0.207X_1 + 0.514X_1^2 + 0.410X_2 + 0.733X_2^2 + 0.412X_3 - 0.371X_3^2 + 0.285X_1X_2 + 0.453X_1X_3 + 0.261X_2X_3$	0.785	0.592
b*	$Y = 23.07 + 0.749X_1 - 1.646X_1^2 - 1.425X_2^2 + 1.000X_3 - 2.140X_3^2 - 1.004X_1X_2 - 0.810X_2X_3$	0.588	0.348
WRC	$Y = 5.784 - 2.229X_1 + 2.566X_1^2 + 2.467X_2^2 + 2.377X_3^2 - 1.996X_1X_3$	0.714	0.612
ORC	$Y = 6.989 - 1.174X_1 + 1.985X_1^2 + 1.449X_2^2 + 0.609X_3^2 - 1.580X_1X_2 - 2.489X_1X_3 + 1.379X_2X_3$	0.875	0.801

[1] X_1 = Time; $X_2 = C_{H_2O_2}$; $X_3 = C_{NaOH}$.

Table 2. Factor-variable correlations (factor loadings), based on correlations.

	Factor 1	Factor 2	Factor 3
Total Sugars	0.946	−0.167	−0.054
GlcNH2	0.861	0.326	−0.059
Glc	0.825	−0.463	−0.065
Xyl	0.837	0.376	−0.061
Man	0.607	0.551	0.219
GalA	0.358	0.686	0.037
GlcA	0.458	−0.801	0.063
Fuc	−0.819	0.213	0.166
Fat	−0.000	−0.284	−0.501
Ash	−0.484	−0.383	0.004
Protein	−0.938	0.002	−0.129
WRC	0.801	−0.030	0.192
ORC	0.652	−0.083	0.205
L*	0.068	0.090	−0.924
a*	−0.072	−0.226	0.922
b*	−0.717	0.311	0.151

References

1. Chang, S.T. World production of edible and medicinal mushrooms in 1997 with emphasis on *Lentinus edods* (Berk). Sing. in China. *Int. J. Med. Mushrooms* **1999**, *1*, 291–301. [CrossRef]
2. Chakravarty, B. Trends in mushroom cultivation and breeding. *Aust. J. Agric. Eng.* **2011**, *2*, 102–109.
3. Wani, B.A.; Bodha, R.H.; Wani, A.H. Nutritional and medicinal importance of mushrooms. *J. Med. Plants Res.* **2010**, *4*, 2598–2604. [CrossRef]
4. Kalač, P. A review of chemical composition and nutritional value of wild-growing and cultivated mushrooms. *J. Sci. Food Agric.* **2013**, *93*, 209–218. [CrossRef]
5. Carbonero, E.R.; Gracher, A.H.P.; Komura, D.L.; Marcon, R.; Freitas, C.S.; Baggio, C.H.; Santos, A.R.S.; Torri, G.; Gorin, P.A.J.; Iacomini, M. *Lentinus edodes* heterogalactan: Antinociceptive and anti-inflammatory effects. *Food Chem.* **2008**, *111*, 531–537. [CrossRef]
6. Chang, C.-W.; Lur, H.-S.; Lu, M.-K.; Cheng, J.-J. Sulfated polysaccharides of *Armillariella mellea* and their anti-inflammatory activities via NF-κB suppression. *Food Res. Int.* **2013**, *54*, 239–245. [CrossRef]
7. Komura, D.L.; Carbonero, E.R.; Gracher, A.H.P.; Baggio, C.H.; Freitas, C.S.; Marcon, R. Structure of *Agaricus* spp. fucogalactans and their anti-inflammatory and antinociceptive properties. *Bioresour. Technol.* **2010**, *101*, 6192–6199. [CrossRef]
8. Lindequist, U.; Niedermeyer, T.H.J.; Jülich, W.-D. The pharmacological potential of mushrooms. *Evid. Based Complement. Altern. Med.* **2005**, *2*, 285–299. [CrossRef]
9. Wessels, G.H. Developmental regulation of fungal cell wall formation. *Annu. Rev. Phytopathol.* **1994**, *32*, 413–437. [CrossRef]
10. Michalenko, G.O.; Hohl, H.R.; Rast, D. Chemistry and Architecture of the Mycelial Wall of *Agaricus bisporus*. *J. Gen. Microbiol.* **1976**, *92*, 251–256. [CrossRef]
11. Berecochea-Lopez, A.; Decordé, K.; Ventura, E.; Godard, M.; Bornet, A.; Teissèdre, P.L.; Cristol, J.P.; Rouanet, J.M. Fungal chitin-glucan from *Aspergillus niger* efficiently reduces aortic fatty streak accumulation in the high-fat fed hamster, an animal model of nutritionally induced atherosclerosis. *J. Agric. Food Chem.* **2009**, *57*, 1093–1098. [CrossRef] [PubMed]
12. Bays, H.E.; Evans, J.L.; Maki, K.C.; Evans, M.; Maquet, V.; Cooper, R.; Anderson, J.W. Chitin-glucan fiber effects on oxidized low-density lipoprotein: A randomized controlled trial. *Eur. J. Clin. Nutr.* **2013**, *67*, 2–7. [CrossRef] [PubMed]
13. Zacour, A.C.; Silva, M.E.; Cecon, P.R.; Bambirra, E.A.; Vieira, E.C. Effect of dietary chitin on cholesterol absorption and metabolism in rats. *J. Nutr. Sci. Vitaminol.* **1992**, *38*, 609–613. [CrossRef] [PubMed]
14. Mathew, P.T.; Ramachandran-Nair, K.G. Hyphocholesterolemic effect of chitin and its hydrolysed products in albino rats. *Fish. Technol.* **1998**, *35*, 46–49.

15. Cao, Y.; Zou, S.; Xu, H.; Li, M.; Tong, Z.; Xu, M.; Xu, X. Hypoglycemic activity of the Baker's yeast β-glucan in obese/type 2 diabetic mice and the underlying mechanism. *Mol. Nutr. Food Res.* **2016**, *60*, 2678–2690. [CrossRef]
16. Synytsya, A.; Míčková, K.; Synytsya, A.; Jablonský, I.; Spěváček, J.; Erban, V.; Kováříková, E.; Čopíková, J. Glucans from fruit bodies of cultivated mushrooms *Pleurotus ostreatus* and *Pleurotus eryngii*: Structure and potential prebiotic activity. *Carbohydr. Polym.* **2009**, *76*, 548–556. [CrossRef]
17. Xu, X.; Yang, J.; Ning, Z.; Zhang, X. *Lentinula edodes*-derived polysaccharide rejuvenates mice in terms of immune responses and gut microbiota. *Food Funct.* **2015**, *6*, 2653–2663. [CrossRef]
18. Xu, X.; Zhang, X. *Lentinula edodes*-derived polysaccharide alters the spatial structure of gut microbiota in mice. *PLoS ONE* **2015**, *10*, e0115037. [CrossRef]
19. Giannenas, I.; Tsalie, E.; Chronis, E.F.; Mavridis, S.; Tontis, D.; Kyriazakis, I. Consumption of *Agaricus bisporus* mushroom affects the performance, intestinal microbiota composition and morphology and antioxidant status of turkey poults. *Anim. Feed Sci. Technol.* **2011**, *165*, 218–229. [CrossRef]
20. Pallav, K.; Dowd, S.E.; Villafuerte, J.; Yang, X.; Kabbani, T.; Hansen, J.; Dennis, M.; Leffler, D.A.; Newburg, D.S.; Kelly, C.P. Effects of polysaccharopeptide from *Trametes versicolor* and amoxicillin on the gut microbiome of healthy volunteers A randomized clinical trial. *Gut Microbes* **2014**, *5*, 458–467. [CrossRef]
21. Zhao, J.; Cheung, P.C.K. Fermentation of β-Glucans derived from different sources by bifidobacteria: Evaluation of their bifidogenic effect. *J. Agric. Food Chem.* **2011**, *59*, 5986–5992. [CrossRef] [PubMed]
22. Rodrigues, D.; Walton, G.; Sousa, S.; Rocha-Santos, T.A.P.; Duarte, A.C.; Freitas, A.C.; Gomes, A.M.P. In vitro fermentation and prebiotic potential of selected extracts from seaweeds and mushrooms. *LWT Food Sci. Technol.* **2016**, *73*, 131–139. [CrossRef]
23. Zivanovic, S. Identification of Opportunities for Production of Ingredients Based on Further Processed Fresh Mushrooms, Off-Grade Mushrooms, By-Products, and Waste Materials. Project Report Prepared for Mushroom Council. Available online: http://mushroomcouncil.org/wp-content/uploads/2012/02/2006_09IndustryReport.pdf (accessed on 20 December 2012).
24. Wani, A.M.; Hussain, P.R.; Meena, R.S.; Dar, M.A.; Mir, M.A. Effect of gamma irradiation and sulphitation treatments on keeping quality of white button mushroom *Agaricus bisporus* (J. Lge). *Int. J. Food Sci. Technol.* **2009**, *44*, 967–973. [CrossRef]
25. Jolivet, S.; Arpin, N.; Wichers, H.J.; Pellon, G. *Agaricus bisporus* browning: A review. *Mycol. Res.* **1998**, *102*, 1459–1483. [CrossRef]
26. European Commission. *The European Regulation of Waste Management, Directive 2008/98/ EC ('Waste Framework Directive')*; European Commission: Brussels, Belgium, 2008.
27. Wu, T.; Zivanovic, S.; Draughon, F.A.; Sams, C.E. Chitin and Chitosan Value-Added Products from Mushroom Waste. *J. Agric. Food Chem.* **2004**, *52*, 7905–7910. [CrossRef]
28. Dallies, N.; Francois, J.; Paquet, V. A new method for quantitative determination of polysaccharides in the yeast cell wall. Application to the cell wall defective mutants of *Saccharomyces cerevisiae*. *Yeast* **1998**, *14*, 1297–1306. [CrossRef]
29. Aguilar-Uscanga, B.; Francois, J.M. A study of the yeast cell wall composition and structure in response to growth conditions and mode of cultivation. *Lett. Appl. Microbiol.* **2003**, *37*, 268–274. [CrossRef]
30. Baker, L.G.; Specht, C.A.; Donlin, M.J.; Lodge, J.K. Chitosan, the deacetylated form of chitin, is necessary for cell wall integrity in *Cryptococcus neoformans*. *Eukaryot. Cell* **2007**, *6*, 855–867. [CrossRef]
31. Roca, C.; Chagas, B.; Farinha, I.; Freitas, F.; Mafra, L.; Aguiar, F.; Oliveira, R.; Reis, M.A.M. Production of yeast chitin–glucan complex from biodiesel industry byproduct. *Process Biochem.* **2012**, *47*, 1670–1675. [CrossRef]
32. Ivshin, V.P.; Artamonova, S.D.; Ivshina, T.N.; Sharnina, F.F. Methods for isolation of chitin-glucan complexes from higher fungi native biomass. *Polym. Sci. Ser. B* **2007**, *49*, 305–310. [CrossRef]
33. Rodríguez, R.; Jiménez, A.; Fernández-Bolaños, J.; Guillén, R.; Heredia, A. Dietary fibre from vegetable products as source of functional ingredients. *Trends Food Sci. Technol.* **2006**, *17*, 3–15. [CrossRef]
34. Guillon, F.; Champ, M. Structural and physical properties of dietary fibres, and consequences of processing on human physiology. *Food Res. Int.* **2000**, *33*, 233–245. [CrossRef]
35. Englyst, H.N.; Wiggims, H.S.; Cummings, J.H. Determination of the non-starch polysaccharides in plant foods by gas-liquid chromatography of constituent sugars as alditol acetates. *Analyst* **1982**, *107*, 307–318. [CrossRef] [PubMed]

36. Englyst, H.N.; Hudson, G.J. The classification and measurement of dietary carbohydrates. *Food Chem.* **1996**, *57*, 15–21. [CrossRef]
37. Abraão, A.S.; Lemos, A.M.; Vilela, A.; Sousa, J.M.; Nunes, F.M. Influence of osmotic dehydration process parameters on the quality of candied pumpkins. *Food Bioprod. Process.* **2013**, *91*, 481–494. [CrossRef]
38. AOAC. *Official Methods of Analysis*, 15th ed.; AOAC International: Arlington, VA, USA, 1996.
39. Buchholz, A.C.; Schoeller, D.A. Is a calorie a calorie? *Am. J. Clin. Nutr.* **2004**, *79*, 899S–906S. [CrossRef]
40. Robertson, J.A.; de Monredon, F.D.; Dysseler, P.; Guillon, F.; Amado, R.; Thibault, J.-T. Hydration properties of dietary fibre and resistant starch: A European collaborative study. *LWT Food Sci. Technol.* **2000**, *33*, 72–79. [CrossRef]
41. Box, G.E.P.; Wilson, K.B. On the experimental attainment of optimum conditions. *J. R. Stat. Soc. Ser. B* **1951**, *13*, 1–45. [CrossRef]
42. Montgomery, D.C. *Introduction to Statistical Quality Control*, 3rd ed.; John Wiley and Sons, Inc.: New York, NY, USA, 1996.
43. Vandeginste, B.G.; Massart, L.; Buydens, L.M.; De Jong, S.; Lewi, P.J.; Smeyers-Verbeke, J. *Handbook of Chemometrics and Qualimetrics*; Elsevier: Amsterdam, The Netherlands, 1998.
44. Massiot, P.; Renard, C.M.G.C. Composition, physicochemical properties and enzymatic degradation of fibers prepared from different tissues of apple. *LWT Food Sci. Technol.* **1997**, *30*, 800–806. [CrossRef]
45. Thomas, M.; Crepeau, M.J.; Rumpunen, K.; Thibault, J.-F. Dietary fiber and cell-wall polysaccharides in the fruits of Japanese quince (*Chaenomeles japonica*). *LWT Food Sci. Technol.* **2000**, *33*, 124–131. [CrossRef]
46. Wong, K.H.; Cheung, P.C. Dietary fibers from mushroom sclerotia: 1. Preparation and physicochemical and functional properties. *J. Agric. Food Chem.* **2005**, *53*, 9395–9400. [CrossRef] [PubMed]
47. FAO/WHO. Joint FAO/WHO food standards programme. In *Report of the 30th Session of the Codex Committee on Nutrition and Foods for Special Dietary Uses, Proceedings of the Codex Alimentarius Commission 32nd Session, Rome, Italy, 29 June–4 July 2009*; ALINORM 09/332/26, Part B Provisions on Dietary Fibre; FAO/WHO: Rome, Italy, 2009.
48. Bernardo, D.; Mendoza, C.G.; Calonje, M.; Novaes-Ledieu, M. Chemical analysis of the lamella walls of *Agaricus bisporus* fruit bodies. *Curr. Microbiol.* **1999**, *38*, 364–367. [CrossRef] [PubMed]
49. Novaes-Ledieu, M.; Mendoza, G.C. The cell walls of *Agaricus bisporus* and *Agaricus campestris* fruiting body hyphae. *Can. J. Microbiol.* **1981**, *27*, 779–787. [CrossRef] [PubMed]
50. Focher, B.; Najji, A.; Torri, G.; Cosani, A.; Terbojevich, M. Structural differences between chitin polymorphs and their precipitates from solutions-evidence from CP-MAS ^{13}C NMR, FT-IR and FT-Raman spectroscopy. *Carbohydr. Res.* **1992**, *17*, 97–102. [CrossRef]
51. Kumirska, J.; Czerwicka, M.; Kaczyński, Z.; Bychowska, A.; Brzozowski, K.; Thöming, J.; Stepnowski, P. Application of spectroscopic methods for structural analysis of chitin and chitosan. *Mar. Drugs* **2010**, *8*, 1567–1636. [CrossRef]
52. Cheung, P.C.-K. Dietary fibre content and composition of some edible fungi determined by two methods of analysis. *J. Sci. Food Agric.* **1997**, *73*, 255–260. [CrossRef]
53. Hammond, J.B.W. Changes in composition of harvested mushrooms (*Agaricus bisporus*). *Phytochemistry* **1979**, *18*, 415–418. [CrossRef]
54. Ramírez, L.; Muez, V.; Alfonso, M.; Barrenechea, A.G.; Alfonso, L.; Pisabarro, A.G. Use of molecular markers to differentiate between commercial strains of the button mushroom *Agaricus bisporus*. *FEMS Microbiol. Lett.* **2001**, *198*, 45–48. [CrossRef]
55. Vetter, J. Chitin content of cultivated mushrooms *Agaricus bisporus*, *Pleurotus ostreatus* and *Lentinula edodes*. *Food Chem.* **2007**, *102*, 6–9. [CrossRef]
56. Monahan, F.J.; German, J.B.; Kinsella, J.E. Effect of pH and temperature on protein unfolding and thiol/disulfide interchange reactions during heat-induced gelation of whey proteins. *J. Agric. Food Chem.* **1995**, *43*, 46–52. [CrossRef]
57. Rice, R.H.; Lee, Y.M.; Brown, W.D. Interactions of heme proteins with hydrogen peroxide: Protein crosslinking and covalent binding of benzo[a]pyrene and 17P-estradiol. *Arch. Biochem. Biophys.* **1983**, *221*, 417–427. [CrossRef]
58. Friedman, M. Chemistry, biochemistry, nutrition, and microbiology of lysinoalanine, lanthionine, and histidinoalanine in food and other proteins. *J. Agric. Food Chem.* **1999**, *47*, 1295–1319. [CrossRef] [PubMed]

59. Thebaudin, J.Y.; Lefebvre, A.C.; Harrington, M.; Bourgeois, C.M. Dietary fibres: Nutritional and technological interest. *Trends Food Sci. Technol.* **1997**, *8*, 41–48. [CrossRef]
60. Grigelmo-Miguel, N.; Martin-Belloso, O. Comparison of dietary fibre from by-products of processing fruits and greens and from cereals. *LWT Food Sci. Technol.* **1999**, *32*, 503–508. [CrossRef]
61. Larrauri, J.A.; Rupérez, P.; Borroto, B.; Saura-Calixto, F. Mango peels as a new tropical fibre: Preparation and characterization. *LWT Food Sci. Technol.* **1996**, *29*, 729–733. [CrossRef]
62. Robertson, J.A.; Eastwood, M.A. An examination of factors which may affect the water holding capacity of dietary fibre. *Br. J. Nutr.* **1981**, *45*, 83–88. [CrossRef]
63. Figuerola, F.; Hurtado, M.L.; Estévez, A.M.; Chiffelle, I.; Asenjo, F. Fibre concentrates from apple pomace and citrus peel as potential fibre sources for food enrichment. *Food Chem.* **2005**, *91*, 395–401. [CrossRef]
64. Rodríguez-Ambriz, S.L.; Islas-Hernández, J.J.; Agama-Acevedo, E.; Tovar, J.; Bello-Pérez, L.A. Characterization of a fibre-rich powder prepared by liquefaction of unripe banana flour. *Food Chem.* **2008**, *107*, 1515–1521. [CrossRef]
65. Garau, M.C.; Simal, S.; Rosselló, C.; Femenia, A. Effect of air drying temperature on physico-chemical properties of dietary fibre and antioxidant capacity of orange (*Citrus aurantium* v. Canoneta) by-products. *Food Chem.* **2007**, *104*, 1014–1024. [CrossRef]
66. Fuentes-Alventosa, J.M.; Rodríguez-Gutiérrez, G.; Jaramillo-Carmona, S.; Espejo-Calvo, J.A.; Rodríguez-Arcos, R.; Fernández-Bolaños, J.; Guillén-Bejarano, R.; Jiménez-Araujo, A. Effect of extraction method on chemical composition and functional characteristics of high dietary fibre powders obtained from asparagus by-products. *Food Chem.* **2009**, *113*, 665–671. [CrossRef]
67. Chaplin, M.F. Fibre and water binding. *Proc. Nutr. Soc.* **2003**, *62*, 223–227. [CrossRef] [PubMed]
68. Elhardallou, S.B.; Walker, A.F. The water-holding capacity of three starchy legumes in the raw, cooked and fibre-rich fraction forms. *Plant Food Hum. Nutr.* **1993**, *44*, 171–179. [CrossRef] [PubMed]
69. Chau, C.F.; Huang, Y.L. Comparison of the chemical composition and physicochemical properties of different fibers prepared from the peel of *Citrus sinensis* L. Cv. Liucheng. *J. Agric. Food Chem.* **2003**, *51*, 2615–2618. [CrossRef] [PubMed]
70. Biswas, A.K.; Kumar, V.; Bhosle, S.; Sahoo, J.; Chatli, M.K. Dietary fibers as functional ingredients in meat products and their role in human health. *Int. J. Livest. Prod.* **2011**, *2*, 45–54.
71. Volman, J.J.; Helsper, J.P.F.G.; Wei, S.; Baars, J.J.P.; van Griensven, L.J.L.D.; Sonnenberg, A.S.M.; Mensink, R.P.; Plat, J. Effects of mushroom-derived β-glucan-rich polysaccharide extracts on nitric oxide production by bone marrow-derived macrophages and nuclear factor-κB transactivation in Caco-2 reporter cells: Can effects be explained by structure? *Mol. Nutr. Food Res.* **2010**, *54*, 268–276. [CrossRef]
72. Smiderle, F.R.; Ruthes, A.C.; van Arkel, J.; Chanput, W.; Iacomini, M.; Wichers, H.J.; Van Griensven, L.J. Polysaccharides from *Agaricus bisporus* and *Agaricus brasiliensis* show similarities in their structures and their immunomodulatory effects on human monocytic THP-1 cells. *BMC Complement. Altern. Med.* **2011**, *11*, 58. [CrossRef]
73. Smiderle, F.R.; Alquini, G.; Tadra-Sfeir, M.Z.; Iacomini, M.; Wichers, H.J.; Van Griensven, L.J. *Agaricus bisporus* and *Agaricus brasiliensis* (1→6)-β-D-glucans show immunostimulatory activity on human THP-1 derived macrophages. *Carbohydr. Polym.* **2013**, *94*, 91–99. [CrossRef]
74. Kozarski, M.; Klaus, A.; Niksic, M.; Jakovljevic, D.; Helsper, J.P.F.G.; Van Griensven, L.J.L.D. Antioxidative and immunomodulating activities of polysaccharide extracts of the medicinal mushrooms *Agaricus bisporus*, *Agaricus brasiliensis*, *Ganoderma lucidum* and *Phellinus linteus*. *Food Chem.* **2011**, *129*, 1667–1675. [CrossRef]
75. Tian, Y.; Zeng, H.; Xu, Z.; Zheng, B.; Lin, Y.; Gan, C.; Lo, Y.M. Ultrasonic-assisted extraction and antioxidant activity of polysaccharides recovered from white button mushroom (*Agaricus bisporus*). *Carbohydr. Polym.* **2012**, *88*, 522–529. [CrossRef]
76. Jeong, S.C.; Koyyalamudi, S.R.; Jeong, Y.T.; Song, C.H.; Pang, G. Macrophage immunomodulating and antitumor activities of polysaccharides isolated from *Agaricus bisporus* white button mushrooms. *J. Med. Food* **2012**, *15*, 58–65. [CrossRef]
77. Pires, A.D.R.A.; Ruthes, A.C.; Cadena, S.M.; Acco, A.; Gorin, P.A.; Iacomini, M. Cytotoxic effect of *Agaricus bisporus* and *Lactarius rufus* β-D-glucans on HepG2 cells. *Int. J. Biol. Macromol.* **2013**, *58*, 95–103. [CrossRef] [PubMed]
78. Pires, A.D.R.A.; Ruthes, A.C.; Cadena, S.M.S.C.; Iacomini, M. Cytotoxic effect of a mannogalactoglucan extracted from Agaricus bisporus on HepG2 cells. *Carbohydr. Polym.* **2017**, *170*, 33–42. [CrossRef] [PubMed]

79. Ruthes, A.C.; Rattmann, Y.D.; Malquevicz-Paiva, S.M.; Carbonero, E.R.; Córdova, M.M.; Baggio, C.H.; Santos, A.R.; Gorin, P.A.; Iacomini, M. *Agaricus bisporus* fucogalactan: Structural characterization and pharmacological approaches. *Carbohydr. Polym.* **2013**, *92*, 184–191. [CrossRef] [PubMed]
80. Ruthes, A.C.; Rattmann, Y.D.; Carbonero, E.R.; Gorin, P.A.J.; Iacomini, M. Structural characterization and protective effect against murine sepsis of fucogalactans from *Agaricus bisporus* and *Lactarius rufus*. *Carbohydr. Polym.* **2012**, *87*, 1620–1627. [CrossRef]
81. Neyrinck, A.M.; Possemiers, S.; Verstraete, W.; De Backer, F.; Cani, P.D.; Delzenne, N.M. Dietary modulation of clostridial cluster XIVa gut bacteria (*Roseburia* spp.) by chitin-glucan fiber improves host metabolic alterations induced by high fat-diet in mice. *J. Nutr. Biochem.* **2012**, *23*, 51–59. [CrossRef]
82. Jaime, L.; Mollá, E.; Fernández, A.; Martín-Cabrejas, M.; López-Andréu, F.; Esteban, R. Structural carbohydrates differences and potential source of dietary fiber of onion (*Allium cepa* L.) tissues. *J. Agric. Food Chem.* **2000**, *50*, 122–128. [CrossRef]
83. Kethireddipalli, P.; Hung, Y.-C.; Phillips, R.O.; Mc Watters, K.H. Evaluating the role of cell material and soluble protein in the functionality of cowpea (*Vigna unguiculata*) pastes. *J. Food Sci.* **2002**, *67*, 53–59. [CrossRef]
84. Roehrig, K.L. The physiological effects of dietary fiber-a review. *Food Hydrocoll.* **1988**, *2*, 1–18. [CrossRef]
85. Faivre, J.; Doyon, F.; Boutron, M. The ECP calcium fibre polyp prevention study. The ECP colon group. *Eur. J. Cancer Prev.* **1993**, *2* (Suppl. 2), 99–106. [CrossRef]
86. Reddy, B.S.; Engle, A.; Katsifis, S.; Simi, B.; Bartram, H.P.; Perrino, P.; Mahan, C. Biochemical epidemiology of colon cancer: Effect of types of dietary fibre on fecal mutagens, acid and neutral sterols in healthy subjects. *Cancer Res.* **1989**, *49*, 4629–4635.

9

Eucalyptus globulus Essential Oil as a Natural Food Preservative: Antioxidant, Antibacterial and Antifungal Properties *In Vitro* and in a Real Food Matrix (Orangina Fruit Juice)

Mohamed Nadjib Boukhatem [1,2,*], Asma Boumaiza [2], Hanady G. Nada [1,3], Mehdi Rajabi [1] and Shaker A. Mousa [1,*]

[1] The Pharmaceutical Research Institute, Albany College of Pharmacy and Health Sciences, Rensselaer, NY 12144, USA; hanadynada@hotmail.com (H.G.N.); m.rajabi.s@gmail.com (M.R.)

[2] Département de Biologie et Physiologie Cellulaire, Faculté des Sciences de la Nature et de la Vie, Université–Saad Dahlab–Blida 1, BP 270, Route de Soumaa, Blida 9000, Algeria; boumaiza.asma@laposte.net

[3] Drug Radiation Research Department, National Center for Radiation Research and Technology (NCRRT), Atomic Energy Authority (AEA), Cairo 11762, Egypt

* Correspondence: mn.boukhatem@yahoo.fr (M.N.B.); shaker.mousa@acphs.edu (S.A.M.)

Abstract: The potential application of *Eucalyptus globulus* essential oil (EGEO) as a natural beverage preservative is described in this research. The chemical composition of EGEO was determined using gas chromatography analyses and revealed that the major constituent is 1,8-cineole (94.03% ± 0.23%). The *in vitro* antioxidant property of EGEO was assessed using different tests. Percentage inhibitions of EGEO were dose-dependent. In addition, EGEO had a better metal ion chelating effect with an IC_{50} value of 8.43 ± 0.03 mg/mL, compared to ascorbic acid (140.99 ± 3.13 mg/mL). The *in vitro* antimicrobial effect of EGEO was assessed against 17 food spoilage microorganisms. The diameter of the inhibitory zone (DIZ) ranged from 15 to 85 mm for Gram-positive bacteria and from 10 to 49 mm for yeast strains. *Candida albicans, C. parapsilosis* and *Saccharomyces cerevisiae* were the most sensitive fungal species to the EGEO vapor with DIZ varying from 59 to 85 mm. The anti-yeast effectiveness of EGEO alone and in association with heat processing was estimated in a real juice matrix (Orangina fruit juices) in a time-dependent manner. The combination of EGEO-heat treatment (70 °C for 2 min) at different concentrations (0.8 to 4 μL/mL) was effective at reducing *S. cerevisiae* growth in the fruit juice of Orangina, compared to juice preserved with synthetic preservatives. Current findings suggest EGEO as an effective and potent inhibitor of food spoilage fungi in a real Orangina juice, and might be a potential natural source of preservative for the food industry.

Keywords: natural food preservative; *Eucalyptus globulus* essential oil; eucalyptol; antioxidant effect; vapor phase; Orangina fruit juice

---

1. Introduction

Food spoilage by fungi, yeasts and bacteria is a major problem in food production, and it considerably impacts the price and availability of the food [1]. The use of synthetic and chemical antibacterial and antifungal compounds and food preservatives is considered as one of the ancient methods for reducing foodborne pathogens and contamination. The addition of synthetic antioxidant and antimicrobial food preservatives is an active way for storage to slow down food alteration and oxidation [2]. Nevertheless, due to increasing confirmation of the dangerous properties of synthetic food additives, there is constant pressure from consumers to decrease the quantity of these chemicals in food [3] and deliver minimally processed foodstuffs without compromising food preservation, safety and quality [4].

Thus, other sources of nontoxic, bioactive and suitable natural food preservatives need to be discovered and investigated, such as plant secondary metabolites, phytochemicals and volatile oils or essential oils (EOs). A new approach to prevent and avoid the proliferation of microorganisms or protect food from oxidation is the use of EOs as antifungal, antibacterial and antioxidant preservatives. The potential application of EOs as functional components in drinks and beverages is gaining force because of growing anxiety about possibly dangerous and toxic synthetic additives [5,6]. Within the context of the extensive variety of the aforementioned foodstuffs, a collective need is the accessibility of phytochemical extracts and EOs with an agreeable flavor or scent associated with a conserving effect and that can avoid lipid alteration, oxidation and contamination by food spoilage microorganisms and pathogens [7–9].

Therefore, there has been growing attention to the discovery and investigation of safe, effective and natural antioxidant bioactive molecules because they can defend the human body from free radicals and delay the development of several chronic or acute illnesses [10]. The antimicrobial molecules found in aromatic and medicinal plants are of interest because multidrug resistant bacteria are now becoming a global community health alarm, particularly in terms of foodborne infections and nosocomial contaminations [11–13]. Several studies have reported antiseptic, anti-inflammatory, wound-healing, analgesic, antioxidant and free radical-scavenging activities [14] from aromatic and medicinal plants, herbs, spices and EOs and, in most cases, a direct food-related application has been verified [15].

The *Eucalyptus* genus is a tall shrub belonging to the family of Myrtaceae. Although some papers about *Eucalyptus globulus* essential oils (EGEOs) have been done [16–20], only a limited of them estimated *Eucalyptus* oil's effect against pathogens and food spoilage species [7]. In spite of the well-reported *in vitro* antibacterial and antifungal effects, food manufacturing has used *Eucalyptus* EOs principally as flavoring agents. Consequently, the application of EOs and phytochemical extracts as natural food additives has been restricted [16].

Despite the great efficacy of EOs and their phytochemical compounds against food-related and spoilage pathogens with *in vitro* methods, a similar result in a food matrix is only accomplished with a greater dose of EOs [3]. This statement suggests a sensorial and organoleptic influence from changing the ordinary flavor of the food and beverages by surpassing suitable taste thresholds [7]. Therefore, to reduce the dose of EO in a real juice matrix, studies on the associated effect of EOs with traditional conservation methods such as heat processing are required. In the current research, the chemical composition of EGEO was analyzed with gas chromatography-mass spectrometry (GC-MS). Then, the *in vitro* antioxidant effect was carried out using DPPH radical scavenging and metal ion chelating activity. The inhibitory effects of Algerian EGEO against several food spoilage bacterial and fungal strains were assessed *in vitro* (disc diffusion and disc volatilization tests) and in a real food matrix (inhibition of *Saccharomyces cerevisiae* strain for the preservation of Orangina fruit juices) and stored at laboratory temperature for 6 days. Further, for reducing the dose of EGEO in the Orangina fruit juice, the associated effect of EGEO with moderate heat treatment was evaluated.

2. Materials and Methods

2.1. Material

2.1.1. Distillation of *Eucalyptus globulus* Essential Oil

Eucalyptus globulus EO was purchased from "Ziphee-Bio" company of essential oils (Lakhdaria, Bouira, Algeria). EGEO was extracted from the aerial part with alembic steam distillation (SD). SD is a method used to obtain EOs from *Eucalyptus globulus* by passing steam generated in a pot still through the plant material. A quantity of fresh plant (leaves and small branches of the tree) was loaded in the still and stacked in layers to allow the appropriate delivery of the steam. When the steam passed through the *Eucalyptus globulus*, tiny pockets that hold the EOs opened to release the volatile compounds. This is referred to as the distillate. The distillate will contain a mix of hydrosol (aromatic water) and EO which return to their liquid form in the condenser and are separated using a Florentine separator. EGEO was stored in air-tight sealed glass bottles at 4 °C until further use.

2.1.2. Food Spoilage Microorganisms

Different food-spoilage bacterial strains (*Escherichia coli, Enterobacter sakazakii, Pseudomonas aeruginosa, Klebsiella ornithinolytica, Bacillus cereus* and *Staphylococcus aureus*), fungal strains (*Aspergillus niger, Aspergillus flavus, Aspergillus fumigatus* and *Aspergillus brasiliensis*) and yeasts (*Saccharomyces cerevisiae, Candida parapsilosis, Candida albicans* and *Trichosporon* sp.) were collected and identified from different food matrices (water, milk, juices and honey) in the Laboratory of Food Microbiology (Laboratoire d'Hygiène, Blida, Algeria) and used to evaluate the microbial inhibitory effect of EGEO.

The identification of microorganisms was carried out using morphologic and biochemical characterization tests. After cell identification through Gram staining and microscopic observation was done, the traditional biochemical tests (using API 20E) were carried out to assess the tested bacteria classification following the Gram-negative bacterial identification method [21]. Different biochemical assays were used such as oxidase, TSI medium, gelatin hydrolysis, sugar assimilation, amino acid degradation, hydrogen sulfide production, citrate and Voges-Proskauer.

The fungal species were identified based on their morphological arrangements such as pigmentation, diameter of the mycelia, and microscopic determination of formation of the germ tube, spores and chlamydoconidias. Yeast strains were identified using the Auxacolor™ kit which is an identification method based on sugar digestion [22]. The growth of yeasts is assessed by the color change of a pH indicator. The Auxacolor™ system contains 16 wells in a plastic microplate. All assays with the Auxacolor™ method were carried out following the manufacturer's guidelines. The Auxacolor™ system was stored at 4 °C and was carried to laboratory temperature before use. The fungal and bacterial species were identified with standard microbiology assays and stored in mueller-hinton agar (MHA) and sabouraud dextrose agar (SDA) for bacteria and fungi, respectively.

2.1.3. Chemicals and Reagents

Dimethyl sulfoxide (DMSO), gallic acid, butylated hydroxyanisole (BHA), L-ascorbic acid (vitamin C.), ethanol, tween 80, FerroZine™ iron reagent, 1,1-diphenyl-2-picrylhydrazyl (DPPH) and iron (II) chloride ($FeCl_2$) were obtained from Sigma Aldrich (St. Louis, MO, USA). Isosaline (0.9% NaCl), MHA and SDA medium were purchased from the Ideal-Labo company (Blida, Algeria). Filter paper discs (9 mm in diameter) were provided by Schleicher and Schull GmbH (Dassel, Germany). Antibiotic discs of amoxicillin-clavulanic acid (AMC, 20/10 μg), erythromycin (E, 15 μg), chloramphenicol (C, 30 μg) (Bio-Rad Laboratories, France) and antiseptic solution of Isomedine® 0.1% (Hexamidine dermal solution, Isopharma, Algiers, Algeria) were used to assess the sensitivity of isolated microorganism species.

2.2. Methods

2.2.1. Chemical Composition of *Eucalyptus globulus* Essential Oil by GC-MS Analysis

Analysis of *Eucalyptus globulus* volatile oil was done using GC-MS. Analyses were carried out on an HP 6890 gas chromatograph (Agilent Technologies, Wilmington, DE, USA) fitted with an HP-5MS fused silica column (30 m × 0.25 mm, 0.25 μm film thickness), interfaced with an HP mass selective detector 5790A (Agilent Technologies) operated by HP Enhanced ChemStation software. The oven temperature program was 45–280 °C (2 °C/min). The injector temperature was 250 °C; the carrier gas was helium, adjusted to a linear velocity of 30 cm/s; the splitting ratio was 1:20 and the detector temperature was 250 °C. Separate peaks were recognized by comparison of their Retention Index (RI) to RI of authentic models, and by comparing their mass spectra with the NIST 2007 (National Institute of Standards and Technology, Gaithersburg, MD, USA) and Wiley 6.0 library (New York, NY, USA) mass spectral database and the literature [23].

2.2.2. *In Vitro* Antioxidant Activity

DPPH Radical Scavenging Assay

The radical scavenging effect was evaluated with a spectrophotometric assay based on the reduction of an ethanol solution of DPPH [24]. Briefly, a series of dilutions of EGEO was made. Then, 1.5 mL of each concentration was mixed with 1.5 mL of a 30 μg/L ethanoic DPPH solution that was incubated at laboratory temperature in a dark storeroom for 40 min. Afterward, the absorbance at 520 nm (maximum absorbance of DPPH) was noted spectrophotometrically. Separately, a negative control was made comprising all reagents except the EGEO. The free radical scavenging effect of each solution was then measured and calculated as percentage inhibition in accordance to the following equation:

$$\% \text{ inhibition} = 100 - \left(\frac{\text{DPPHs}}{\text{DPPHb}}\right) * 100$$

where DPPHs corresponds to the absorbance of DPPH with the sample and DPPHb to the absorbance of DPPH without sample (blank).

The antioxidant ability was recorded as the IC_{50} (medium inhibitory concentration). The IC_{50} is defined as the quantity of antioxidant required to reduce the primary DPPH quantity by 50%. The results are expressed as the mean ± standard deviation (SD) of three tests. Ascorbic acid and BHA were used as positive standards.

Metal Chelating Activity

Briefly, different concentrations of 1 mL of EGEO were dissolved in DMSO and added to a solution of 0.05 mL of 2 mM $FeCl_2$ in H_2O. The reaction was started by adding 0.02 mL of 5 mM ferrozine. The mixture was vigorously shaken and incubated at room temperature for 15 min. The absorbance of the EGEO sample was then estimated and determined at 565 nm using a spectrophotometer [24]. The metal chelating activity was expressed according to the following formula:

$$\% \text{ inhibition} = 1 - \left(\frac{\text{Abs Control} - \text{Abs Sample}}{\text{Abs Control}}\right) * 100$$

Gallic acid, ascorbic acid and BHA were used as positive standards. The amount of inhibition by the test samples was expressed as the percentage of concentration required to do 50% inhibition (IC_{50}).

2.2.3. *In Vitro* Antimicrobial Effect of EGEO

Disc Diffusion Method

Microbial media used for culture and growth of bacterial and fungal strains were MHA and SDA, respectively. Inoculum of each bacterial and fungal species to be tested was prepared with fresh cultures by suspending the strain in isosaline (0.9% NaCl). In the first step, the antimicrobial potential of EGEO was explored with the disc diffusion assay [7]. Antibiotic discs of amoxicillin-clavulanic acid, erythromycin, chloramphenicol and antiseptic solution of hexamidine were used to control the antibacterial of isolated micro-organisms strains according to the NCCLS guidelines [25]. Discs without EGEO were considered as a negative control. Filter paper discs (diameter 9 mm) were saturated with three different quantities (20, 40 and 60 μL per disc) of *Eucalyptus* EO and sited in the inoculated microbial media (MH for bacteria and SDA for fungi). After keeping at laboratory temperature for 40 min, the Petri dishes were incubated at 37 °C/24 h for bacterial strains and at 25 °C/72 h for fungal strains. The microbial inhibitory effect was calculated by measuring the diameter of the growth-inhibition zone (DIZ) in mm (including filter diameter of 9 mm) for the tested species and compared to the antibiotic standards.

Disc Volatilization Assay

The usual assay setup as designated by Tyagi et al. [7] was followed. Briefly, a 0.1 mL portion of each suspension was spread over the surface of MHA (bacteria) or SDA (fungi) plates. A filter disc was placed on the inside external of the upper lid and 10 μL EGEO was placed on each disc. The Petri dish inoculated with strains was directly overturned on top of the lid and wrapped with parafilm to avoid the escape of EGEO vapor. Petri dishes were incubated at 37 °C/24 h for bacterial strains and at 25 °C/72 h for fungal strains. The microbial inhibitory effect of *Eucalyptus* volatile oil was estimated by calculating the DIZ of bacterial and fungal growth above the disc. Blank discs were used as a negative control. The quantity of EGEO used was varied (20, 40 or 60 μL) by using a suitable number of sterile discs.

2.2.4. Orangina Juice Preservation by *Eucalyptus globulus* Oil and Moderate Heat Processing

Preparation of Orangina Juice Inoculated with a Yeast Strain (*Saccharomyces cerevisiae*)

Orangina fruit juices were purchased from a local company (Djgaguen Company, Blida city, Algeria). The suspension of *Saccharomyces cerevisiae* was added to Orangina beverage, and the inoculated juices were moved into 250 mL sterilized glass flasks.

Orangina juice is a lightly carbonated beverage made from carbonated water, 12% citrus juice (10% from concentrated orange, 2% from an association of concentrated grapefruit, lemon, and mandarin juices), as well as 2% orange pulp. Orangina juice is sugared with high fructose corn syrup and natural orange flavors are added. Preservatives such as benzoate sodium (E211), potassium sorbate (E202) and citric acid (E330) are also added. All Orangina bottles were kept at 4 °C.

Influence of *Eucalyptus globulus* Essential Oil Alone

Tween 80 solution (0.5%) of EGEO was added in the inoculated Orangina at different doses (0.8, 2 and 4 μL/mL). The Orangina sample inoculated with *Saccharomyces cerevisiae* alone was considered as a positive standard. Afterward, the flasks were kept at laboratory temperature for up to 6 days and juices were drawn on days 0, 2, 4, and 6.

The microbiological method used for yeast counts was the standard plate count (SPC) agar method. This method is used by the food industry for estimating the microbial populations in most types of juices products and samples and for determining the quality and sources of contamination at successive stages of processing. All Orangina fruit juices were successively diluted and plated on SDA medium. The petri dishes were incubated for 48 h at 25 °C and CFU counts were estimated. The effect of different doses of EGEO treatment was measured in a time-dependent way by the difference in log CFU/mL of the inoculated *S. cerevisiae* [7].

Influence of *Eucalyptus globulus* Essential Oil and Moderate Heat Processing: Combined Action

Three different doses (0.8, 2 and 4 μL/mL) of EGEO were added and mixed to inoculated Orangina fruit juice vials and were exposed to a medium heat treatment (70 °C) for 2 min [7]. Then, the flasks were deposited at laboratory temperature for up to 6 days and juices were drawn on day 0, 2, 4, and 6. All Orangina fruit juices were successively diluted and plated on SDA medium. The Petri dishes were incubated for 48 h at 25 °C and CFU counts were estimated. The effects of different doses of EGEO in association with medium heat treatment were measured in a time-dependent way by the difference in log CFU/mL of the inoculated *S. cerevisiae*.

2.3. Statistical Analysis

The significance of variances was analyzed using the test of one-way ANOVA followed by Tukey's post hoc multiple comparison test. Differences with $p < 0.05$ between experimental groups were considered statistically significant. Statistical data analysis was performed using XLstat 2014 software, Addinsoft, Paris, France. For all tests, three replicates were done and the final results represent the mean of these repeats with standard deviation. The IC_{50} (median inhibitory concentration) was calculated from the dose-response curve obtained by plotting percentage inhibition versus concentrations.

3. Results

3.1. Chemical Composition of *Eucalyptus globulus* Essential Oil

Six compounds were identified with GC-MS (Table 1). The major constituent of the EGEO was 1,8-cineole or eucalyptol (94.03% ± 0.23%), followed by α-pinene (94.03% ± 0.23%) and γ-terpinene (94.03% ± 0.23%). The concentration of other compounds in the EGEO was less than 1%.

Table 1. Chemical profile of EO from *Eucalyptus globulus* analyzed with GC-MS.

Retention Time (RT, min)	RI §	Name #	Concentration (%)
8.777	925	α-Pinene	2.93 ± 0.1
9.685	969	β-Pinene	0.20 ± 0.02
10.110	983	Myrcene	0.19 ± 0.07
10.282	1000	α-Phellandrene	0.59 ± 0.02
10.886	1033	Eucalyptol (1,8-Cineole)	94.03 ± 0.23
11.282	1053	γ-Terpinene	1.93 ± 0.17
		Oxygenated monoterpenes	94.03
		Monoterpene hydrocarbons	05.86

Compounds listed in order of elution from a non-polar column. § RI (retention index) calculated relative to C6–C17 n-alkanes.

3.2. Antioxidant Effect of the EGEO

The antioxidant effect was determined by DPPH radical scavenging and metal ion chelating activity (Table 2). The capacity of the EGEO to scavenge DPPH radical and its reducing ability was assessed on the basis of its dose giving 50% inhibition (IC_{50}). In addition, its ability to chelate Fe^{2+} metal ions was evaluated and calculated using different doses. The radical scavenging activities of positive controls (BHA and ascorbic acid) were more active than those obtained from EGEO. However, EGEO had a superior metal ion chelating activity with an IC_{50} value of 8.43 ± 0.03 mg/mL, followed by BHA (104.73 ± 7.30 mg/mL) and gallic acid (136.97 ± 9.09 mg/mL). Current results show that EGEO has the best chelating activity.

Table 2. Antioxidant property of *Eucalyptus globulus* volatile oil *in vitro*.

Sample	DPPH Radical Scavenging IC_{50} (mg/mL)	Chelation IC_{50} (mg/mL)
Eucalyptus globulus Essential Oil	2.48 ± 2.24 ^{C}	8.43 ± 0.03 ^{A}
Positive Control (BHA)	0.13 ± 0.05 ^{B}	104.73 ± 7.30 ^{B}
Positive Control (Ascorbic acid)	0.018 ± 0.004 ^{A}	140.99 ± 3.13 ^{C}
Positive Control (Gallic Acid)	—	136.97 ± 9.09 ^{C}

IC_{50} = medium inhibitory concentration; values are given as mean ± SD (n = 3). Means within the same column followed by the same capital letters are significantly not different ($p > 0.05$) from one another according to the ANOVA test followed by Tukey's comparison tests.

3.3. *In vitro Antibacterial and Antifungal Effects*

3.3.1. Disc Diffusion Assay

The microbial inhibitory effect of EGEO was assessed against different food spoilage microorganisms: six yeast, six bacteria and five fungal strains. The results of the antibacterial tests of EGEO are presented in Table 3. The EGEO displayed a dose-dependent inhibition effect. EGEO was found to be active against all the Gram-positive bacteria species. The EGEO inhibited the growth of *Staphylococcus aureus*, *Bacillus cereus* and *Escherichia coli* with DIZ ranging from 11 to 18 mm at the lower volume of EGEO (20 μL/mL) and from 19 to 85 mm at the higher amount (60 μL/mL). The DIZ increased with the increasing quantity (20, 40 and 60 μL) of EGEO in each paper disc. However, no inhibitory action was found in the case of *Pseudomonas aeruginosa*. For the fungal strains, the DIZ varied from 10 to 49 mm (Table 4). The highest DIZs were shown by *Candida albicans* ATCC (40 mm) and *Saccharomyces cerevisiae* (49 mm) at a greater volume of EGEO (60 μL). The sensitivity of these bacteria to chloramphenicol and EGEO can be explicated by the fact that they have a similar mechanism of action on Gram-negative strains.

The highest susceptible yeast was *Saccharomyces cerevisiae* (49 mm), followed by *Candida albicans* ATCC (40 mm), *Trichosporon* sp. (39 mm) and *Candida parapsilosis* (20 mm) (Table 4). Further, the DIZ due to the *Eucalyptus* volatile oil was bigger for yeast and Gram-positive strains than for mycelial species and Gram-negative bacteria.

3.3.2. Disc Volatilization Method

The *in vitro* antifungal and antibacterial effects of EGEO were assessed according to the absence or the presence of inhibition zones. The DIZ resulting from the exposure to EGEO vapors is shown in Tables 3 and 4. The DIZ due to the same quantity of EGEO was larger for yeast than for mycelial species (Figure 1A,B).

Table 3. Susceptibility of bacterial strains to *Eucalyptus globulus* essential oil and to classic antibiotics (positive controls).

	DIZ (mm) [a]								
	Disc Diffusion Technique			**Disc Vapor Technique**					
Bacterial Strains	**Volume of EGEO (μL) per Disc**						**Positive Control** [b]		
Gram-negative bacteria	20	40	60	20	40	60	AMC	E	C
Pseudomonas aeruginosa	-	-	-	-	-	-	-	16	14
Enterobacter sakazakii	12	15	25	-	85	85	-	19	27
Klebsiella ornithinolytica	-	10	19	-	-	-	-	22	12
Escherichia coli	11	19	34	-	-	36	12	19	7
Gram-positive bacteria									
Bacillus cereus	15	35	50	24	40	59	25	35	24
Staphylococcus aureus	18	48	85	41	85	85	26	R	16

[a] Diameter of inhibition zone (mm) comprising a disc diameter of 9 mm; [b] Amoxicillin-clavulanic acid (AMC, 20/10 μg), erythromycin (E, 15 μg) and chloramphenicol (C, 30 μg) were tested as a positive control for microbial species. EGEO: *Eucalyptus globulus* essential oil. (-) No activity.

Table 4. Susceptibility of fungal strains to *Eucalyptus globulus* essential oil and antiseptic solution.

	DIZ (mm) [a]						
	Disc Diffusion Assay			**Disc Volatilization Assay**			
Fungal Strains	**Quantity of EGEO (μL) per Disc**						**Hex** [b]
Yeasts	20	40	60	20	40	60	40
Candida albicans ATCC	-	11	40	-	-	-	30
Candida albicans (Ca1)	10	25	27	-	-	53	85
Candida albicans (Ca2)	14	19	24	85	85	85	13
Candida parapsilosis	12	17	20	85	85	85	30
Saccharomyces cerevisiae	11	37	49	-	-	59	-
Trichosporon sp.	16	34	39	21	85	85	42
Molds							
Aspergillus niger (An1)	12	21	29	-	-	-	-
Aspergillus niger (An2)	-	10	15	-	-	-	-
Aspergillus fumigatus	-	-	-	-	-	-	-
Aspergillus flavus	-	-	-	-	-	-	-
Aspergillus brasiliensis ATCC	-	-	14	-	43	85	14

[a] Diameter of inhibition zone (mm) including a disc diameter of 9 mm; [b] Antiseptic solution (Hoxamidine 0.1%) used as a positive control for fungal strains. EGEO: *Eucalyptus globulus* essential oil; (-) No inhibitory effect; ATCC: American Type Culture Collection.

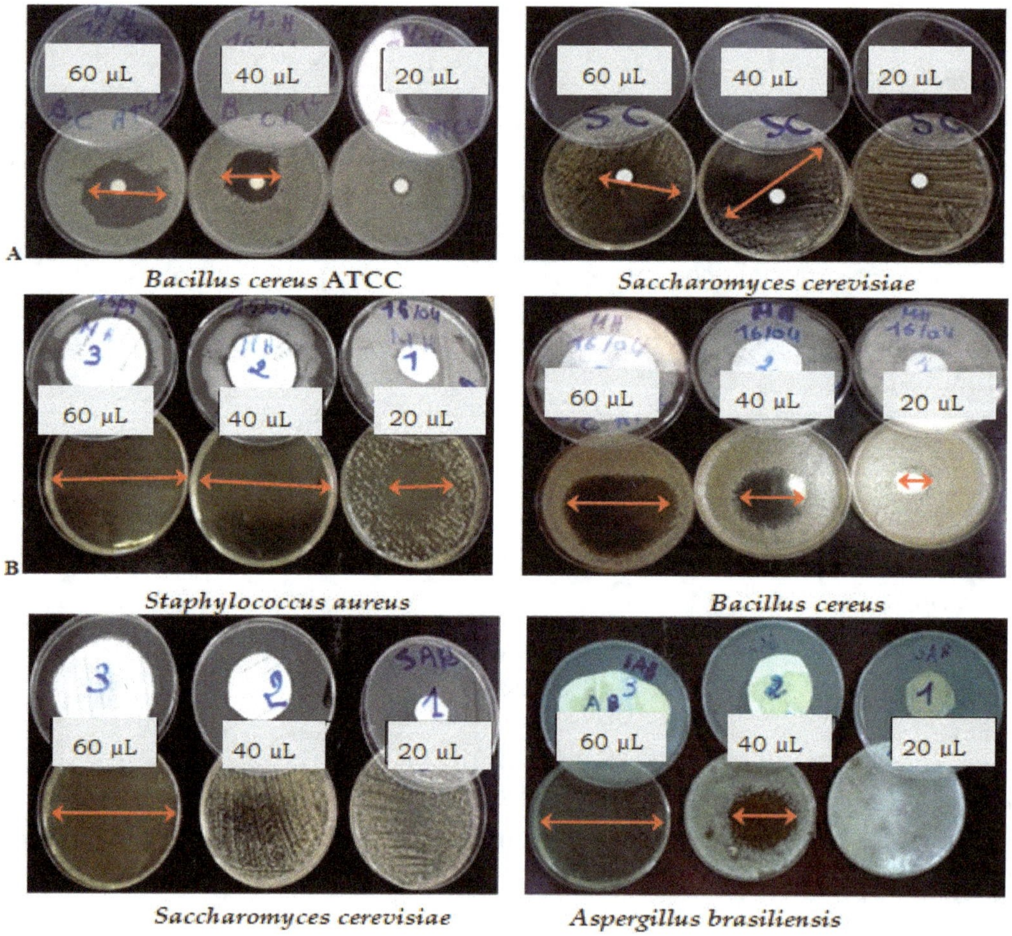

Figure 1. *In vitro* inhibitory activity of *Eucalyptus globulus* essential oil against bacterial and fungal species: Disc diffusion (**A**) versus vapor diffusion (**B**) methods using three different quantities of EO (20, 40 and 60 μL/disc). Red arrows are the diameter of the inhibitory zone (DIZ).

As detected in the previous analyses using EGEO in the liquid phase, the DIZ due to EGEO vapors augmented with an increasing amount of the EGEO and followed a similar tendency with respect to the different microbial species. Nevertheless, in comparison with the liquid phase, the EGEO vapors resulted in considerably superior DIZ in all the yeast strains tested, except *Candida albicans* ATCC. In addition, a total inhibitory effect (85 mm) of EGEO vapors was found in the case of *Staphylococcus aureus* and *Enterobacter sakazakii* bacterial strains. However, no inhibitory action was found for *Aspergillus* species, *Pseudomonas aeruginosa* and *Klebsiella ornithinolytica*. *Candida albicans* (Ca2) and *Candida parapsilosis* were the most sensitive yeasts to EGEO vapors because total inhibition zones were generated using 20, 40 and 60 μL of EO per disc.

3.4. *Orangina Fruit Juice Preservation*

3.4.1. Effect of Varying Dose of EGEO

As EGEO was active to inhibit different food-borne spoilage bacteria and fungi in *in vitro* methods, its effect in a fruit juice matrix (Orangina juice) was also studied (Figure 2). The reduction in viability of *Saccharomyces cerevisiae* due to EGEO use in a concentration-dependent way (0.8, 2 and 4 μL/mL) and a time-dependent manner (i.e., 0, 1, 2, and 6 days) was evaluated. Complete growth inhibition was observed in Orangina fruit juice only when a high concentration of EGEO (4 μL/mL) was used. However, the doses of 2 and 4 μL/mL did not show an important decrease in the final amount of yeasts (2.8 log CFU/mL and 2 log CFU/mL, respectively) in comparison to untreated Orangina juice (2.3 log CFU/mL).

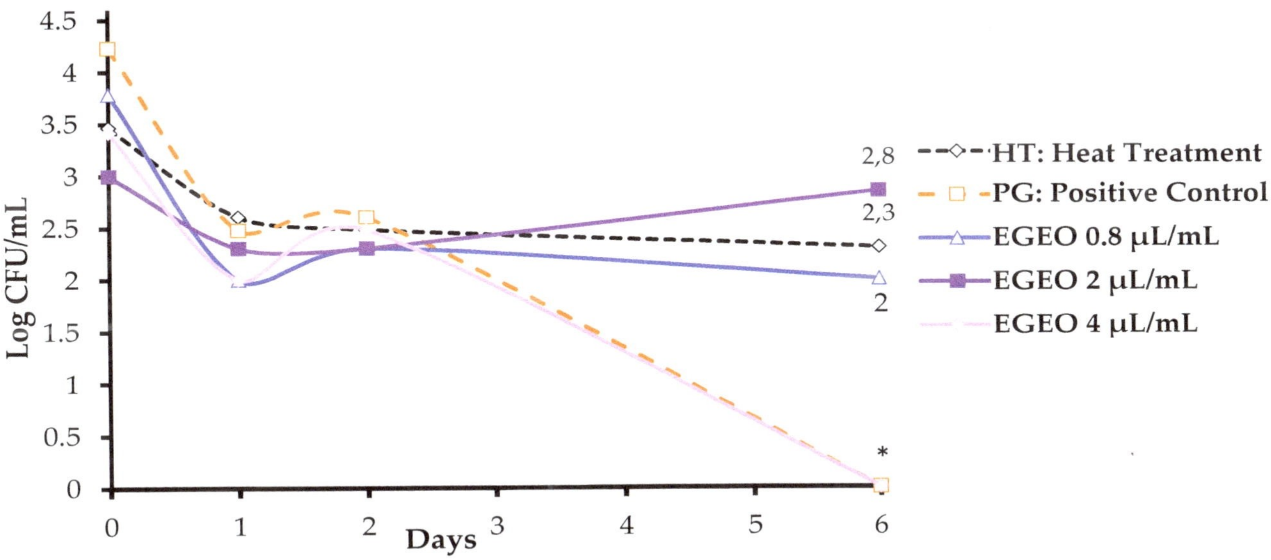

Figure 2. Effect of different doses of EGEO (0.8, 2 and 4 μL/mL) on the viability of *Saccharomyces cerevisiae* cells in Orangina beverage during storage. The fungal growth was followed up to 6 days after the application. HT: Heat treatment at 70 °C for 2 min; PG: Positive control or juice with synthetic antimicrobial additives (sodium benzoate and potassium sorbate); EGEO: *Eucalyptus globulus* essential oil; CFU: Colony-forming unit. * significant difference ($p < 0.05$) according to ANOVA one-way analysis followed by Tukey's *post hoc* multiple comparison tests.

3.4.2. Combined Effect of EGEO and Moderate Heat Processing

The log decrease in CFU count of the *Saccharomyces cerevisiae* due to the associated action of EGEO at different doses along with medium heat treatment at 70 °C for 2 min of Orangina juices was calculated for a specific time interval (0, 1, 2 and 6 days). In juices treated using an association of medium heat processing and all EGEO doses, total fungal inhibition of *Saccharomyces cerevisiae* was recorded on first sampling after 2 days (Figure 3). Therefore, the association of medium heat processing with EGEO reduced the EGEO concentration requirement considerably. Even in the Orangina juices treated with a lower quantity of EGEO, the association of medium heat processing at 70 °C for 2 min improved the log reduction by 3.5 log CFU/mL in comparison to EGEO-treated juices. Therefore, the application of moderate heat processing with EGEO can offer improved Orangina juice preservative.

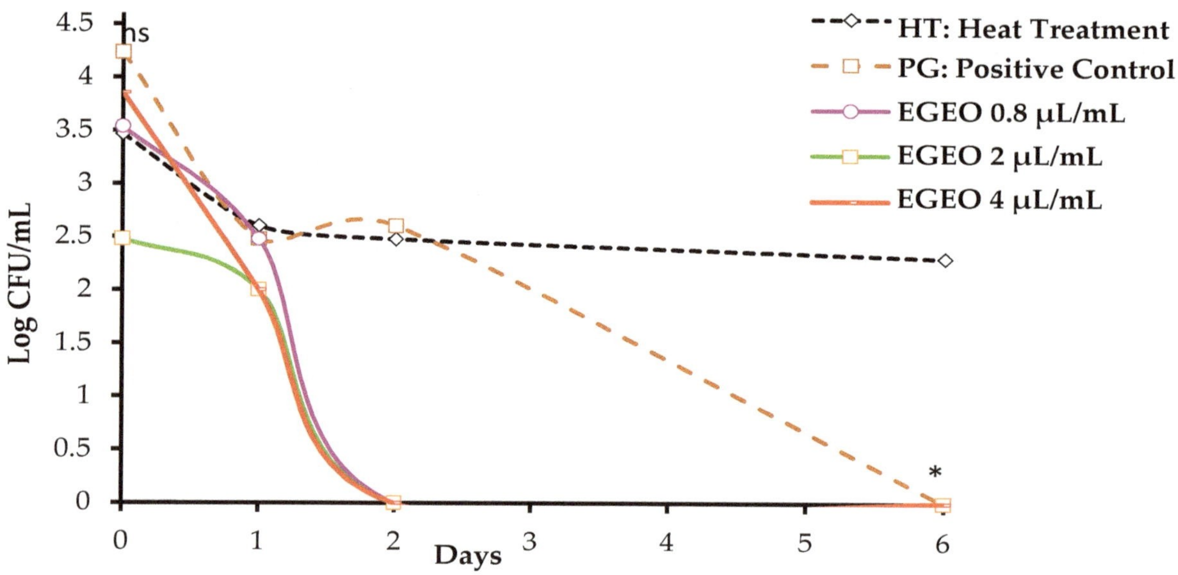

Figure 3. Effect of EGEO at different doses (0.08, 0.2 and 0.4 μL/mL) in association with moderate heat processing (70 °C for 2 min) on the viability of *Saccharomyces cerevisiae* cells in Orangina beverage during storage. The fungal growth was followed up to 6 days after the heat processing. HT: Heat treatment at 70 °C for 2 min; PG: Positive control or juice with synthetic antimicrobial additives (sodium benzoate and potassium sorbate); EGEO: *Eucalyptus globulus* essential oil; CFU: Colony-forming unit. * significant difference ($p < 0.05$) according to ANOVA one-way analysis followed by Tukey's post hoc multiple comparison tests.

4. Discussion

As published in previous reports, the EO of the *Eucalyptus* genus was described by a great quantity of 1,8-cineole (eucalyptol). Current data are in accordance with those published by Elaissi et al. [18] and Goldbeck et al. [26], who found that the principal chemical element of EGEO was eucalyptol. The chemical composition of a diversity of other *Eucalyptus* species have been reported [7,19,27] and are also in accordance with our data.

Different percentages of eucalyptol in *Eucalyptus globulus* leaf EO have been shown: 53.7% in Tunisia, 14.5% in Germany, 33.6% to 66.7% in India and 71% in Brazil. The majority of EO extracted from *Eucalyptus* trees contains at least 10% to as high as 97% eucalyptol (1,8-cineole). Ecological position (Table 5), climatic conditions and extraction methods have been invoked as reasons for the chemical composition disparities and variations [18,20].

Table 5. Comparison of the chemical composition of *Eucalyptus* essential oil from different countries.

Plants	Country	Period	Method	Composition (%)	Authors
E. globulus	Spain		Hydrodistillation of leaves and small branches of the tree. Certified as biological products to be used in humans.	**Eucalyptol = 63.81** α-Pinene = 16.06 Aromadendrene = 3.68 o-Cymene = 2.35	Luís et al. [28]
E. radiata	Australia			**Limonene = 68.51** α-Terpineol = 8.60 α-Terpinyl acetate = 6.07 α-Pinene = 3.01	
E. globulus leaves	Alentejo (Portugal)	Spring 2014	Hydrodistillation in a modified Clevenger-type apparatus	**Eucalyptol** = 4.6% Metileugenol = 3.5 α-Pinene = 2.9 Globulol = 3.2 Terpinene-4-ol = 2	Vieira et al. [29]
E. globulus fruits	Bejaia (Algeria)	2013	Hydrodistillation using a Clevenger type apparatus	**Globulol = 23.6** Eucalyptol = 19.8 α-Pinene = 3.8 iso-Valeradehyde = 2.4 α-Phellandrene = 1.9	Si Said et al. [30]
E. globulus aerial parts	Takelsa (Tunisia)	Vegetative stages (Feb. 2017)	Hydrodistillation by Clevenger apparatus	**Eucalyptol = 13.2** *p*-Cymene = 12.5 α-Pinene = 12.1 β-Pinene = 10.6	Salem et al. [31]
		Full Flowering Stages (March 2017)		***p*-Cymene = 32.1** α-Pinene = 10.4 Eucalyptol = 7.7 β-Pinene = 7.4	
		Fructification stages (May 2017)		***p*-Cymene = 37.8** α-Pinene = 13.3 Eucalyptol = 10.3 L-Phellandrene = 8.2	
Fresh leaves	Ankober Ethiopia		Hydrodistilled in a Clevenger-type apparatus	**Eucalyptol = 63.001** α-Pinene 16.101 Camphor 3.422	Mekonnen et al. [32]
Fresh stems and leaves	Nakhon Nayok, (Thailand)	Rainy Season June–Aug. 2018	Hydrodistilled	**Eucalyptol = 44.54** α-terpinene = 19.83 α-Pinene = 4.95 Terpinene-4-ol = 3.49	Soonwera and Sittichok [33]

A few investigations have been completed to study the antioxidant activity of different *Eucalyptus* EO such as *E. globulus* [28,30,34–37]. Our IC_{50} values are not in agreement with those published for the DPPH radical scavenging method [34]. The scavenging activity on the DPPH radical reported as IC_{50} value was 57 μg/mL for Tunisian EGEO, but this result is inferior as compared to the BHT value obtained with the same test (11.5 μg/mL) [34]. *E. tereticornis* EO presented powerful DPPH, OH and O^{2-} radical scavenging activity [35]. In opposition, *E. camaldulensis* and *E. radiata* EOs have been reported to display a medium DPPH scavenging effect [38]. This variance in antioxidant power may be related to the variation in chemical composition, distillation methods and environmental aspects, age of the trees, storage conditions and geo-climatic situations [12].

In addition, Singh et al. [35] tested the *Eucalyptus* EO and its three main oxygenated terpenes (isopulegol, β-citronellol and citronellal) for antioxidant and scavenging effect. The authors reported that the EO extracted from *Eucalyptus* displayed medium to powerful antioxidant effect in terms of metal chelating (877.3% ± 9.27% inhibition), DPPH radical (IC_{50} = 425.4 ± 6.79 mg/mL) and lipid peroxidation inhibition. This research revealed that *Eucalyptus* EO leaves contain oxygenated monoterpenes rich EO presenting antioxidant action.

The chelating property on metal ions is one of the important mechanisms of antioxidant activity. *Eucalyptus* EO showed a better chelating effect (8.43 ± 0.03 mg/mL) on ferrous ions in comparison with standards (BHA = 104.73 ± 7.30 mg/mL and ascorbic acid = 140.99 ± 3.13 mg/mL). Analysis of metal ion chelating activities revealed that all EOs extracted from *Eucalyptus* species were capable of chelating iron (II) in a dose-dependent way [9]. Another study reported that the antioxidant action of phytochemicals in lemon eucalyptus oil may be due to their redox activities of the phenolic compounds and oxygenated terpenes and that make them good reducing, scavenging and chelating EO [8]. One of the probable modes of action of the antioxidative effect is the chelation of transition metals.

There are very limited published studies about the antioxidant property of eucalyptol as the principal chemical compound of the EGEO [36]. Consequently, antioxidant property detected for the volatile oil could be linked to the remaining compounds [35]. El-Ghorab et al. [37] revealed a medium antioxidant property by preventing the oxidative alteration of linoleic acid (20%) for 12 days for the EO of *Eucalyptus camaldulensis*. Instead, EOs extracted from aerial parts of *Eucalyptus camaldulensis*, growing wild in different regions of Sardinia Island (Italy), have exhibited an *in vitro* antioxidant potential that varied between 0.5 and 5.8 mM [38]. The mode of action involved in the lipid peroxidation and inhibition of DPPH assay is not analogous, thus, the results of the current experiment are not similar to those formerly published by El-Ghorab et al. [37] and Barra et al. [38] because the positive controls and units used in both assays for the determination of the IC_{50} values are not identical.

Numerous published reports have assessed and confirmed the *in vitro* antibacterial, anti-yeast and antifungal potential of EGEO against a varied collection of pathogens [39,40]. For example, *Eucalyptus citriodora* EO has been demonstrated to have a wide range of anti-yeast action. Moreover, *Eucalyptus urophylla* and *Eucalyptus camaldulensis* EOs are also recognized for their microbial inhibitory effect [38]. Though much research has been dedicated to the antifungal and anti-yeast effects of EGEO [40], only a limited number of studies have estimated their bio-activity against foodborne bacteria and fungi [7]. Damjanović-Vratnica et al. [41] reported 85.8% of eucalyptol in EGEO from Montenegro and demonstrated its important and significant effect in the inhibition of different yeast and bacteria growth. Furthermore, another study [18] revealed powerful antiviral, antiseptic and antimicrobial activities of eight EGEOs from Tunisia.

The microbial inhibitory action of EGEO has been shown to diverge considerably within microorganisms and species. The higher antiseptic potential could be directly linked to their main chemical constituents detected in the EGEO (such as eucalyptol and α-pinene) or with the interaction among the minor and major components [18]. Previously published studies revealed that Gram-positive strains are more vulnerable than Gram-negative bacteria; the inhibitory effect against yeasts (*C. albicans* and *S. cerevisiae*) and fungi (*Aspergillus*, *Mucor*, and *Penicillium* species) has also been investigated [7]. According to one of the reports, *Eucalyptus odorata* volatile oil presented the strongest *in vitro* inhibitory effect against micro-organisms and *Eucalyptus bicostata* EOs possess the greatest antiviral action [18].

The EGEO vapor could be extremely active against food spoilage microorganisms in minor doses in comparison with the liquid diffusion, thus producing less influence on the organoleptic and sensorial food properties [42]. Hence, estimating the *in vitro* antifungal and antibacterial actions of EGEO vapor might open up a promising dimension with many possible uses, especially in the food industry.

Current data obtained by both vapor diffusion and agar disc diffusion tests were not similar. The efficiency of the EGEO had previously been described but their use in the vapors phase requires an advanced approach [20]. This could be related to the variance in the chemical composition profile of the vapors and liquid oil because the oil must be enriched in terms of its volatile compounds [7]. A supplementary clarification that has been proposed for the vapor phase being more active is that the hydrophobic compounds in the aqueous phase associate to create micelles and thus restrain that connection of the EO to the microorganism, while the vapor phase permits free attachment [43]. Despite published papers on the *in vitro* antibacterial and antifungal properties of EGEO, few published articles exist on the bioactivity of EGEO vapors. The research done by Goni et al. [44] showed that the *in vitro* antibacterial activity of a combination of cinnamon and clove volatile oils presented a greater inhibitory action with less active doses in the vapor phase in comparison to the liquid phase.

Current results revealed that Algerian EGEO was effective against all yeast and Gram-positive bacteria strains. Previous data already showed that EGEO has *in vitro* inhibitory activity against several microorganisms [7,18]. For example, EGEO displayed powerful action (with 14.3 to 18.2 mm

DIZ) against different bacterial species (*S. aureus*, *E. coli*, and *A. faecalis*) and no inhibitory effect was reported against yeast strain (*C. albicans*) [45]. Vilela et al. [42] tested the *in vitro* antifungal property of both the EGEO and its main compound (eucalyptol) against two *Aspergillus* strains. They obtained complete inhibition when using the EGEO, while less antifungal activity was obtained when testing eucalyptol alone. This proves that the potential synergistic influence of minor and main chemical compounds defines the final *in vitro* inhibitory potential of the volatile oils [3]. Based on the chemical profile of EGEO, it can be suggested that the *in vitro* antiseptic potential is seemingly due to its great concentration of oxygenated monoterpenes (94.09%).

Tserennadmid et al. [46] assessed the antifungal activity of different volatile EOs such as lemon, clary sage, marjoram and juniper in fruit juices. The minimum inhibitory concentration (MIC) of these EOs in fruit juices was considerably greater than *in vitro* MIC values. As great doses of several EOs are necessary to accomplish a suitable fungal inhibitory activity, undesirable levels of unsuitable tastes and smells may exist [47]. To more decrease the necessary EGEO dose for monitoring the *S. cerevisiae* load in Orangina juices, the interaction between EO and heat processing was evaluated.

To avoid the development of spoilage bacteria and yeasts in foods, numerous protection methods, such as thermal processing, the additions of acids or salts, and drying have been investigated in food production [48–52]. In this background, several volatile molecules and EOs containing oxygenated monoterpenes (linalool, geraniol, citronellol, citral, limonene and pinene), combined with moderate thermal processing, were tested to decrease the growth of *S. cerevisiae* in beverages [48].

In the last decade, numerous reports have revealed the incidence of additional activities when associating EOs with moderate heat and high hydrostatic pressure actions [49,50,53,54]. Synergistic effects between EOs with high hydrostatic pressure or moderate heat have been linked to the existence of lethal damages in the external membrane of surviving microorganisms, which may help the entrance of oil's compounds into the cells.

The research of Cherrat et al. [50] revealed the superior effect of EOs extracted from *Myrtus communis* and *Laurus nobilis* in association with medium thermal processing and high hydrostatic pressure to accomplish a greater level of bacterial inhibition of food spoilage microorganisms, and as result, decrease undesirable effects on sensorial food properties. Belletti et al. [48] have proved that the addition of citral and *Citrus* EO to soft juices in association with moderate heat processing can avoid yeast spoilage in beverages. In addition, the bacterial growth of *Listeria innocua* in orange juice was inactivated by the addition of vanillin in relation to the entity of heat processing [51].

As the required EO concentration against foodborne and spoilage bacteria and yeast is affected by the interactions of the EO chemical constituents with the food medium and ingredients, higher quantities are necessary to achieve appropriate food preservative action. This undesirably influences the organoleptic and sensorial properties of the foodstuff [7,52]. To resolve this problem, an interesting alternative is the application of an association of moderate heat treatment with EOs, which improves the antibacterial and antifungal effects of the EO influencing the vapor pressure of the compounds [55–57]. Consequently, the association of EOs with medium heat processing can be investigated for emerging food conservation technologies. Few studies have focused on the association of EOs (*Eucalyptus* and *Mentha*) with thermal processing at 55 °C [7,52]. This approach considerably decreases the EOs concentration necessity, offers a very valuable interaction, as the rise of heating increases the quantity of EO in the vapor phase, thus it improves its anti-yeast effect.

Belletti et al. [58] detected that neither the presence of the EO at their greater doses alone nor the heat treatment alone, was able to maintain or decrease the yeast and fungal stability of the drinks against *Saccharomyces cerevisiae*. In opposition, when applied in association, moderate heat processing (55 °C, 15 min) improved the activity of EO compounds (pinene, linalool and citral) and made an increase in their vapor pressure, which in turn amplified their chance to solubilize in the fungal cell membrane. The current research also revealed the improvement in the antifungal effect of EGEO on association with moderate heat action. The association of medium heat treatment with EGEO application has not been formerly published for avoiding Orangina juice contamination. Current findings demonstrated that EGEO can be used with moderate heat action for the food protections of Orangina juices.

5. Conclusions

Current findings revealed that EGEO could be used as a possible antifungal and antibacterial agent against foodborne and food spoilage microorganisms. The chemical composition of the different compounds characterizing the EGEO showed the predominance of oxygenated terpenes responsible for the microbial inhibitory effect against pathogens. The use of the EGEO in association with moderate heat processing effectively reduced the growth of spoilage yeast strain in Orangina fruit juices. Current data offer an outstanding record of EGEO as an antifungal agent and propose its possible use for beverage preservation. Supplementary research should be done to determine the effectiveness of EGEO in order to use it as a natural additive in different food matrices and/or improvement of food shelf life.

Author Contributions: Conceptualization, M.N.B.; methodology, M.N.B., A.B., H.G.N.; GC-MS analysis, M.N.B., M.R.; formal analysis, M.N.B., A.B., H.G.N.; resources, S.A.M.; writing—original draft preparation, M.N.B., S.A.M.; writing—review and editing, M.N.B., S.A.M.; All authors have read and agreed to the published version of the manuscript.

Acknowledgments: The authors would like to thank Kelly Keating (The Pharmaceutical Research Institute (PRI), Albany College of Pharmacy and Health Sciences, Rensselaer, NY, USA) for proofreading, constructive criticism and English editing of the manuscript. Also, we would like to thank the "Laboratoire d'Hygiène de Blida (Blida, Algeria)", especially Djamel Teffahi and Abdenacer Hmida for their help and making the facilities available for carrying out this research. M.N.B. sincerely thanks Noureldien Darwish and Thangirala Sudha from the PRI for their continuous support, advice and scientific interactions.

References

1. Tomar, R.S.; Sharma, B.; Kaushik, S.; Mishra, R.K. Potential Antifungal Activity of Essential Oils and their Application in Food Preservation. *Asian J. Pharm. Clin. Res.* **2018**, *11*, 54–57. [CrossRef]
2. Carocho, M.; Barreiro, M.F.; Morales, P.; Ferreira, I.C. Adding Molecules to Food, Pros and Cons: A Review on Synthetic and Natural Food Additives. *Compr. Rev. Food Sci. Food Saf.* **2014**, *13*, 377–399. [CrossRef]
3. Burt, S. Essential Oils: Their Antibacterial Properties and Potential Applications in Foods—A Review. *Int. J. Food Microbiol.* **2004**, *94*, 223–253. [CrossRef]
4. Valdés, A.; Mellinas, A.C.; Ramos, M.; Burgos, N.; Jiménez, A.; Garrigós, M.D.C. Use of Herbs, Spices and Their Bioactive Compounds in Active Food Packaging. *RSC Adv.* **2015**, *5*, 40324–40335. [CrossRef]
5. Prakash, B.; Kedia, A.; Mishra, P.K.; Dubey, N.K. Plant Essential Oils as Food Preservatives to Control Moulds, Mycotoxin Contamination and Oxidative Deterioration of Agri-Food Commodities–Potentials and Challenges. *Food Control* **2015**, *47*, 381–391. [CrossRef]
6. Pandey, A.K.; Kumar, P.; Singh, P.; Tripathi, N.N.; Bajpai, V.K. Essential Oils: Sources of Antimicrobials and Food Preservatives. *Front. Microbiol.* **2017**, *7*, 2161. [CrossRef]
7. Tyagi, K.A.; Bukvicki, D.; Gottardi, D.; Tabanelli, G.; Montanari, C.; Malik, A.; Guerzoni, M.E. Eucalyptus Essential Oil as a Natural Food Preservative: *In Vivo* and *In Vitro* Antiyeast Potential. *BioMed Res. Int.* **2014**, *2014*, 969143. [CrossRef]
8. Jirovetz, L.; Bail, S.; Buchbauer, G.; Stoilova, I.; Krastanov, A.; Stoyanova, A.; Schmidt, E. Chemical Composition, Olfactory Evaluation and Antioxidant Effects of the Leaf Essential Oil of *Corymbia citriodora* (Hook) from China. *Nat. Prod. Commun.* **2007**, *2*, 1934578X0700200518. [CrossRef]
9. Bhagat, M.; Gupta, S.; Jamwal, V.S.; Sharma, S.; Kattal, M.; Dawa, S.; Bindu, K. Comparative Study on Chemical Profiling and Antimicrobial Properties of Essential Oils from Different Parts of *Eucalyptus lanceolatus*. *Indian J. Tradit. Knowl.* **2016**, *15*, 425–432.
10. Maqsood, S.; Benjakul, S.; Abushelaibi, A.; Alam, A. Phenolic Compounds and Plant Phenolic Extracts as Natural Antioxidants in Prevention of Lipid Oxidation in Seafood: A Detailed Review. *Compr. Rev. Food Sci. Food Saf.* **2014**, *13*, 1125–1140. [CrossRef]

11. Mostafa, A.A.; Al-Askar, A.A.; Almaary, K.S.; Dawoud, T.M.; Sholkamy, E.N.; Bakri, M.M. Antimicrobial Activity of Some Plant Extracts Against Bacterial Strains Causing Food Poisoning Diseases. *Saudi J. Biol. Sci.* **2018**, *25*, 361–366. [CrossRef] [PubMed]
12. Ušjak, L.; Petrović, S.; Drobac, M.; Soković, M.; Stanojković, T.; Ćirić, A.; Niketić, M. Essential Oils of Three Cow Parsnips–Composition and Activity Against Nosocomial and Foodborne Pathogens and Food Contaminants. *Food Funct.* **2017**, *8*, 278–290. [CrossRef] [PubMed]
13. Gelmini, F.; Belotti, L.; Vecchi, S.; Testa, C.; Beretta, G. Air Dispersed Essential Oils Combined with Standard Sanitization Procedures for Environmental Microbiota Control in Nosocomial Hospitalization Rooms. *Complement. Ther. Med.* **2016**, *25*, 113–119. [CrossRef] [PubMed]
14. Biswas, N.N.; Saha, S.; Ali, M.K. Antioxidant, Antimicrobial, Cytotoxic and Analgesic Activities of Ethanolic Extract of *Mentha arvensis* L. *Asian Pac. J. Trop. Biomed.* **2014**, *4*, 792–797. [CrossRef]
15. Perricone, M.; Arace, E.; Corbo, M.R.; Sinigaglia, M.; Bevilacqua, A. Bioactivity of Essential Oils: A Review on their Interaction with Food Components. *Front. Microbiol.* **2015**, *6*, 76. [CrossRef]
16. Boukhatem, M.N.; Ferhat, M.A.; Kameli, A.; Mekarnia, M. *Eucalyptus globulus* (Labill.): Un Arbre à Essence aux Mille Vertus. *Phytothérapie* **2018**, *16*, 203–214. [CrossRef]
17. Goetz, P.; Ghedira, K. *Phytothérapie Anti-Infectieuse*; Springer: Paris, France, 2012; pp. 271–279.
18. Elaissi, A.; Rouis, Z.; Salem, N.A.B.; Mabrouk, S.; Ben Salem, Y.; Salah, K.B.H.; Khouja, M.L. Chemical composition of 8 *Eucalyptus* species' essential oils and the evaluation of their antibacterial, antifungal and antiviral activities. *BMC Complement. Altern. Med.* **2012**, *12*, 81. [CrossRef]
19. Kumar, P.; Mishra, S.; Malik, A.; Satya, S. Compositional Analysis and Insecticidal Activity of *Eucalyptus globulus* (Family: Myrtaceae) Essential Oil against Housefly (*Musca domestica*). *Acta Trop.* **2012**, *122*, 212–218. [CrossRef]
20. Boukhatem, M.N.; Ferhat, M.A.; Kameli, A.; Fairouz, S.; Mekarnia, M. Liquid and vapour phase antibacterial activity of *Eucalyptus globulus* essential oil: Susceptibility of selected respiratory tract pathogens. *Am. J. Infect. Dis.* **2014**, *10*, 105.
21. Cowan, S.T.; Steel, K.J. *Manual for the Identification of Medical Bacteria*, 3rd ed.; Cambridge University Press: Cambridge, UK, 1993; 216p.
22. Davey, K.G.; Chant, P.M.; Downer, C.S.; Campbell, C.K.; Warnock, D.W. Evaluation of the AUXACOLOR System, a New Method of Clinical Yeast Identification. *J. Clin. Pathol.* **1995**, *48*, 807–809. [CrossRef]
23. Adams, R.P. *Identification of Essential Oil Components by Gas Chromatography/Mass Spectrometry*, 4th ed.; Allured Publ.: Carol Stream, IL, USA, 2007.
24. Ye, C.L.; Dai, D.H.; Hu, W.L. Antimicrobial and Antioxidant Activities of the Essential Oil From Onion (*Allium cepa* L.). *Food Control* **2013**, *30*, 48–53. [CrossRef]
25. NCCLS (National Committee for Clinical Laboratory Standards). *Performance Standards for Antimicrobial Disc Susceptibility Tests: Approved Standard M2-A8*; NCCLS: Wayne, PA, USA, 2003.
26. Goldbeck, J.C.; do Nascimento, J.E.; Jacob, R.G.; Fiorentini, Â.M.; da Silva, W.P. Bioactivity of essential oils from Eucalyptus globulus and *Eucalyptus urograndis* against planktonic cells and biofilms of *Streptococcus mutans*. *Ind. Crops Prod.* **2014**, *60*, 304–309. [CrossRef]
27. Manika, N.; Chanotiya, C.S.; Negi, M.P.S.; Bagchi, G.D. Copious Shoots as a Potential Source for the Production of Essential Oil in *Eucalyptus globulus*. *Ind. Crops Prod.* **2013**, *46*, 80–84. [CrossRef]
28. Luís, Â.; Duarte, A.; Gominho, J.; Domingues, F.; Duarte, A.P. Chemical composition, antioxidant, antibacterial and anti-quorum sensing activities of *Eucalyptus globulus* and *Eucalyptus radiata* essential oils. *Ind. Crops Prod.* **2016**, *79*, 274–282. [CrossRef]
29. Vieira, M.; Bessa, L.J.; Martins, M.R.; Arantes, S.; Teixeira, A.P.; Mendes, A.; Belo, A.D. Chemical Composition, Antibacterial, Antibiofilm and Synergistic Properties of Essential Oils from *Eucalyptus globulus* Labill. and seven Mediterranean Aromatic Plants. *Chem. Biodivers.* **2017**, *14*, e1700006. [CrossRef]
30. Si Said, Z.B.; Haddadi-Guemghar, H.; Boulekbache-Makhlouf, L.; Rigou, P.; Remini, H.; Adjaoud, A.; Madani, K. Essential Oil Composition, Antibacterial and Antioxidant Activities of Hydrodistillated Extract of *Eucalyptus globulus* fruits. *Ind. Crops Prod.* **2016**, *89*, 167–175. [CrossRef]
31. Salem, N.; Kefi, S.; Tabben, O.; Ayed, A.; Jallouli, S.; Feres, N.; Sghaier, A. Variation in Chemical Composition of *Eucalyptus globulus* Essential Oil under Phenological Stages and Evidence Synergism with Antimicrobial Standards. *Ind. Crops Prod.* **2018**, *124*, 115–125. [CrossRef]

32. Mekonnen, A.; Yitayew, B.; Tesema, A.; Taddese, S. *In vitro* Antimicrobial Activity of Essential Oil of *Thymus schimperi, Matricaria chamomilla, Eucalyptus globulus,* and *Rosmarinus officinalis*. *Int. J. Microbiol.* **2016**. [CrossRef]
33. Soonwera, M.; Sittichok, S. Adulticidal Activities of *Cymbopogon citratus* (Stapf.) and *Eucalyptus globulus* (Labill.) Essential Oils and of their Synergistic Combinations against *Aedes aegypti* (L.), *Aedes albopictus* (Skuse), and *Musca domestica* (L.). *Environ. Sci. Pollut. Res.* **2020**, *27*, 20201–20214. [CrossRef]
34. Noumi, E.; Snoussi, M.; Hajlaoui, H.; Trabelsi, N.; Ksouri, R.; Valentin, E.; Bakhrouf, A. Chemical Composition, Antioxidant and Antifungal Potential of *Melaleuca alternifolia* (Tea Tree) and *Eucalyptus globulus* Essential Oils Against Oral *Candida* Species. *J. Med. Plants Res.* **2011**, *5*, 4147–4156.
35. Singh, H.P.; Kaur, S.; Negi, K.; Kumari, S.; Saini, V.; Batish, D.R.; Kohli, R.K. Assessment of In Vitro Antioxidant Activity of Essential Oil Of *Eucalyptus citriodora* (Lemon-Scented Eucalypt; Myrtaceae) and its Major Constituents. *LWT-Food Sci. Technol.* **2012**, *48*, 237–241. [CrossRef]
36. Horvathova, E.; Navarova, J.; Galova, E.; Sevcovicova, A.; Chodakova, L.; Snahnicanova, Z.; Slamenova, D. Assessment of Antioxidative, Chelating, and DNA-Protective Effects of Selected Essential Oil Components (Eugenol, Carvacrol, Thymol, Borneol, Eucalyptol) of Plants and Intact *Rosmarinus officinalis* Oil. *J. Agric. Food Chem.* **2014**, *62*, 6632–6639. [CrossRef] [PubMed]
37. El-Ghorab, A.H.; El-Massry, K.F.; Marx, F.; Fadel, H.M. Antioxidant Activity of Egyptian *Eucalyptus camaldulensis* var. *Brevirostris Leaf Extracts. Food* **2003**, *47*, 41–45. [PubMed]
38. Barra, A.; Coroneo, V.; Dessi, S.; Cabras, P.; Angioni, A. Chemical Variability, Antifungal and Antioxidant Activity of *Eucalyptus camaldulensis* Essential Oil From Sardinia. *Nat. Prod. Commum.* **2010**, *5*, 329–335. [CrossRef]
39. Su, Y.C.; Ho, C.L.; Wang, E.I.C.; Chang, S.T. Antifungal Activities and Chemical Compositions of Essential Oils From Leaves of four *Eucalyptus*. *Taiwan J. For. Sci.* **2006**, *21*, 9–61.
40. Tolba, H.; Moghrani, H.; Benelmouffok, A.; Kellou, D.; Maachi, R. Essential Oil of Algerian *Eucalyptus citriodora*: Chemical Composition, Antifungal Activity. *J. Mycol. Med.* **2015**, *25*, e128–e133. [CrossRef]
41. Damjanović-Vratnica, B.; Đakov, T.; Šuković, D.; Damjanović, J. Antimicrobial Effect of Essential Oil Isolated From *Eucalyptus globulus* Labill. From Montenegro. *Czech J. Food Sci.* **2011**, *29*, 277–284. [CrossRef]
42. Vilela, G.R.; de Almeida, G.S.; D'Arce, M.A.B.R.; Moraes, M.H.D.; Brito, J.O.; da Silva, M.F.D.G.; da Gloria, E.M. Activity of Essential Oil and its Major Compound, 1, 8-Cineole, from *Eucalyptus globulus* Labill., Against the Storage Fungi *Aspergillus flavus* Link and *Aspergillus parasiticus* Speare. *J. Stored Prod. Res.* **2009**, *45*, 108–111. [CrossRef]
43. Inouye, S.; Takizawa, T.; Yamaguchi, H. Antibacterial Activity of Essential Oils and Their Major Constituents Against Respiratory Tract Pathogens by Gaseous Contact. *J. Antimicrob. Chemother.* **2001**, *47*, 565–573. [CrossRef]
44. Goni, P.; López, P.; Sánchez, C.; Gómez-Lus, R.; Becerril, R.; Nerín, C. Antimicrobial Activity in the Vapour Phase of a Combination of Cinnamon and Clove Essential Oils. *Food Chem.* **2009**, *116*, 982–989. [CrossRef]
45. Wilkinson, J.M.; Cavanagh, H.M. Antibacterial Activity of Essential Oils From Australian Native Plants. *Phytother. Res.* **2005**, *19*, 643–646. [CrossRef] [PubMed]
46. Tserennadmid, R.; Takó, M.; Galgóczy, L.; Papp, T.; Pesti, M.; Vágvölgyi, C.; Krisch, J. Anti Yeast Activities of Some Essential Oils in Growth Medium, Fruit Juices and Milk. *Int. J. Food Microbiol.* **2011**, *144*, 480–486. [CrossRef] [PubMed]
47. Gutierrez, J.; Barry-Ryan, C.; Bourke, P. Antimicrobial Activity of Plant Essential Oils using Food Model Media: Efficacy, Synergistic Potential and Interactions with Food Components. *Food Microbiol.* **2009**, *26*, 142–150. [CrossRef] [PubMed]
48. Belletti, N.; Kamdem, S.S.; Patrignani, F.; Lanciotti, R.; Covelli, A.; Gardini, F. Antimicrobial Activity of Aroma Compounds against *Saccharomyces cerevisiae* and Improvement of Microbiological Stability of Soft Drinks as Assessed by Logistic Regression. *Appl. Environ. Microbiol.* **2007**, *73*, 5580–5586. [CrossRef] [PubMed]
49. Espina, L.; Gelaw, T.K.; de Lamo-Castellvi, S.; Pagán, R.; Garcia-Gonzalo, D. Mechanism of Bacterial Inactivation by (+)-Limonene and its Potential Use in Food Preservation Combined Processes. *PLoS ONE* **2013**, *8*, 0056769. [CrossRef] [PubMed]
50. Cherrat, L.; Espina, L.; Bakkali, M.; García-Gonzalo, D.; Pagán, R.; Laglaoui, A. Chemical Composition and Antioxidant Properties of *Laurus nobilis* L. and *Myrtus communis* L. Essential Oils from Morocco and Evaluation of Their Antimicrobial Activity Acting Alone or in Combined Processes for Food Preservation. *J. Sci. Food Agric.* **2014**, *94*, 1197–1204. [CrossRef] [PubMed]

51. Char, C.; Guerrero, S.; Alzamora, S.M. Survival of *Listeria innocua* in Thermally Processed Orange Juice as Affected by Vanillin Addition. *Food Control* **2009**, *20*, 67–74. [CrossRef]
52. Tyagi, A.K.; Gottardi, D.; Malik, A.; Guerzoni, M.E. Anti-Yeast Activity of Mentha Oil and Vapours Through *In Vitro* and *In Vivo* (Real Fruit Juices) Assays. *Food Chem.* **2013**, *137*, 108–114. [CrossRef]
53. Somolinos, M.; García, D.; Pagán, R.; Mackey, B. Relationship Between Sublethal Injury and Microbial Inactivation by the Combination of High Hydrostatic Pressure and Citral or Tert-Butyl Hydroquinone. *Appl. Environ. Microbiol.* **2008**, *74*, 7570–7577. [CrossRef]
54. Ait-Ouazzou, A.; Espina, L.; Gelaw, T.K.; de Lamo-Castellví, S.; Pagán, R.; García-Gonzalo, D. New Insights in Mechanisms of Bacterial Inactivation by Carvacrol. *J. Appl. Microbiol.* **2013**, *114*, 173–185. [CrossRef]
55. Hyldgaard, M.; Mygind, T.; Meyer, R.L. Essential Oils in Food Preservation: Mode of Action, Synergies, and Interactions with Food Matrix Components. *Front. Microbiol.* **2012**, *3*, 12. [CrossRef] [PubMed]
56. Gottardi, D.; Bukvicki, D.; Prasad, S.; Tyagi, A.K. Beneficial Effects of Spices in Food Preservation and Safety. *Front. Microbiol.* **2016**, *7*, 1394. [CrossRef] [PubMed]
57. Boukhatem, M.N. Scientific Findings: The Amazing Use of Essential Oils and Their Related Terpenes as Natural Preservatives to Improve the Shelf-Life of Food. *Food Sci. Nutr. Technol.* **2020**, *5*, 00021.
58. Belletti, N.; Kamdem, S.S.; Tabanelli, G.; Lanciotti, R.; Gardini, F. Modeling of Combined Effects of Citral, Linalool and β-Pinene Used Against *Saccharomyces cerevisiae* in Citrus-Based Beverages Subjected to a Mild Heat Treatment. *Int. J. Food Microbiol.* **2010**, *136*, 283–289. [CrossRef]

10

Dietary Supplementation with Pioglitazone Hydrochloride and Resveratrol Improves Meat Quality and Antioxidant Capacity of Broiler Chickens

Fan Zhang [1], Chenglong Jin [1], Shiguang Jiang [1], Xiuqi Wang [1], Huichao Yan [1], Huize Tan [2] and Chunqi Gao [1,*]

1 College of Animal Science, South China Agricultural University/Guangdong Provincial Key Laboratory of Animal Nutrition Control, Guangzhou 510642, China; fz@stu.scau.edu.cn (F.Z.); jin@stu.scau.edu.cn (C.J.); sgjiang@stu.scau.edu.cn (S.J.); xqwang@scau.edu.cn (X.W.); yanhc@scau.edu.cn (H.Y.)

2 WENS Foodstuff Group Co., Ltd., Guangzhou 527439, China; Tanhuize5@163.com

* Correspondence: cqgao@scau.edu.cn

Abstract: The study aimed to investigate the effects of pioglitazone hydrochloride (PGZ) and resveratrol (RES) on yellow-feathered broiler chickens. A total of 500 broiler chickens were randomly divided into four groups and fed a basic diet (control group) or a basic diet supplemented with 15 mg/kg PGZ, 400 mg/kg RES, or 15 mg/kg PGZ plus 400 mg/kg RES for 28 days. Compared with the control group, the PGZ and PGZ plus RES groups presented a significantly higher average daily gain and a decreased feed-to-gain ratio. Increases in the dressing percentage, semi-eviscerated yield, muscle intramuscular fat content, and C18:1n-9c, C18:3n-6, C20:3n-3, and monounsaturated fatty acid (MUFA) percentages were found in the PGZ plus RES group. Moreover, the diet supplemented with RES or PGZ plus RES increased the activities of catalase, glutathione peroxidase, and superoxide dismutase, and decreased the levels of reactive oxygen species of thigh muscle. Additionally, the mRNA abundance of peroxisome proliferator-activated receptor γ coactivator 1α, fatty acid-binding protein 3, nuclear factor erythroid-2-related factor 2, and superoxide dismutase 1 was increased in the PGZ plus RES group. In conclusion, this study suggested that dietary supplementation of PGZ combined with RES improved the growth performance, the muscle intramuscular fat content, and antioxidant ability of yellow-feathered broiler chickens.

Keywords: resveratrol; pioglitazone hydrochloride; fatty acid; meat quality; antioxidant ability; yellow-feathered broiler chicken

---

1. Introduction

In recent years, the demands of consumers have shifted from quantity to quality and, as a result, the intramuscular fat (IMF) content and fatty acid profile of poultry meat have become important to both producers and consumers [1]. Due to its relatively higher proportion of polyunsaturated fatty acids, poultry meat is usually better than other meats [2]. However, unsaturated fatty acids are susceptible to oxidation, and malonaldehyde (MDA) is well known as one of the end products of this process [3]. Thus, lipid oxidation is one of the main factors leading to the deterioration of meat quality, which can occur both before and after death [4]. Furthermore, lipid oxidation causes adverse changes in glycolysis that increase the drip loss and thereby lead to meat spoilage and a shorter shelf life [5,6]. Thus, an effective approach for improving the IMF and protecting intramuscular lipids against oxidative damage is needed.

Thiazolidinediones (TZDs) are a class of medicines currently been used to treat type 2 diabetes [7]. Although TZDs have beneficial effects on glycemic control, insulin sensitivity, inflammation and oxidative stress, and reduction of triglycerides [8–10], TZDs are clinically at risk for hepatic insufficiency, thus the use of TZDs in the animal diet is prohibited in some countries [11]. However, regarding the effects of TZDs on skeletal muscle lipid metabolism, many studies have found that intramuscular lipid content and the proportion of unsaturated fatty acids are increased after TZD treatment [12–14]. As adipogenic compounds, TZDs play a crucial role in adipocyte differentiation and have the potential to alter the formation of intramuscular or marbled fat [15,16]. As one of the TZDs, pioglitazone hydrochloride (PGZ) is a high-affinity ligand for peroxisome proliferator-activated receptor gamma (*PPARγ*) [17], and previous study has found that PGZ can promote adipocyte differentiation to modify intramuscular adipogenesis [15]. More adipocytes and larger cell sizes have been observed in mice supplemented with PGZ [13,14,18]. According to previous reports, PGZ has the potential to promote fat deposition in animal muscle [19,20]. Consistent with these findings, our previous studies confirmed that dietary supplementation with 15 mg/kg PGZ can increase the IMF in the longissimus thoracis muscle of pigs [21,22]. Therefore, PGZ has potential as a new feed additive for improving meat quality of animals. However, few studies have explored the effects of PGZ on poultry, such as chickens.

The inclusion of an antioxidant additive in broiler chicken diets is necessary to protect the PGZ supplementation-induced increase in the IMF of the thigh muscle from oxidation. Resveratrol (RES) is a botanical polyphenolic compound, and previous studies have indicated that dietary supplemental with RES could promote antioxidant activity in quail eggs and broiler chickens [23,24]. Furthermore, the impairment in the antioxidant status caused by heat stress is attenuated in chickens fed a diet supplemented with RES [25]. As an important plant-derived bioactive polyphenol, RES can eliminate reactive oxygen species (ROS) and thereby improve antioxidant activity [26]. Consequently, RES has the potential to work as an antioxidant and preservative to extend the shelf life of meat and thereby avoid huge economic losses.

Because RES can improve the antioxidant capacity and PGZ can enhance the IMF and proportions of unsaturated fatty acids, the aim of this study was to explore whether the combination of PGZ and RES exerts effects on the muscle antioxidant status, IMF content, and fatty acid profile of broiler chickens.

2. Materials and Methods

The protocols used for the feeding and management of broiler chickens in this study were approved by the Animal Ethics Committee of South China Agricultural University and were in accordance to the Guidelines for the Care and Use of Laboratory Animals of South China Agricultural University (Guangzhou, China).

2.1. Materials

PGZ (purity ≥ 99%) and RES (purity ≥ 98%) was obtained from Sichuan Jisheng Biopharmaceutical Co., Ltd. (Leshan, China).

2.2. Experimental Design, Diets and Growth Performance

A total of 500 female yellow-feathered broiler chickens, approximately 72 days of age (28 days before slaughter), were randomly assigned to four groups: a control group (fed with basic diet, Table S1), and the PGZ, RES, or PGZ+RES groups, which were fed the basic diet and supplemented with 15 mg/kg PGZ, 400 mg/kg RES, or 15 mg/kg PGZ + 400 mg/kg RES, respectively, for 28 days. The basic diet was formulated according to the Nutrient Requirements of Poultry (Ministry of Agriculture of the People's Republic of China 2004).

Prior to the experiment, the experimental room was cleaned and disinfected. Immunization was performed using a routine procedure. The broiler chickens were housed in a room with a concrete floor covered with wheat shavings and allowed access to feed and water ad libitum. The room was illuminated for 23 h, and the temperature was maintained at approximately 25 ± 2 °C. Before the experiment, the animals were pre-fed with the assigned diet for 5 days, and all weak broiler chickens were eliminated. The weight and feed intake of weak broiler chickens were recorded, and these data were excluded in the final statistics. The experiment spanned 28 days, and the average daily feed intake (ADFI) was recorded. All broiler chickens were weighed at 1, 14, and 28 days to calculate the average daily gain (ADG) and feed/gain (F/G) ratio.

2.3. Serum Biochemical Indices

After feeding for 28 days, 3 broiler chickens were selected from each replicate (totaling 15 broiler chickens per diet group) and fasted overnight for 12 h. The broiler chickens were bled from the jugular vein, and the blood samples from the broiler chickens of the formal experiment were collected, then maintained at an oblique position for 30 min. The serum samples were then collected after centrifugation of blood samples at 3000 rpm for 10 min and stored at −20 °C. Various serum biochemical indices, including total protein (TP), triglyceride (TG), cholesterol (CHO), low-density lipoprotein cholesterol (LDL-C), serum urea nitrogen (SUN), and high-density lipoprotein cholesterol (HDL-C), were then detected using kits (Nanjing Jiancheng Bioengineering Institute, Nanjing, China). The kits and their sensitivity and detection limits used in this study were as follows: TP assay kit A045-2-2, 5.0-122.1 U/mL; TG assay kit A110-1-1; Total CHO assay kit A111-1-1; LDL-C assay kit A113-1-1; SUN assay kit C013-2-1; and HDL-C assay kit A112-1-1.

2.4. Carcass Performance and Meat Quality

After blood was harvested and feathers were removed, carcass weights were calculated. The carcass traits and meat quality were measured as previously described [27]. Dressing percentage was calculated by dividing carcass weight by live weight. The semi-eviscerated yield (feet, head, and all the organs except the lungs and kidneys were removed), eviscerated yield (lung and kidney were removed), breast muscle yield (2 × right left muscle), thigh muscle yield (2 × left thigh muscle), and abdominal fat were expressed relative to carcass weight.

The entire left breast muscle and thigh muscle (the skin was removed) were collected immediately after slaughter and used for detection of the meat quality. The pH was detected using a meter (HI99161, HANNA, Rome, Italy) equipped with an insertion glass electrode, and the color was detected at the same part of the front of all muscle using a colorimeter (CR410, MINOLTA, Tokyo, Japan) after 45 min and 24 h slaughter. The drip loss was determined with the muscle samples were suspended in a zip-lock bag and stored at 4 °C for 24 h. The cooking loss was determined using muscle samples sealed in a zip-lock bag; the muscle samples were cooked in a 75 °C water bath and maintained at 72 °C for 20 min. The shear force was detected using the muscle cooked in a water bath at 70 °C for 30 min with a digital muscle tenderness tester (C-LM3B, TENOVO, Beijing, China) at 24 h after slaughter. A piece of muscle from the same location on the right side of the body was obtained and stored in liquid nitrogen for histological analysis, determination of the fatty acid composition, and RT-PCR assay. The remaining of the thigh muscle samples of each chicken were divided into 5 sections and stored at 4 °C. They were then collected for the detection of the total volatile basic nitrogen (TVB-N) at 0, 3, 5, 7, and 9 days. As a crucial indicator used for evaluating the shelf life of meat, the TVB-N values were detected using the procedure described by Goulas [28] and expressed as mg of TVB-N/100 g.

Six sections of thigh muscle were cut at 8 μm and embedded in 4% paraformaldehyde to protect against dehydration. The sections were then stained with Oil Red O. The whole staining procedure lasted approximately 10 min. Specifically, the slices were immersed in isopropanol for 2 min, washed under running tap water for 1 min, covered with working solution for 5 min, and then washed in clean isopropanol for 2 min to adjust the slice color. A working solution composed of 0.5 g of Oil Red O diluted with 100 mL of isopropanol was prepared and stored at 4 °C [29].

2.5. Determination of the Fatty Acid Composition

The fatty acid contents and compositions were measured as previously described [30,31]. Samples of 30 g thigh muscle were baked at constant temperature (at 70 °C). 2 g portion of each sample was weighed and then placed in a degreasing filter paper bag and dried to constant weight for extraction. After extraction, 2 mL methylation reagent (DongYing HeYi Chemical Co., LTD., Shandong, China) was taken in a 10 mL screw cap centrifuge tube, and accurately added to 200 mL of fat and gently mixed by pipetting. After sealing, the screw cap centrifuge tube was placed in a boiling water bath at 100 °C for 30 min. The upper organic phase was transferred to a 2 mL centrifuge tube for centrifuge. The upper organic phase was transferred to a 1.5 mL gas chromatography sample vial (Jinpu Analytical Instrument Co., Ltd., Shandong, China) for later use. The fatty acid profile was detected by GC 7890A gas chromatograph (Agilent, Santa Clara, CA, USA). Nitrogen was used as carrier gas (2 mL/min). Injector and detector temperature were 270 °C. The temperature of the column was operated as follows: 75 °C for 0.5 min, from 75 °C to 190 °C at 20 °C/min, and from 190 °C to 250 °C at 5 °C/min. The types of fatty acids were identified by comparing the retention times with FAME Mix 37 (18919–1 AMP, Supelco, Bellefonte, PA, USA). Contents of various fatty acids were calculated by calculating retention times and peak area percentages.

2.6. Determination of Muscle Antioxidant Abilities and ROS

The MDA, catalase (CAT), total superoxide dismutase (T-SOD) activity, glutathione peroxidase (GSH-Px), and total antioxidant capacity (T-AOC) of thigh muscle were determined using commercial kits (Nanjing Jiancheng Bioengineering Institute, Nanjing, China). The thigh muscles slaughtered within two hours were cut into frozen sections of 5 μm, washed twice with phosphate buffer saline, and returned to room temperature for incubation with 10 μM dihydroethidium (DHE, 50102ES02, YEASEN, Shanghai, China) at 37 °C for 60 min. Fluorescence intensity was measured using Varioskan LUX (Thermo Fisher Scientific, Waltham, MA, USA).

2.7. Determination of mRNA Abundances

Total RNA from the thigh muscle was extracted using TRIzol (Ambion, Austin, TX, USA) [32]. A quantity of 50–100 mg of frozen thigh muscle tissue was cut and placed in a mortar, poured into liquid nitrogen, and crushed. A quantity of 1 mL TRIZOL was added to separate the nucleoprotein complex. A quantity of 0.2 mL of chloroform was then added and the upper aqueous phase was transferred into 1.5 mL centrifuge tubes, to which were added 0.5 mL of isopropanol. A quantity of 98 μL of Rnase-free water was then added after washing the RNA pellet (GeneStar, Beijing, China). The concentration of RNA was determined by NanoDrop 2000 (Waltham, MA, USA), and first-strand cDNA was synthesized with Primer Script™ (GeneStar, Beijing, China) and used for PCR amplification with T100™ Thermal Cycler (Bio-Rad, Hercules, CA, USA). The IQ5 Real-Time PCR Detection System (Bio-Rad, CA, USA) was used to determine the mRNA abundances, and the sequences of the primers used in this study are listed in Table S2.

2.8. Statistical Analysis

All the data are shown as means. SPSS software (version 20.0) was used for the statistical analyses, and the statistical significance levels ($p < 0.05$) were determined by one-way analysis of variance (ANOVA) followed by Duncan's multiple range test.

3. Results

3.1. Growth Performance

The growth performances of the broiler chickens are shown in Table 1. After feeding for 28 days, the broiler chickens belonging to the PGZ and PGZ + RES groups presented heavier weights compared to the control group ($p < 0.05$). Moreover, the PGZ and PGZ + RES groups exhibited 8.92% and 9.86% lower F/G ratios ($p < 0.05$) and 12.14% and 13.64% higher ADG values ($p < 0.05$), respectively.

Table 1. Effects of dietary supplemental with pioglitazone hydrochloride (PGZ) and resveratrol (RES) on the growth performance of broilers.

Item	Treatment				SEM	p-Value
	Control	PGZ	RES	PGZ + RES		
IBW (g)	1623.6	1624.2	1623.7	1624.1	8.24	0.303
FBW (g)	2112.3 [b]	2163.1 [a]	2119.6 [b]	2168.5 [a]	10.32	<0.05
ADFI (g)	93.4	94.2	94.8	94.9	2.01	0.647
ADG (g)	17.4 [b]	19.2 [a]	17.7 [b]	19.4 [a]	0.51	<0.05
F/G (g/g)	5.37 [a]	4.91 [b]	5.34 [a]	4.89 [b]	0.09	<0.05

[a,b] Values with different letters within the line mean significant differences ($p < 0.05$). $n = 5$. Abbreviations: SEM, standard error of the means; PGZ, pioglitazone hydrochloride; RES, resveratrol; IBW, initial body weight; FBW, final body weight; F/G, feed/gain ratio; ADG, average daily gain; and ADFI, average daily feed intake.

3.2. Serum Biochemical Indices

As indicated by the results shown in Table 2, compared with the control group, the serum LDL-C level was significantly decreased in the broiler chickens fed with PGZ, RES, or PGZ + RES ($p < 0.05$). In addition, the broiler chickens fed with PGZ and PGZ + RES presented decreased serum CHO levels ($p < 0.05$) and increased HDL-C levels ($p < 0.05$).

Table 2. Effects of dietary supplemental with PGZ and RES on serum biochemical indices of broilers.

Item	Treatment				SEM	p-Value
	Control	PGZ	RES	PGZ + RES		
SUN (mmol/L)	0.61	0.50	0.51	0.59	0.06	0.331
LDL-C (mmol/L)	0.91 [a]	0.71 [b]	0.64 [b]	0.36 [c]	0.04	<0.05
CHO (mmol/L)	3.30 [a]	2.97 [b]	3.20 [a]	2.86 [b]	0.11	<0.05
TP (g/L)	45.53	46.96	46.70	48.07	1.45	0.251
TG (mmol/L)	1.73	1.62	1.78	1.89	0.57	0.734
HDL-C (mmol/L)	1.73 [b]	2.31 [a]	1.67 [b]	2.56 [a]	0.08	<0.05

[a–c] Values with different letters within the line mean significant differences ($p < 0.05$). $n = 5$. Abbreviations: SEM, standard error of the means; PGZ, pioglitazone hydrochloride; RES, resveratrol; SUN, serum urea nitrogen; LDL-C, low-density lipoprotein cholesterol; CHO, cholesterol; TP, total protein; TG, triglyceride; and HDL-C, high-density lipoprotein cholesterol.

3.3. Carcass Performance and Meat Quality

The results of carcass performance are shown in Table 3. The dressing percentages of the PGZ and PGZ + RES groups were higher than that in control group ($p < 0.05$). Moreover, the semi-eviscerated yield was significantly increased ($p = 0.045$ and $p = 0.037$, respectively) and the abdominal fat was decreased in PGZ, RES, and PGZ + RES supplemental groups ($p < 0.05$).

Table 3. Effects of dietary supplemental with PGZ and RES on the carcass performance of broilers.

Item	Treatment				SEM	p-Value
	Control	PGZ	RES	PGZ + RES		
Dressing percentage (%)	90.96 [b]	91.71 [a]	91.54 [a]	91.73 [a]	0.20	<0.05
Semi-eviscerated yield (%)	86.53 [b]	87.28 [a]	87.24 [a]	87.25 [a]	0.19	<0.05
Eviscerated yield (%)	69.75	69.80	70.33	70.81	0.33	0.817
Breast muscle yield (%)	14.98	14.67	14.84	14.12	0.78	0.520
Thigh muscle yield (%)	17.46	16.71	16.88	16.2	0.56	0.793
Abdominal fat (%)	11.15 [a]	10.13 [b]	10.12 [b]	9.40 [b]	0.14	<0.05

[a,b] Values with different letters within the line mean significant differences ($p < 0.05$). $n = 5$. Abbreviations: SEM, standard error of the means; PGZ, pioglitazone hydrochloride; and RES, resveratrol.

Relative to the control treatment, RES and PGZ + RES supplementation reduced the cooking loss and drip loss of breast muscle (Table S3) and thigh muscle (Table 4) ($p < 0.05$). In addition, the thigh muscle of broiler chickens fed RES and PGZ + RES exhibited an increased muscle A^* (red) ($p < 0.05$) and pH ($p < 0.05$) at 24 h after slaughter. Furthermore, the breast muscle of broiler chickens fed RES and PGZ + RES displayed a tendency toward an improved pH ($p = 0.08$) at 24 h after slaughter. As expected, increases in the IMF values of breast muscle and thigh muscle were observed in broilers fed PGZ or PGZ + RES-supplemented diet ($p < 0.01$), as evidenced by Oil Red O staining (Figure 1).

Table 4. Effects of dietary supplemental with PGZ and RES on the meat quality in the thigh muscle of broilers.

Item		Treatment				SEM	*p*-Value
		Control	PGZ	RES	PGZ + RES		
Shear force (N)		23.42	23.44	23.58	23.23	0.47	0.935
Drip loss (%)		1.43 [a]	1.41 [a]	1.23 [b]	1.20 [b]	0.05	<0.05
Cooking loss (%)		22.25 [a]	22.85 [a]	19.83 [b]	19.35 [b]	0.76	<0.05
$pH_{45\ min}$		6.02	5.94	6.06	5.98	0.06	0.305
$pH_{24\ h}$		5.82 [b]	5.80 [b]	5.91 [a]	5.94 [a]	0.03	<0.05
Color at 45 min	L^*	52.44	51.93	51.10	52.21	0.51	0.532
	A^*	12.69	12.82	12.32	12.71	0.44	0.891
	B^*	7.39	7.49	8.17	8.10	0.67	0.589
Color at 24 h	L^*	51.01	50.33	50.11	50.36	0.78	0.354
	A^*	11.04 [b]	10.87 [b]	11.76 [a]	11.84 [a]	0.16	<0.05
	B^*	8.23	8.45	8.56	10.29	0.43	0.197
Intramuscular fat (%)		3.18 [b]	3.88 [a]	3.22 [b]	4.21 [a]	0.15	<0.01

[a,b] Values with different letters within the line mean significant differences ($p < 0.05$). $n = 5$. Abbreviations: SEM, standard error of the means; L^*, lightnesss; A^*, redness; B^*, yellowness; PGZ, pioglitazone hydrochloride; and RES, resveratrol.

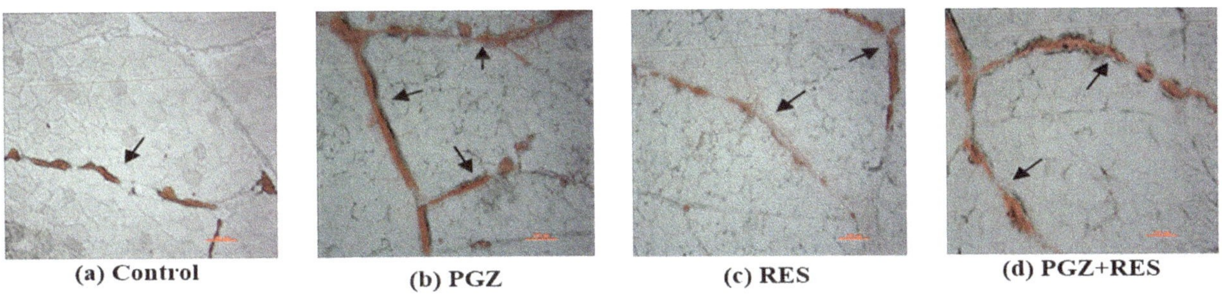

Figure 1. Effects of PGZ and RES on Oil Red O staining in thigh muscle of broilers. The sections were visualized under a light microscope with 100× magnification. $n = 5$. The red areas indicated by the arrows in the figure represent intramuscular fat.

3.4. Determination of the Fatty Acid Composition

Because of the 215.69%–240.35% higher IMF contents of thigh muscle compared to breast muscle (Table S3 and Table 4), we determined the fatty acid compositions of thigh muscle; results are listed in Table 5. Compared with the control group, diet supplemented with PGZ, RES, and PGZ + RES exhibited higher proportions of C18:1ω-9 ($p = 0.009$, $p = 0.008$ and $p = 0.005$, respectively) and monounsaturated fatty acid (MUFA) ($p < 0.05$). Meanwhile, the proportions of C20:3ω-3 were increased in PGZ and PGZ + RES groups ($p < 0.05$).

Table 5. Effects of diet supplemented with PGZ and RES on the fatty acid composition in the thigh muscle of broilers.

Item	Treatment				SEM	*p*-Value
	Control	PGZ	RES	PGZ + RES		
C14:0	0.60	0.64	0.59	0.59	0.02	0.174
C16:0	23.16	23.01	22.76	23.03	0.42	0.527
C16:1	2.91	2.83	2.91	3.01	0.17	0.314
C18:0	8.58	8.39	8.18	8.16	0.33	0.937
C18:1ω9	37.25 [b]	38.90 [a]	39.03 [a]	39.09 [a]	0.37	<0.05
C18:2ω6	20.99	20.87	20.39	21.08	0.25	0.149
C18:3ω6	0.15 [b]	0.18 [a]	0.15 [b]	0.19 [a]	0.01	<0.05
C18:3ω3	1.50	1.51	1.49	1.48	0.03	0.537
C22:0	0.24	0.21	0.22	0.21	0.01	0.217
C20:3ω3	0.30 [b]	0.39 [a]	0.32 [b]	0.41 [a]	0.15	<0.05
C20:4ω6	1.73	1.69	1.74	1.67	0.15	0.111
SFA	32.59	32.25	31.75	31.99	0.28	0.218
MUFA	40.16 [b]	41.73 [a]	41.94 [a]	42.10 [a]	0.33	<0.01
PUFA	24.67	24.64	24.09	24.83	0.35	0.379

[a,b] Values with different letters within the line mean significant differences ($p < 0.05$). $n = 5$. Abbreviations: SEM, standard error of the means; PGZ, pioglitazone hydrochloride; RES, resveratrol; SFA, saturated fatty acid; MUFA, monounsaturated fatty acid; and PUFA, polyunsaturated fatty acid.

3.5. Determination of Muscle Antioxidant Abilities and ROS

The results from the analysis of the lipid antioxidant capacities are presented in Table 6. ROS levels in RES and PGZ + RES groups were significantly decreased compared with the control group ($p < 0.05$), meaning that oxidative stress in thigh muscle was attenuated by RES addition. The broiler chickens belonging to the RES and PGZ + RES groups exhibited higher thigh muscle CAT, GSH-Px, and SOD activities, and lower MDA values ($p < 0.05$) compared with the control chickens. As displayed in Figure 2, the RES group had lower TVB-N values at 5, 7, and 9 days in thigh muscle ($p < 0.05$), and the combination of PGZ with RES substantially reduced the TVB-N values of thigh muscle meat at 7 and 9 days relative to the control levels ($p < 0.05$).

Table 6. Effects of dietary supplemental with PGZ and RES on antioxidant activity in the thigh muscle of broilers.

Item	Treatment				SEM	*p*-Value
	Control	PGZ	RES	PGZ + RES		
ROS (% of Control)	1.00 [a]	0.83 [a]	0.41 [b]	0.35 [b]	0.12	<0.05
T-AOC (U/mg prot)	0.20	0.21	0.21	0.25	0.07	0.978
CAT (U/mg prot)	2.01 [b]	2.05 [b]	2.63 [a]	2.65 [a]	0.15	<0.05
GSH-Px (U/mg prot)	8.43 [b]	8.27 [b]	12.33 [a]	12.78 [a]	0.43	<0.05
T-SOD (U/mg prot)	34.01 [b]	33.10 [b]	39.26 [a]	40.23 [a]	0.37	<0.05
MDA (nmol/mg prot)	5.03 [a]	4.71 [a]	3.85 [b]	3.72 [b]	0.27	<0.05

[a,b] Values with different letters within the line mean significant differences ($p < 0.05$). $n = 5$. Abbreviations: SEM, standard error of the means; PGZ, pioglitazone hydrochloride; RES, resveratrol; T-AOC, total antioxidant capacity; MDA, malonaldehyde; T-SOD, total superoxide dismutase; GSH-Px, glutathione peroxidase; CAT, catalase; ROS, reactive oxygen species; and prot, protein.

3.6. Determination of mRNA Abundances

The mRNA expression levels of antioxidation- and lipogenesis-related genes in thigh muscle are shown in Figure 3. Compared with the control group, the mRNA abundances of the lipogenesis-related genes, such as PGC-1α and FABP3, were greater in the PGZ and PGZ + RES groups ($p < 0.05$). Furthermore, RES and PGZ + RES supplementation resulted in an upregulation of the mRNA abundances of antioxidation-related genes, such as Nrf2 ($p < 0.05$) and SOD1 ($p < 0.05$). In addition, a trend toward an increased GPX 4 mRNA abundance ($p = 0.07$) was found in the PGZ + RES group.

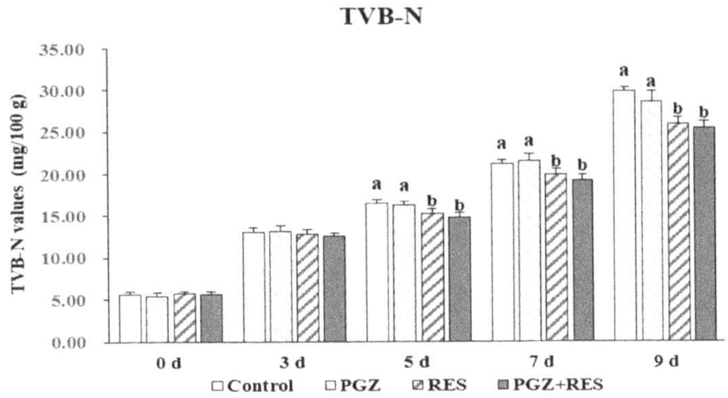

Figure 2. Effects of PGZ and RES on the TVB-N values of the thigh muscle of broilers. [a,b] Values with different letters within the line mean significant differences ($p < 0.05$). $n = 5$. Abbreviations: SEM, standard error of the means; PGZ, pioglitazone hydrochloride; RES, resveratrol; and TVB-N, total volatile basic nitrogen.

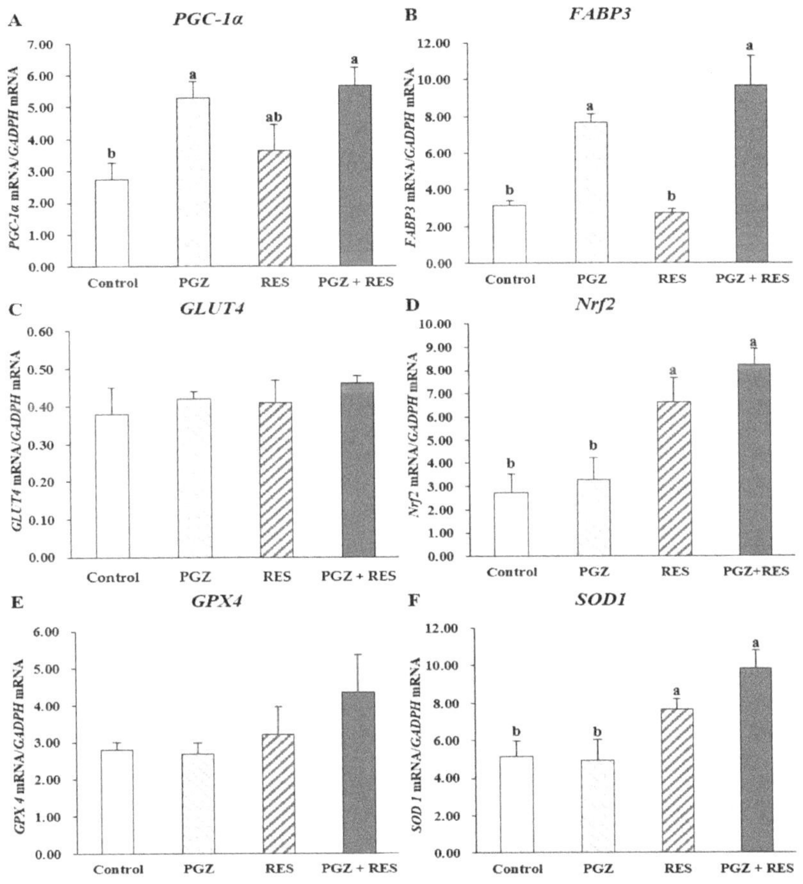

Figure 3. Effects of PGZ and RES on the mRNA abundances ($\times 10^{-4}$) of lipogenesis-related genes, such as (**A**) *PGC-1α*, (**B**) *FABP3*, and (**C**) *GLUT4*, and antioxidant genes, such as (**D**) *NRF2*, (**E**) *GPX4*, and (**F**) *SOD1*, in the thigh muscle of broilers. [a,b] Values with different letters within the line mean significant differences ($p < 0.05$). $n = 5$. Abbreviations: PGZ, pioglitazone hydrochloride; RES, resveratrol; *PGC-1α*, peroxisome proliferator-activated receptor γ coactivator 1α; *FABP3*, fatty acid-binding protein 3; *GLUT4*, glucose transporter 4; *SOD1*, superoxide dismutase 1; *GPX4*, glutathione peroxidase 4; and *NRF2*, nuclear factor erythroid-2-related factor 2.

4. Discussion

The yellow-feathered broiler chicken is highly accepted in the local market of Asian countries due to its delicious meat [33]. However, the yellow-feathered broiler chicken is a slow-growing breed. The ADG and feed/gain of yellow feather broilers are approximately 18.0 g/d and 4.8 (feed/gain, g/g), respectively [27,34]. Therefore, optimization of their feed nutrients is important for improving the growth performance of these slow-growing broiler chickens.

Our previous studies in pigs showed that dietary PGZ and PGZ + RES supplementation improved the ADG and reduced the F/G ratio, the results being consistent with this study [21,22]. The increased ADG of pig may be due to the ability of PGZ to promote adipocyte differentiation and store more fat in the body [35]. In the present study, we used low dose of PGZ as an adipogenic additive rather than as a drug, and in order to minimize the impact of PGZ on the liver and prevent drug residue in chicken products, we started to add a low dose (15 mg/kg) of PGZ to the diets one month before the chicken was released. Furthermore, broiler chickens supplemented with PGZ + RES exhibited an increased dressing percentage and a decreased abdominal fat percentage. Previous studies showed RES reduced the subcutaneous fat mass of pigs and obese rats through the inhibition of fat formation and lipolysis, which was due to the enhanced expression of silent information regulator 1 in adipocytes [36,37]. Our results show that the PGZ and PGZ + RES groups present decreased CHO and LDL-C levels but increased HDL-C concentrations, indicating that these broiler chickens exhibit an increased lipid utilization and an improved fat metabolism in vivo, which is more beneficial for IMF deposition rather than simply shifting toward abdominal fat [22,38,39].

The cooking loss and drip loss are significantly decreased by PGZ + RES supplementation, which suggests an improved water holding capacity [40]. The enhanced antioxidant capacity of the PGZ + RES group is beneficial for reducing glycolysis and increasing the water storage capacity. In addition, the glycogen level largely affects the pH value, and we thus find that PGZ + RES supplementation increases A^* and pH at 24 h after slaughter [21,30]. During storage, most nutrients, such as carbohydrates, proteins, and fats, decompose into various volatile organic compounds following microbial spoilage and biochemical reactions, and these basic nitrogenous compounds increase the TVB-N value, which is an important index for evaluating the shelf life of meat [41,42]. We find that the TVB-N values at 5, 7, and 9 days are decreased in the RES and PGZ + RES groups, which indicates that PGZ+RES addition has positive effects on extending the meat shelf life and improving the meat quality. PGZ targets the adipose tissue through *PPARγ* and *PGC-1α*, and the latter is used to measure the effect of PGZ [12,43]. Moreover, PGZ has potential as a new feed additive for improving meat quality because it can increase the meat IMF [30]. In this study, PGZ activates *PGC-1α* and its downstream genes, such as *FABP3*, and may thus induce a more active fat metabolism. In addition, the Oil Red O staining results shown in Figure 1 also confirm that increased amounts of IMF are deposited in the muscles of the chickens belonging to the PGZ and PGZ + RES groups.

Higher unsaturated fatty acid proportions in meat are beneficial for human health [1]. Early studies had demonstrated that PGZ could enhance the proportions of polyunsaturated fatty acids in serum phospholipids and longissimus thoracis muscle, and MUFAs in rodent muscle [12,21,30,44]. Similar to previous studies, our present study finds that both the PGZ and PGZ+RES supplementation can increase the C18:1ω-9, C18:3ω-6, and C20:3ω3 proportions in thigh muscle, and the latter supplementation results in higher proportions. The changes may be associated with the roles of PGZ as an affinity ligand of *PPARγ*, and PGZ affects several specific genes, not only *PPARγ*, but also *PGC-1α* and *FABP3*, to ensure its normal function [45,46]. Our results support the hypothesis that PGZ improves the IMF contents and MUFA proportions by activating critical genes involved in fat metabolism. In addition, free radicals in meat can attack unsaturated fatty acids, and MDA is well known as one of the end products [3]. Our study demonstrates that dietary supplementation with RES and PGZ + RES decreases the MDA content and enhances the proportion of MUFAs in thigh muscle, which indicates that unsaturated fatty acids are protected from oxidation [47].

Antioxidant enzyme defensive systems, composed of SOD, GSH-Px, and CAT, can directly eliminate ROS in meat [36,44]. The content of ROS determines the degree of oxidative stress response [48]. Excessive ROS can cause cholesterol peroxidation, which in turn reduces membrane fluidity and receptor activity, thereby impairing membrane function [49]. In general, decreased lipid peroxidation or improved antioxidant ability in muscle is beneficial to meat quality. Mujahid et al. showed that excessive MDA accumulation could inhibit the activities of antioxidant enzymes and accelerate oxidative damage to proteins and DNA [50]. RES is a naturally occurring polyphenol compound, and its biological activities, including antioxidant and lipogenesis regulation, have been well researched in vitro and in vivo [51,52]. Numerous studies on the functionality of RES in poultry and pigs have confirmed its efficacy as a feed additive for improving animal production and health [12,29]. RES facilitates the inactivation and subsequent elimination of oxide precursors and mobilizes the expression of antioxidation-related proteins [53,54]. In our present study, the activities of the CAT, T-SOD, and GSH-Px enzymes are increased by RES and PGZ+RES supplementation, and ROS is reduced in the cells of thigh muscle. The mechanism underlying this effect may involve increased mRNA expression of *NRF2*, *SOD1*, and *GPX4*. *NRF2* is a redox-sensitive transcription factor that can initiate the transcription of antioxidant genes, and the synthesis of CAT, SOD, and GSH-Px is regulated by *NRF2* [55,56]. The above results of antioxidant enzyme activities are confirmed through an analysis of the antioxidant gene expression. Indeed, a strong positive correlation is found between antioxidant enzyme activities and the corresponding mRNA levels, which suggests that activities of antioxidant enzymes may be mainly regulated by their transcriptional levels [43].

From the present and some previous studies [13–22], we can conclude that dietary PGZ can increase muscle fat deposition and improve the meat quality of food animals. It has potential as a new functional feed additive. However, in many countries PGZ is a human drug and it is not allowed to be used in feeds or foods. Dietary supplementation with PGZ has the potential to generate residues in animal-derived products. There is limited information on the magnitude of PGZ residue worldwide. Therefore, extensive work has to be carried out to investigate the effects of dietary supplementation with PGZ on food-producing animals, and to prevent the occurrence of PGZ residues.

5. Conclusions

In conclusion, this study indicated that dietary supplementation with 15 mg/kg PGZ and 400 mg/kg RES improved the growth and carcass performances, meat quality, and antioxidant ability of yellow-feathered broiler chickens and prolonged the shelf life of the meat. Importantly, the IMF contents and MUFA proportions were improved and oxidative stress was reduced by PGZ and RES supplementation, and the mechanisms underlying these effects likely involve increases in the mRNA expression of *PGC-1α*, *FABP3*, *Nrf2*, and *SOD1*.

Author Contributions: Conceptualization, H.Y. and H.T.; investigation, C.G. and X.W.; resources, C.G. and X.W.; data curation, F.Z.; formal analysis, F.Z.; writing—original draft preparation, F.Z.; writing—review and editing, C.G., C.J. and F.Z.; visualization, C.G. and S.J. All authors have read and agreed to the published version of the manuscript.

Acknowledgments: Thanks for the help of the laboratory and South China Agricultural University.

References

1. Kouba, M.; Mourot, J. A review of nutritional effects on fat composition of animal products with special emphasis on n-3 polyunsaturated fatty acids. *Biochimie* **2011**, *93*, 13–17. [CrossRef] [PubMed]
2. Bonoli, M.; Caboni, M.F.; Rodriguez-Estrada, M.T.; Lercker, G. Effect of feeding fat sources on the quality and composition of lipids of precooked ready-to-eat fried chicken patties. *Food Chem.* **2007**, *101*, 1327–1337. [CrossRef]
3. Kim, J.E.; Clark, R.M.; Park, Y.; Lee, J.; Fernandez, M.L. Lutein decreases oxidative stress and inflammation in liver and eyes of guinea pigs fed a hypercholesterolemic diet. *Nutr. Res. Pract.* **2012**, *6*, 113–119. [CrossRef] [PubMed]
4. Engel, E.J.; Ratel, J.; Bouhlel, C.; Planche, C.; Meurillon, M. Novel approaches to improving the chemical safety of the meat chain towards toxicants. *Meat Sci.* **2015**, *109*, 75–85. [CrossRef]
5. Fung, D.Y.; Toldra, F. Microbial hazards in food: Food-borne infections and intoxications. In *Handbook of Meat Processing*; Blackwell Publishing: Hoboken, NJ, USA, 2010; pp. 481–500. [CrossRef]
6. Dave, D.; Ghaly, A.E. Meat spoilage mechanisms and preservation techniques: A critical review. *Am. J. Agric. Biol. Sci.* **2011**, *6*, 486–510. [CrossRef]
7. Fürrnsinn, C.; Waldhausl, W. Thiazolidinediones: Metabolic actions in vitro. *Diabetologia* **2002**, *45*, 1211–1223. [CrossRef]
8. American Diabetes Association. Standards of medical care in diabetes–2014. *Diabetes Care* **2014**, *37* (Suppl. S1), S14–S80. [CrossRef]
9. Mirmiranpour, H.; Mousavizadeh, M.; Noshad, S.; Ghavami, M.; Ebadi, M.; Ghasemiesfe, M. Comparative effects of pioglitazone and metformin on oxidative stress markers in newly diagnosed type 2 diabetes patients: A randomized clinical trial. *J. Diabetes Complicat.* **2013**, *27*, 501–507. [CrossRef]
10. Rodriguez, A.; Reviriego, J.; Karamanos, V.; del Canizo, F.J.; Vlachogiannis, N.; Drossinos, V. Management of cardiovascular risk factors with pioglitazone combination therapies in type 2 diabetes: An observational cohort study. *Cardiovasc. Diabetol.* **2011**, *10*, 18. [CrossRef]
11. Shibuya, A.; Watanabe, M.; Fujita, Y.; Saigenji, K.; Kuwao, S.; Takahashi, H. An autopsy case of troglitazone-induced fulminant hepatitis. *Diabetes Care* **1998**, *21*, 2140–2143. [CrossRef]
12. Chabowski, A.; Endzian-Piotrowska, M.; Nawrocki, A.; Górski, J. Not only accumulation, but also saturation status of intramuscular lipids is significantly affected by pparγ activation. *Acta Physiol.* **2012**, *205*, 145–158. [CrossRef] [PubMed]
13. Muurling, M.; Mensink, R.P.; Pijl, H.; Romijn, J.A.; Havekes, L.M.; Voshol, P.J. Rosiglitazone improves muscle insulin sensitivity, irrespective of increased triglyceride content, in ob/ob mice. *Metabolism* **2003**, *52*, 1078–1083. [CrossRef]
14. Lessard, S.J.; Lo Giudice, S.L.; Lau, W.; Reid, J.J.; Turner, N.; Febbraio, M.A.; Hawley, J.A.; Watt, M.J. Rosiglitazone enhances glucose tolerance by mechanisms other than reduction of fatty acid accumulation within skeletal muscle. *Endocrinology* **2004**, *145*, 5665–5670. [CrossRef] [PubMed]
15. Poulos, S.; Hausman, G. A comparison of thiazolidinedione-induced adipogenesis and myogenesis in stromal-vascular cells from subcutaneous adipose tissue or semitendinosus muscle of postnatal pigs. *J. Anim. Sci.* **2006**, *84*, 1076–1082. [CrossRef]
16. George, R.B.; Natasha, B.K.; Gary, F.B.; Corinne, E.C.; Yiming, L.; Laura, M.G.; Joselita, S.; Limin, P.; Francisco, P.; Denise, U. The effects of thiazolidinediones on human bone marrow stromal cell differentiation in vitro and in thiazolidinedione-treated patients with type 2 diabetes. *Transl. Res.* **2012**, *161*, 145–155. [CrossRef]
17. Machado, M.M.; Bassani, T.B.; Cóppola-Segovia, V.; Moura, E.L.; Zanata, S.M.; Andreatini, R.; Vital, M.A. PPAR-γ agonist pioglitazone reduces microglial proliferation and nf-κb activation in the substantia nigra in the 6-hydroxydopamine model of parkinson's disease. *Pharmacol. Rep.* **2019**, *71*, 556–564. [CrossRef]
18. MacKellar, J.; Cushman, S.W.; Periwal, V. Differential effects of thiazolidinediones on adipocyte growth and recruitment in zucker fatty rats. *PLoS ONE* **2009**, *4*, e8196. [CrossRef]
19. Arevalo-Turrubiarte, M.; Gonzalez-Davalos, L.; Yabuta, A.; Garza, J.D.; Davalos, J.L.; Mora, O.; Shimada, A. Effect of 2, 4-thiazolidinedione on limousin cattle growth and on muscle and adipose tissue metabolism. *PPAR Res.* **2012**. [CrossRef]

20. Schoenberg, K.M.; Overton, T.R. Effects of plane of nutrition and 2, 4-thiazolidinedione on insulin responses and adipose tissue gene expression in dairy cattle during late gestation. *J. Dairy Sci.* **2011**, *94*, 6021–6035. [CrossRef]
21. Jin, C.L.; Gao, C.Q.; Wang, Q.; Zhang, Z.M.; Xu, Y.L.; Li, H.C.; Yan, H.C.; Wang, X.Q. Effects of pioglitazone hydrochloride and vitamin E on meat quality, antioxidant status and fatty acid profiles in finishing pigs. *Meat Sci.* **2018**, *145*, 340–346. [CrossRef]
22. Chen, X.; Feng, Y.; Yang, W.J.; Shu, G.; Jiang, Q.Y.; Wang, X.Q. Effects of dietary thiazolidinedione supplementation on growth performance, intramuscular fat and related genes mRNA abundance in the longissimus dorsi muscle of finishing pigs. *Asian Australas. J. Anim. Sci.* **2013**, *26*, 1012–1020. [CrossRef] [PubMed]
23. Ognik, K.; Cholewińska, E.; Sembratowicz, I.; Grela, E.; Czech, A. The potential of using plant antioxidants to stimulate antioxidant mechanisms in poultry. *Worlds Poult. Sci. J.* **2016**, *72*, 291–298. [CrossRef]
24. Sahin, K.; Akdemir, F.; Orhan, C.; Tuzcu, M.; Hayirli, A.; Sahin, N. Effects of dietary resveratrol supplementation on egg production and antioxidant status. *Poult. Sci.* **2010**, *89*, 1190–1198. [CrossRef] [PubMed]
25. Liu, L.L.; He, J.H.; Xie, H.B.; Yang, Y.S.; Li, J.C.; Zou, Y. Resveratrol induces antioxidant and heat shock protein mRNA expression in response to heat stress in black-boned chickens. *Poult. Sci.* **2014**, *93*, 54–62. [CrossRef]
26. Rubiolo, J.A.; Vega, F.V. Resveratrol protects primary rat hepatocytes against necrosis induced by reactive oxygen species. *Biomed. Pharmacother.* **2008**, *62*, 606–612. [CrossRef]
27. Chen, X.; Jiang, W.; Tan, H.Z.; Xu, G.F.; Zhang, X.B.; Wei, S.; Wang, X.Q. Effects of outdoor access on growth performance, carcass composition, and meat characteristics of broiler chickens. *Poult. Sci.* **2013**, *92*, 435–443. [CrossRef]
28. Goulas, A.E.; Kontominas, M.G. Effect of salting and smoking-method on the keeping quality of chub mackerel (Scomber japonicus): Biochemical and sensory attributes. *Food Chem.* **2005**, *93*, 511–520. [CrossRef]
29. Sullivan, K.; El-Hoss, J.; Quinlan, K.G.; Deo, N.; Garton, F.; Seto, J.T. NF1 is a critical regulator of muscle development and metabolism. *Hum. Mol. Genet.* **2014**, *23*, 1250–1259. [CrossRef]
30. Jin, C.L.; Wang, Q.; Zhang, Z.M. Dietary Supplementation with Pioglitazone Hydrochloride and Chromium Methionine Improves Growth Performance, Meat Quality, and Antioxidant Ability in Finishing Pigs. *J. Agric. Food Chem.* **2018**, *66*, 4345–4351. [CrossRef]
31. Slover, H.T.; Lanza, E. Quantitative analysis of food fatty acids by capillary gas chromatography. *J. Am. Oil Chem. Soc.* **1979**, *56*, 933–943. [CrossRef]
32. Wan, X.; Ahmad, H.; Zhang, L.; Wang, Z.; Wang, T. Dietary enzymatically treated *Artemisia annua* L. improves meat quality, antioxidant capacity and energy status of breast muscle in heat-stressed broilers. *J. Sci. Food Agric.* **2018**, *98*, 3715–3721. [CrossRef] [PubMed]
33. Gou, Z.Y.; Jiang, S.Q.; Jiang, Z.Y.; Zheng, C.T.; Li, L.; Ruan, D.; Lin, X.J. Effects of high peanut meal with different crude protein level supplemented with amino acids on performance, carcass traits and nitrogen retention of Chinese Yellow broilers. *J. Anim. Physiol. Anim. Nutr.* **2016**, *100*, 657–664. [CrossRef] [PubMed]
34. Wang, X.Q.; Jiang, W.; Tan, H.Z.; Zhang, D.X.; Zhang, H.J.; Wei, S.; Yan, H.C. Effects of breed and dietary nutrient density on the growth performance, blood metabolite, and genes expression of target of rapamycin (TOR) signaling pathway of female broiler chickens. *J. Anim. Physiol. Anim. Nutr.* **2013**, *97*, 797–806. [CrossRef] [PubMed]
35. De Souza, C.J.; Eckhardt, M.; Gagen, K.; Dong, M.; Chen, W.; Laurent, D. Effects of pioglitazone on adipose tissue remodeling within the setting of obesity and insulin resistance. *Diabetes* **2001**, *50*, 1863–1871. [CrossRef]
36. Zhang, C.; Luo, J.; Yu, B.; Zheng, P.; Huang, Z.; Mao, X.; He, J.; Yu, J.; Chen, J.; Chen, D. Dietary resveratrol supplementation improves meat quality of finishing pigs through changing muscle fiber characteristics and antioxidative status. *Meat Sci.* **2015**, *102*, 15–21. [CrossRef] [PubMed]
37. Wang, B.; Sun, J.; Li, L.; Zheng, J.; Shi, Y.; Le, G. Regulatory effects of resveratrol on glucose metabolism and T-lymphocyte subsets in the development of high-fat diet-induced obesity in C57BL/6 mice. *Food Funct.* **2014**, *5*, 1452–1463. [CrossRef]
38. Khan, M.A.; Peter, J.V.; Xue, J.L. A prospective, randomized comparison of the metabolic effects of pioglitazone or rosiglitazone in patients with type 2 diabetes who were previously treated with troglitazone. *Diabetes Care* **2002**, *25*, 708–711. [CrossRef]

39. Boyle, P.J.; King, A.B.; Olansky, L. Effects of pioglitazone and rosiglitazone on blood lipid levels and glycemic control in patients with type 2 diabetes mellitus: A retrospective review of randomly selected medical records. *Clin. Ther.* **2002**, *24*, 378–396. [CrossRef]
40. Mazur-Kuśnirek, M.; Antoszkiewicz, Z.; Lipiński, K.; Fijałkowska, M.; Purwin, C.; Kotlarczyk, S. The effect of polyphenols and vitamin E on the antioxidant status and meat quality of broiler chickens fed diets naturally contaminated with ochratoxin A. *Arch. Anim. Nutr.* **2019**, *73*, 431–444. [CrossRef]
41. Cai, J.R.; Chen, Q.S.; Wan, X.M.; Zhao, J.W. Determination of total volatile basic nitrogen (TVB-N) content and Warner–Bratzler shear force (WBSF) in pork using Fourier transform near infrared (FT-NIR) spectroscopy. *Food Chem.* **2011**, *126*, 1354–1360. [CrossRef]
42. Rukchon, C.; Nopwinyuwong, A.; Trevanich, S.; Jinkarn, T.; Suppakul, P. Development of a food spoilage indicator for monitoring freshness of skinless chicken breast. *Talanta* **2014**, *130*, 547–554. [CrossRef] [PubMed]
43. Ma, X.; Lin, Y.; Jiang, Z.; Zheng, C.; Zhou, G.; Yu, D.; Cao, T.; Wang, J.; Chen, F. Dietary arginine supplementation enhances antioxidative capacity and improves meat quality of finishing pigs. *Amino Acids* **2010**, *38*, 95–102. [CrossRef] [PubMed]
44. Veleba, J.; Kopecky, J.; Janovska, P.; Kuda, O.; Horakova, O.; Malinska, H.; Hajek, M. Combined intervention with pioglitazone and n-3 fatty acids in metformin-treated type 2 diabetic patients: Improvement of lipid metabolism. *Nutr. Metab.* **2015**, *12*, 52. [CrossRef] [PubMed]
45. Li, F.N.; Yang, H.S.; Duan, Y.H.; Yin, Y.L. Myostatin regulates preadipocyte differentiation and lipid metabolism of adipocyte via ERK1/2. *Cell Biol. Int.* **2011**, *35*, 1141–1146. [CrossRef]
46. Hondares, E.; Mora, O.; Yubero, P.; de la Concepción, M.R.; Iglesias, R.; Giralt, M.; Villarroya, F. Thiazolidinediones and rexinoids induce peroxisome proliferator-activated receptor-coactivator (PGC)-1α gene transcription: An autoregulatory loop controls PGC-1α expression in adipocytes via peroxisome proliferator-activated receptor-α coactivation. *Endocrinology* **2006**, *147*, 2829–2838. [CrossRef]
47. Zhang, C.; Luo, J.; Yu, B.; Chen, J.; Chen, D. Effects of resveratrol on lipid metabolism in muscle and adipose tissues: A reevaluation in a pig model. *J. Funct. Foods* **2015**, *14*, 590–595. [CrossRef]
48. Gill, S.S.; Tuteja, N. Reactive oxygen species and antioxidant machinery in abiotic stress tolerance in crop plants. *Plant Physiol. Biochem.* **2010**, *48*, 909–930. [CrossRef]
49. Arulselvan, P.; Subramanian, S.P. Beneficial effects of Murraya koenigii leaves on antioxidant defense system and ultrastructural changes of pancreatic b-cells in experimental diabetes in rats. *Chem. Biol. Interact.* **2007**, *165*, 155–164. [CrossRef]
50. Mujahid, A.; Akiba, Y.; Warden, C.H.; Toyomizu, M. Sequential changes in superoxide production, anion carriers and substrate oxidation in skeletal muscle mitochondria of heatstressed chickens. *FEBS Lett.* **2007**, *581*, 3461–3467. [CrossRef]
51. Paulo, L.; Ferreira, S.; Gallardo, E.; Queiroz, J.A.; Domingues, F. Antimicrobial activity and effects of resveratrol on human pathogenic bacteria. *World J. Microbiol. Biotechnol.* **2010**, *26*, 1533–1538. [CrossRef]
52. Alagawany, M.M.; Farag, M.R.; Dhama, K.; Abd El-Hack, M.E.; Tiwari, R.; Alam, G.M. Mechanisms and beneficial applications of resveratrol as feed additive in animal and poultry nutrition: A review. *Int. J. Pharmacol.* **2015**, *11*, 213–221. [CrossRef]
53. Liu, Y.; Chan, F.; Sun, H.; Yan, J.; Fan, D.; Zhao, D.; An, J.; Zhou, D. Resveratrol protects human keratinocytes HaCaT cells from uVA-induced oxidative stress damage by downregulating Keap1 expression. *Eur. J. Pharmacol.* **2011**, *650*, 130–137. [CrossRef] [PubMed]
54. Sgambato, A.; Ardito, R.; Faraglia, B.; Boninsegna, A.; Wolf, F.I.; Cittadini, A. Resveratrol, a natural phenolic compound, inhibits cell proliferation and prevents oxidative DNA damage. *Mutat. Res.* **2001**, *496*, 171–180. [CrossRef]
55. Loboda, A.; Damulewicz, M.; Pyza, E.; Jozkowicz, A.; Dulak, J. Role of Nrf2/HO-1 system in development, oxidative stress response and diseases: An evolutionarily conserved mechanism. *Cell. Mol. Life Sci.* **2016**, *73*, 3221–3247. [CrossRef] [PubMed]
56. Balasubramanian, P.; Longo, V.D. Linking Klotho, NRF2, MAP kinases and aging. *Aging* **2010**, *2*, 632. [CrossRef] [PubMed]

11

Formulation Strategies to Improve Oral Bioavailability of Ellagic Acid

Guendalina Zuccari *, Sara Baldassari, Giorgia Ailuno, Federica Turrini, Silvana Alfei and Gabriele Caviglioli

Department of Pharmacy, Università di Genova, 16147 Genova, Italy; baldassari@difar.unige.it (S.B.); ailuno@difar.unige.it (G.A.); turrini@difar.unige.it (F.T.); alfei@difar.unige.it (S.A.); caviglioli@difar.unige.it (G.C.)

* Correspondence: zuccari@difar.unige.it

Featured Application: An updated description of pursued approaches for efficiently resolving the low bioavailability issue of ellagic acid.

Abstract: Ellagic acid, a polyphenolic compound present in fruit and berries, has recently been the object of extensive research for its antioxidant activity, which might be useful for the prevention and treatment of cancer, cardiovascular pathologies, and neurodegenerative disorders. Its protective role justifies numerous attempts to include it in functional food preparations and in dietary supplements, and not only to limit the unpleasant collateral effects of chemotherapy. However, ellagic acid use as a chemopreventive agent has been debated because of its poor bioavailability associated with low solubility, limited permeability, first pass effect, and interindividual variability in gut microbial transformations. To overcome these drawbacks, various strategies for oral administration including solid dispersions, micro and nanoparticles, inclusion complexes, self-emulsifying systems, and polymorphs were proposed. Here, we listed an updated description of pursued micro and nanotechnological approaches focusing on the fabrication processes and the features of the obtained products, as well as on the positive results yielded by in vitro and in vivo studies in comparison to the raw material. The micro and nanosized formulations here described might be exploited for pharmaceutical delivery of this active, as well as for the production of nutritional supplements or for the enrichment of novel foods.

Keywords: ellagic acid; oral administration; bioavailability; microformulations; nanoformulations; solubility enhancement

---

1. Introduction

Pomegranate, *Punica granatum*, is well-known as a traditional medicinal fruit mentioned in the Old Testament of the Bible, the Qur'an, the Jewish Torah, and the Babylonian Talmud as a sacred fruit harbinger of fertility, abundance, and luck. Historically and currently, pomegranate has been used for various purposes [1]. The bioactive compound mainly responsible for the health effects of pomegranate is ellagic acid (EA), as it represents one of the most potent dietary antioxidants.

EA is a polyphenol compound which derives from ellagitannins (ET), a family of molecules in which hexahydroxydyphenic acid residues are esterified with glucose or quinic acid. Following a hydrolytic process, the hexahydroxydyphenic acid group is released, dehydrates and spontaneously lactonizes, forming EA. Punicalagin isomers are the most representative of total tannins extracted from pomegranate (Figure 1).

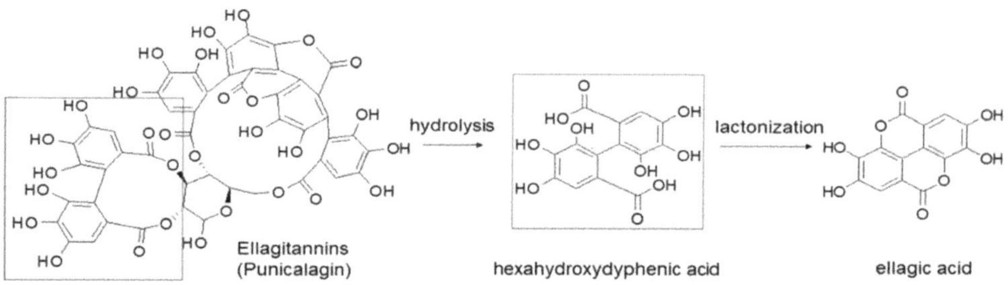

Figure 1. Hydrolysis of punicalagin (a pomegranate ellagitannin) to produce ellagic acid.

Present also in a large variety of tropical fruit, nuts, berries (strawberries, raspberries, blackberries, cranberries, goji berries) and in a type of edible mushroom (Fistulina epatica), EA has recently attracted deep interest, since many research studies showed the role of oxidative stress in different pathologic conditions such as cancer, diabetes, cardiovascular and autoimmune diseases, obesity, and neurodegenerative disorders [2–7]. In this regard, EA may be a useful adjunct in Parkinson's disease treatment, as it proved to protect dopamine from oxidation and, by reducing inflammation and oxidative stress, to exert a neuroprotective effect [8]. Besides being able to reduce the pathological levels of NF-kB, EA may play a beneficial role in diseases associated with CNS inflammation, such as multiple sclerosis. EA has also been proposed as antidepressant and anxiolytic drug for its capability to modulate the monoaminergic system and to increase the endogenous levels of brain-derived neurotrophic factors [6]. In the last decade, several studies investigated EA effects on many types of cancer, showing its ability to arrest cell cycle progression, modulate pathways linked to cell viability, and inhibit angiogenesis via inactivating metalloproteinases [9–18]. For example, EA resulted in inducing apoptosis and modulating gene expression in different colon cancer cell lines at the concentrations achievable in the intestinal lumen from the diet, suggesting a potential role in cancer chemoprevention [19]. Moreover, EA may counterbalance the dangerous side effects of antitumoral drugs such as cisplatin, doxorubicin, and cyclosporine [20–22]. In addition, EA proved to possess antimicrobial properties inhibiting the growth of methicillin-resistant Staphylococcus aureus and Salmonella [23]. These properties were explained through the ability of EA of either coupling with proteins of the bacterial wall or inhibiting gyrase activity, which cleaves the DNA strand during bacterial replication. Furthermore, EA seemed to counteract the HIV-1 virus replication, by binding envelope proteins and inhibiting reverse transcriptase [24]. Pomegranate extract has been traditionally used for treating gastrointestinal bleeding and various types of wounds, due to EA's ability to promote blood coagulation by the activation of the Hageman factor (Factor XII) [25]. Moreover, preliminary results suggest potential anti-inflammatory properties [26,27] and an important role in prevention of cardiovascular diseases [28–30]. Finally, EA finds application also in cosmetic and nutraceutical industries, mainly for antiaging and prophylactic purposes respectively [31–33]. An overview of EA activities is shown in Figure 2.

However, though EA has the potential to become an efficacious agent in the prevention and therapy of several diseases, as supported by several papers present in the literature, the working efficacy of EA dietary and therapeutic formulations have been mainly examined at preclinical level. To date, few clinical studies have been performed to evaluate EA beneficial effects in humans, with often a limited number of patients, and most of them concern the administration of pomegranate juice or extract in cancer patient diet or deal with the evaluation of the enhancement of cognitive/functional recovery after stroke [34,35]. It was suggested that EA'S low water solubility and rapid metabolism might hinder the progress towards translational research. In our opinion, further studies focused on the application of micro and nanotechnology could provide more encouraging data, opening the path to new strategies able to overcome EA's poor biopharmaceutical characteristics. Hence, the goal of this review is to provide to scientists, embarking on the research involving EA, a scenario of all pursued formulation attempts. Therefore, starting from a description of EA bioavailability and solubility, a summary of micro and nanosystem-based strategies suitable for improving orally administered EA efficacy is provided.

2. EA Chemical Structure and Solubility

EA is a chromene-dione derivative (2,3,7,8-tetrahydroxy-chromeno [5,4,3-cde]chromene-5,10-dione), encompassing both a hydrophilic moiety with 4 hydroxyl groups and 2 lactone groups, and a planar lipophilic moiety with 2 biphenyl rings. This particular structure has both hydrogen bonding acceptor (lactone) and donor (–OH) sites (Figure 1). Due to the weak acidic nature of its four phenolic groups (pKa1 = 5.6 at 37 °C), around neutral pH it is mainly deprotonated on positions 8 and 8′, while above pH 9.6 lactone rings open to give a carboxyl derivative [36]. EA low oral bioavailability is mostly due to its poor water solubility (9.7 μg/mL), which increases with pH, as well as the antioxidant action [37]. However, in basic solutions, phenolic compounds lack stability as these molecules, under ionic form, undergo extensive transformations or are converted to quinones as a result of oxidation. A stability study on pomegranate fruit peel extract demonstrated that EA content significantly decreases in few weeks regardless of the pH of the solution, due to the hydrolysis of the ester group with hexahydroxydiphenic acid formation, suggesting that EA should not be stored in aqueous medium [38]; this aspect reinforces the need to develop novel systems also for EA stabilization.

Prior to facing the route of the development of a new delivery system, the knowledge of solvents, co-solvents and substances in which EA could be consistently soluble and stable represents an indispensable step for designing a good formulation. In this regard, with the aim of providing a useful guidance for further research studies, Table 1 gathers published data concerning EA solubility. Concerning organic solvents, EA is slightly soluble in methanol, soluble in DMSO and shows maximum solubility in N-methyl-2-pyrrolidone (NMP), confirming the effect of basic pH on EA dissolution. An analogous trend is also observable in aqueous solutions, where results implied that the solubility of EA depends on the pH values of the media. While EA is almost insoluble in acidic media and distilled water, its water solubility is significantly improved by basic pH. As highlighted further ahead, one of the mostly exploited vehicles is polyethylene glycol (PEG) 400, as it is endowed with satisfactory biocompatibility and, at the same time, is miscible with both aqueous and organic solvents. EA solubility in oils and surfactants is also provided, helpful for developing emulsifying-based techniques.

3. EA Dietary Assumption

In foods and beverages, EA is present in several forms, such as unmodified, glycosylated and/or acetylated or inside the structure of hydrolysable ET polymers, usually esterified with glucose moieties. However, only a small fraction of free EA is absorbed in the stomach, since ET are resistant to acidic pH. ET hydrolysis occurs in the small intestine, leading to the release of EA, which can be absorbed mainly by passive diffusion, although an in vitro experiment on Caco-2 cells monolayer model suggested the involvement of a protein-mediated transport [39]. Once reached the systemic circulation, EA undergoes a massive first pass effect, being transformed in methyl esters, dimethyl esters or glucuronides, detectable in human plasma from 1 to 5 h after ET ingestion [40]. Meanwhile, unabsorbed ET and EA fractions are mostly converted to a family of metabolites called urolithins by colon microflora. Urolithins contain a common structure of dibenzopyranone and are more lipophilic, showing higher absorption rate across colon epithelium compared to EA, thus resulting 25–80 times more bioavailable [41]. Naturally, there is huge variability in microbial metabolism of EA among individuals depending on differences in gut microbiota composition. According to the metabotype (M-0, M-A and M-B), humans may produce no urolithins, highly active urolithins or less active urolithin, so that EA consumption may not exert equal health benefits in all subjects [42–44].

EA oral bioavailability was studied in human subjects after 180 mL of pomegranate juice consumption. In this study, the maximum EA blood concentration (Cmax) was 32 ng/mL which was rapidly metabolized in the next 4 h, confirming the extremely poor intestinal absorption [41]. Other pharmacokinetic studies supported the hypothesis that higher EA-to-ET ratio in the oral dose corresponds to higher EA plasma concentrations, but, intriguingly, no enhancement in bioavailability was observed increasing the dose of free EA up to 524 mg, suggesting that a saturation condition in the absorption process was achieved [45]. In addition to these unfavorable conditions, it must be considered that polyphenols are not consumed in sufficient quantities among population in Western Europe and developing countries, because of inadequate fruit and vegetable intake, though an increased awareness of the benefits of a balanced diet is fostering the assumption of dietary supplements [46].

4. Formulation Strategies for Improving EA Oral Bioavailability

The Biopharmaceutics Classification System (BCS) is a scientific framework for classifying drug substances based on their aqueous solubility and intestinal permeability. It is a drug-development tool that divides drugs into high/low solubility and permeability classes. Based on its low aqueous solubility and low permeability (apparent permeability coefficient = 0.13×10^{-6} cm/s [47]), EA is classified as class IV drug according to the BCS, i.e., endowed with low solubility and low permeability, features that limit a lot its clinical application. Micro and nanotechnology approaches widely demonstrated great potential in modifying pharmacokinetic, bioavailability and stability of several drugs, including phytochemicals used in cancer chemoprevention or in dietary supplements, contributing to preserve the properties of the active ingredients or to mask bad tastes and odors [48–50]. From a formulation point of view, a good EA dosage form would grant easier handling, transport and storage, increase its light resistance, hamper undesirable reactions such as oxidation and hydrolysis, and enhance solubility.

Focusing on preparative methods, features and biological results of the developed EA-loaded formulations, an exhaustive description of the employed strategies is thereafter presented. The various approaches were divided according to the kind of the dosage form and reported in Tables 2 and 3 depending on the micro or nanosize of the final product. Moreover, in the final paragraph, examples of fixed combinations containing EA were also described and discussed.

4.1. Micronized EA (m-EA)

According to Noyes-Whitney law, an effective way to increase dissolution rate and oral absorption of a substance is the size reduction of powder particles [51]. For this purpose, anti-solvent precipitation may represent a valid processing technique. In comparison to more popular micro and nanocarriers that will be discussed in the following sections, this approach presents several advantages, such as easy realization and rapidity. In addition, the process allows the reduction of organic solvents use and the one-step processing favors scalability. The anti-solvent precipitation of a poorly water-soluble substance is simply obtained by dissolving it in a solvent, followed by rapid mixing with a solvent-miscible anti-solvent. After mixing, the substance precipitates in micro-sized particles, since a supersaturated solution forms. The critical step of this method is to produce crystal nuclei rapidly, avoiding their excessive growth. For process optimization, precipitation time and temperature, addition speed of the solution to the anti-solvent, their volume ratio, drug concentration and stirring intensity are the keys parameters that have to be checked.

Li et al. set the best conditions to produce m-EA by anti-solvent precipitation with an accurate preformulative study [52]. An EA solution in NMP (30 mg/mL) was added to water, used as anti-solvent, at a rate of 30 mL/h with 2 min precipitation time, at 3 °C and 2500 rpm stirring. Then, the precipitate was dispersed in a maltodextrin aqueous solution to have a solid concentration of 1 mg/mL and was lyophilized. The authors verified that residual NMP (class 2 residual solvent) in the final product was in agreement with the established International Council for Harmonization of Technical Requirements for Pharmaceuticals for Human Use (ICH) limit [53]. The m-EA freeze-dried powder, whose mean particle diameter was 428 nm, in a comparison to raw EA and to a physical mixture of EA in maltodextrin, showed the fastest dissolution rate. Surely, maltodextrin acted as hydrotrope, but the result could be attributed exclusively to the high specific surface of the lyophilized powder and to the low crystallinity of the incorporated EA. All in all EA water dissolution was improved up to 11.67 μg/mL at 37 °C.

In addition, the 2, 2-diphenyl-1-1-pycrylhydrazyl (DPPH)-scavenging activity was higher than that of not-micronized EA and oral bioavailability in rats increased twice in comparison to raw EA.

In another study, Beshbishy et al. obtained m-EA using the anti-solvent precipitation method by injecting into deionized water a 10 mg/mL ethanolic solution of EA at a fixed flow rate [54]. m-EA particles, collected by filtration and vacuum dried, showed modified morphology with respect to the parent material and appeared as needle-shaped or rod-like structures. In vitro and in vivo experiments, performed by intraperitoneal injection in mice, showed a significantly improved m-EA activity against blood parasites as Babesia and Theileria. However, the authors concluded that EA activity requires further investigations to understand whether EA inhibits parasites grow or causes their death.

A similar approach was performed using supercritical CO_2 as anti-solvent. In this procedure a solution of EA in NMP was sprayed into a vessel where a CO_2 stream was continuously flowed under supercritical conditions. Solution atomization led to a fast mass transfer between supercritical CO_2 and the solution itself, which caused supersaturation and subsequent rapid precipitation of EA in the form of micro-sized particles [55]. The study focused on the influence of process parameters and EA concentration on size, polydispersity index (PDI) and morphology. Moreover, a co-precipitation with Eudragit® L 100 was also carried out and, starting from EA:Eudragit® 1:1 weight ratio, a drug loading (DL) of 49% was achieved. Experimental results showed that EA concentration should be, if possible, close to saturation, thus allowing obtaining particles in the form of sticks and flowers and with a mean diameter of about 3 μm. Also, in this case residual NMP was far lower than the mandatory established limit. m-EA showed higher dissolution rate with respect to raw EA due to the small particle size, reaching higher concentrations even at pH 1.2. Finally, the coprecipitates with Eudragit® showed the fastest dissolution rates, probably because the dispersion of EA within the polymer led to smaller particles and, surprisingly, the presence of the polymer did not delay the pomegranate acid delivery, possibly since EA particles were obtained in crystalline form, confirming that the product was a solid dispersion in which the pomegranate acid particles were not encapsulated.

4.2. *EA in Spray Dried and Lyophilized Powders*

Solid dispersions are semi-crystalline or amorphous dispersions (ASDs) of a molecule in an inert matrix. ASDs represent a valid alternative for the development of microsystems entrapping poorly water-soluble molecules. ASDs can be prepared from a solution by spray drying, freeze drying, co-precipitation, rotary evaporation, film casting, or hot-melt extrusion. In all cases, a suitable polymeric excipient should have functional groups able to form H-bonds with EA, thus allowing the formation of metastable amorphous EA dispersions with adequate stability over time.

In this context, a first attempt was made with maltodextrins, a saccharide-based excipient extensively used in food industry. Using a freeze drying technique, maltodextrin DE5-8 or DE18.5 were applied to form a solid network around a cloudberry phenolic extract [56]. The amorphous matrices were prepared starting from a maltodextrin (9% *w/w*) and a cloudberry extract (1% *w/w*) aqueous solution, mixed under slight heating for about 0.5 h to avoid ET degradation. DE5-8 complexed phenolics in a more efficient way, rationally due to its higher molecular weight. The microencapsulation improved the extract storage stability to hydrolysis, and also in this case the improvement contribution of DE5-8 was better than that of DE18.5. Microencapsulation always resulted in a decrease of EA formation by ET hydrolysis during storage, but the stability was strongly dependent on relative vapor pressure (RVP). At 66% RVP and 25 °C maltodextrin DE5-8 protected phenolics up to 32 days, then the degradation reactions occurred in a major extent. On the contrary, the antioxidant properties did not alter during storage either in the extract alone or in the presence of DE5-8, probably because the loss of original phenolics was compensated by new formed molecules with equal antioxidant activity.

In another study, polymers as the hydrophilic hydroxypropylmethyl cellulose acetate succinate (HPMCAS), the rather hydrophobic carboxymethyl cellulose acetate butyrate (CMCAB), and the very hydrophobic cellulose acetate adipate propionate (CAAdP) were compared with polyvinylpyrrolidone (PVP), taken as reference excipient being widely used in ASD formulations [57]. Mixtures of EA and

PVP, CMCAB or HPMCAS at different weight ratios (1:9 and 1:3), dissolved in acetone:ethanol (1:4 *v/v*), were spray dried with yields of 50%–60%. ASD from CAAdP were instead prepared by co-precipitation method, due to the limited quantity of polymer available. EA was amorphous up to 25% *w/w* in solid dispersions with PVP and HPMCAS, and up to 10% with CMCAB and CAAdP. Consequently, EA-PVP and EA-HPMCAS reached the highest solution concentration of 1500 and 280 μg/mL, respectively. In a stability study performed in aqueous buffer (pH 6.8) for 24 h at room temperature (rt), pure EA showed a degradation degree by lactone ring opening of 20%, while lower values—16% for CMCAB, 14% for CAAdP, 6% for PVP and just 5% for HPMCAS—were found in the ASD samples. Dissolution rate at pH 6.8 was remarkably superior to that of pure EA, both from PVP and HPMCAS ASDs, while from CAAdP or CMCAB ASDs it was very slow and did not achieve adequate EA concentration. As expected, under acidic conditions EA release from PVP was quite fast, whereas from cellulose esters it was minimal, but this advantage was nullified by crystallization of a large amount of the EA released from PVP. Since the 1:9 ASDs with HPMCAS effectively stabilized EA against crystallization and degradation, the authors concluded that this could be considered the most promising formulation.

To prepare an ingredient for functional foods, a fine microdispersed powder containing EA was obtained by spray drying using low methoxyl pectin, characterized by high biocompatibility, good palatability, taste, and prebiotic properties [58]. Pectin represents a common natural food additive (E440) authorized in several food categories [59]. By varying EA:pectin weight ratio, different formulations were prepared. The best microdispersed powder, obtained with 1:4.5 EA:pectin ratio, showed a mean particle diameter of about 10 μm and a DL equal to 21%, allowing solubilizing 63 μg/mL of EA in water. Moreover, the drug loading of EA in the powder remained stable for one year of storage in a desiccator at 25 °C.

Recently, the search for promising systems suitable for dietary supplements enlarged the research field to other natural polymers, such as alginic acid (ALG) [60]. EA-ALG nanoparticles (NPs) were prepared by dissolving both EA and ALG at the concentration of 250 μg/mL in an aqueous medium at pH 8.5. The solution was spray dried and the obtained powder was added to a $CaCl_2$ solution in order to induce reticulation by ionic gelation. The resulting NPs had a mean diameter of 670 nm with zeta potential around −27 mV. Thanks to the high degree of EA solubilization in the basic medium, the encapsulation efficiency (EE) was 50%, much higher than the EE of NPs prepared from a neutral medium. As rational remark to this procedure performed in basic environment, it may be highlighted that the possible degradation of EA in alkaline medium during preparation was not taken into consideration. This EA-ALG system showed a biphasic release profile with a fast phase during the initial 3 h, justified by EA adsorbed on NPs surface, followed by a sustained, complete release until 8 h. A mice model of epilepsy was used to assess in vivo EA-ALG NPs efficacy as anticonvulsant and neuroprotective agent by oral treatment every other day for 33 days. Results indicated that EA contained in this dosage form prevented seizures during the experimental period, and had a more pronounced effect, compared to free EA, by reducing oxidative stress damage, inhibiting apoptosis and down-regulating cytokine levels.

4.3. *Inclusion Complexes*

4.3.1. EA Inclusion in Cyclodextrins (CDs)

CDs are able to form inclusion complexes with a variety of molecules by hosting a guest drug with suitable polarity and dimension inside their lipophilic cavity, thus modifying its physico-chemical behavior. Among CDs, hydroxypropyl-β-CD (HP-β-CD) is characterized by better inclusion ability and higher complex solubility. To investigate the feasibility and the stoichiometry of inclusion complex formation of EA in HP-β-CD, phase solubility studies were carried out in water at 30 °C for 72 h to reach the equilibrium [61]. The obtained solubility curve of EA showed a linear increase with HP-β-CD concentration up to 12 mM, followed by a negative deviation from linearity up to 24 mM. This trend belongs to AN type and was explained through the formation of a soluble 1:2

EA:HP-β-CD inclusion complex with stability constants K1:1 and K1:2 of 201.61 and 18.91 M-1, respectively. A 15 mM HP-β-CD solution allowed to solubilize 54.40 µg/mL of EA in water at 30 °C. Subsequently, the inclusion complex was prepared by freeze drying a solution of EA:HP-β-CD in 1:2 molar ratio upon its filtration. In a dissolution test performed at pH 6.8 and 37 °C, HP-β-CD released about 55% of the loaded drug in 15 min, more than 5-fold the amount dissolved from pure EA powder. Furthermore, the anti-inflammatory effect of complexed EA was tested in a rat model of inflammation. Oral treatment with 10 or 20 mg/kg EA-HP-β-CD resulted more efficacious than the administration of EA alone or of 10 mg/kg indomethacin as indicated by the measure of paw edema volume. The feasibility of using β-CDs as complexing agent for EA was also investigated with less satisfactory results [62]. The complex was less soluble, leading to a total EA concentration up to 39.14 µg/mL, lower than that obtained in the previous study with HP-β-CD, due to the lower β-CD solubility.

By following a different preparative procedure, β-CD was again chosen as EA complexing agent in another study [63]. A saturated aqueous β-CD solution was slowly mixed with 125 mg/mL of EA ethanolic solution and stirred for 2 h at rt, then the mixture was filtered and finally freeze-dried. As highlighted by SEM images, the obtained powder was different from those of the pure components in terms of morphology and dimensions; EE was 35% and in vitro dissolution studies (pH from 6.8 to 7.4) showed a multiphase release profile: a little amount of EA (3%) was released in a slow initial stage during the first 4–8 h, followed by a rapid phase between 8 and 24 h with 73% of drug released, and by a final slow phase. The effect of EA-β-CD complexes on proliferation of human liver carcinoma cells was evaluated by MTT assay and, though the lack of data relating to the treatment of cells with EA alone do not allow a comparison, a remarkable inhibition was observed.

Another study to increase EA solubility regarded EA complexation with β-CD nanosponges (NS) [64]. NS are hyper-cross-linked CDs obtainable either from a mixture of CDs, or CDs conjugated with relevant amounts of linear dextrin. The cross-linking leads to a cage-like structure, where CDs cavities and nanochannels are strictly connected to form a porous network. Consequently, NS are able to incorporate drugs both as inclusion and non-inclusion complexes, thus improving the overall solubilizing ability of the starting CD. In this work the β-CD NS were obtained using dimethyl carbonate as a cross-linker. By a solubility study the authors demonstrated that the β-CD NS solubilized EA in water up to 49.79 µg/mL. The mean particle size of EA-β-CD NS was about 423 nm, PDI was found of 0.409 and the zeta potential equal to −34 mV, thus sufficiently high to produce a stable suspension. In this regard, it has to be remembered that very low Z-potential values (ζ < 5 mV) usually translates in particles with high tendency to agglomerate that means physical instability in solution. On the contrary, increasing the charge associated with the particle i.e., $\zeta \pm 30$ mV or higher, usually prevents particles sticking after collision [65,66].

Moreover, EE was around 69% and, as highlighted by X-ray diffraction, in the polymeric structure EA was present either in the amorphous form or as a solid-state solution. The release profiles showed that only about 20% of loaded EA was released after 24 h, suggesting strong retention of EA in the NS network. A pharmacokinetic study in rabbits indicated that oral administration of EA-β-CD NS increased EA bioavailability by more than 2-fold if compared to the free EA suspension.

In a more recent work, a useful analysis of the preparation processes and experimental conditions for obtaining inclusion complexes was reported [67]. Three inclusion methods were considered, i.e., stirring-ultrasonic, ultrasonic, and grinding. In the first method, which led to the highest EE (84%), EA, dissolved in a small amount of ethanol, was added by slowly dripping into HP-β-CD aqueous solution under stirring, then the mixture was sonicated for 20 min, and finally kept under stirring at rt for further 18 h. The suspension was filtered, concentrated with rotary evaporator and vacuum dried to obtain the inclusion compound. Process conditions were optimized by an orthogonal test design, in which EA:HP-β-CD molar ratio, ethanol concentration, inclusion time and temperature were considered to be experimental parameters. The experimental design showed that EA:HP-β-CD molar ratio of 1:2, ethanol concentration of 60%, inclusion time of 36 h, and inclusion temperature of 20 °C were the best conditions.

Recently, Gontijo et al. failed in realizing an effective complexation in HP-β-CD as the first study did, possibly because in this case the phase solubility studies were performed at rt instead of 30 °C [68]. In fact, a linear increase in EA solubilization was achieved only in alkaline solution, where raising HP-β-CD concentrations up to 300 mM led to a total EA concentration only 2.8-times higher than that without CD. However, the low stability constant of the complex (K1:1 = 4.5 M-1) resulted in a low complexation efficiency with an EA:CD stoichiometric ratio equal to 1:45. Concerning the procedure, the inclusion complex was prepared by spray drying a suspension of EA:CD 1:1 molar ratio in 0.1 M NaOH solution. Furthermore, also methyl-β-CD was used without success, since no complexing ability was found either in water or in basic solution. Finally, Caco-2 cells were employed in an in vitro model of invasive Candida albicans infection to test the bioactivity of EA complexes, but no statistically significant difference was observed in terms of antifungal activity between free or complexed EA, suggesting that complexation apparently did not improve antimycotic efficacy.

4.3.2. EA Inclusion in Metalla-Cages

A recent strategy for allowing EA administration in a more bioavailable form consisted of a self-assembled metallo-supramolecular architecture able to host EA inside three-dimensional cages [69]. These vectors, engineered via coordination-driven self-assembly, present several advantages. In particular, the metal-guest interactions are very strong and highly directed, leading to the formation of a stable rigid complex. In this regard, EA was encapsulated in arene-ruthelium metalla-prism cages with a yield of about 90% and its anticancer activity was investigated. The cytotoxic effect against A549 human lung cancer cells was significant, overall considering that free EA lacked any activity. In an attempt to investigate if EA effect was macrophage-mediated, a study on RAW264.7 murine leukemia monocytes was performed, highlighting that EA encapsulated in metalla-cages exhibited an inhibitory effect for cancer cells via G-CSF induction and Rantes inhibition at both mRNA and protein levels.

4.4. EA Encapsulated in Polymeric Carriers

4.4.1. Eudragit® Microspheres

EA was proposed as a prophylactic agent for the treatment of inflammatory bowel disease. Jeong et al. developed microspheres for EA site-specific delivery to the ileum using Eudragit® P-4135, a copolymer of methacrylic acid, methyl acrylate and methyl methacrylate able to dissolve at pH > 7.2, which corresponds to the pH of the distal part of the small intestine [70]. The adopted preparation method was a solvent evaporation process in oil phase using an acetone/light liquid paraffin system. Different polymer amounts, ranging from 0.5 to 1.5 g, were dissolved in acetone and mixed with 0.5 mg of EA, previously dispersed in the same solvent and sonicated. Then, the resultant solution was added to light liquid paraffin containing Span 80 (3% *v*/*v*), and the emulsion was stirred up to complete evaporation of acetone. The microspheres, harvested by filtration and washed with hexane to remove paraffin, yielded an EE ranging from 57 to 99% and a DL from 33 to 36%. Increasing polymer amounts resulted in higher EE and size increase from 98 to 168 μm. As expected, EA release was pH-dependent and at pH 6.8 an initial burst effect of about 25% was followed by a sustained release, with approx. 40% of loaded drug released after 6 h. In this case, the burst effect would not be critical, as it occurred at the target site, as demonstrated by the negligible EA in vitro release at more acidic pH. For in vivo studies fluorescein was added to the preparative mixture to accurately measure microsphere dissolution rate. The obtained microspheres were orally administered to rats and blood samples were collected every hour. The comparison between collected images of microspheres in small intestine of euthanized rats and fluorescein plasma concentration evidenced that the plasmatic peak occurred 3 h after administration, when microspheres reached the ileocaecal junction. Therefore, this Eudragit®-based system represents an effective vehicle to target EA release to the terminal ileum, providing enhanced absorption in the region and thus preventing the variability connected to EA conversion into urolithins.

4.4.2. Poly (Lactic-Co-Glycolic Acid) (PLGA) and Poly (ε-Caprolactone) (PCL) Nanospheres

Among the various encapsulating polymers, PLGA has been extensively used due to its biocompatibility, biodegradability, and ability to protect the drug from degradation and in obtaining sustained drug release [71]. To increase EA bioavailability, PLGA-based formulations suitable for oral administration were developed [72]. The particles were prepared by using the emulsion-diffusion-evaporation technique. PLGA was dissolved in ethyl acetate under stirring for 2 h, then EA, previously dissolved in PEG 400, was added, and a fine EA dispersion was obtained. The dispersion was emulsified in an aqueous phase containing a stabilizer (1% *w*/*v*), such as polyvinyl alcohol (PVA), PVA:chitosan (CS) in 80:20 ratio, or didodecyldimethylammonium bromide (DMAB). After with stirred the emulsion at 1000 rpm for 3 h, homogenization at 15,000 rpm for 5 min was performed to obtain a more homogeneous and smaller size distribution. Then, the addition of water caused the diffusion of the organic solvent into the aqueous phase, and the evaporation of the organic phase by heating led to EA-polymer precipitation. The use of DMAB yielded smaller particles, while the other two stabilizers led to bigger sizes and higher PDI, probably due to the increased viscosity and irregular entanglement associated with the long polymeric chains. The zeta potential was highly positive for NPs containing DMAB (about +75 mV), equal to +25 mV for the ones with PVA-CS, and slightly negative for those with PVA. The highest EE (55%) was obtained with PVA-CS, the lowest with DMAB (42%). Concerning EA release at pH 7.4, all products exhibited a rapid initial release followed by a slower sustained phase, with PVA NPs being the fastest, because PVA hydrophilic groups favor water penetration into the NPs compared to the more lipophilic DMAB. However, the release study was not performed simulating the pH conditions of the whole gastrointestinal tract. To study the permeability of NPs, an in situ intestinal study was performed on rats based on the close loop method, even though the disappearance of drug from the luminal side, used for determining permeation, not always correlates with the rate of absorption of the drug in the systemic circulation. EA-DMAB NPs showed the highest uptake (87%) in accordance with their smaller size and higher hydrophobicity. The antioxidant activity was assessed in cell free system and in yeast cell culture model, confirming the good scavenging activity of the encapsulated pomegranate acid. The same research group also investigated the feasibility of EA-loaded PCL NPs in comparison to PLGA NPs using the same emulsion-diffusion-evaporation method, but with an important modification: during the primary emulsion step EA underwent a rapid precipitation that caused its low entrapment, so the authors added the stabilizer to the polymer solution to increase EA solubility [22]. As expected, EE increased from 42% to 52% for DMAB-PLGA NPs and from 55% to 62% for PVA-PLGA NPs, not much different from EE of DMAB-PCL and PVA-PCL NPs (47% and 57% respectively). Since PCL is a slower degrading polymer compared to PLGA, its release profiles yielded slower release rates. The antioxidant potential of EA-DMAB NPs was assessed by evaluating their protective action against cyclosporine A-induced nephrotoxicity in rats: both PLGA- and PCL-based NPs were 3-fold more effective than free EA in kidney protection, thus indicating the improved bioavailability of the encapsulated EA.

Unfortunately, PLGA NPs major drawback is rapid opsonization, so that their systemic circulation time is too short. To address this issue, EA was encapsulated in PLGA NPs grafted with poly (ethylene glycol) (PEG) chains to escape to the reticuloendothelial system [73]. In a proof of principle study, NPs were prepared by the double emulsion-solvent evaporation method. Two dichloromethane stock solutions, containing PLGA-PEG and EA respectively, were mixed, added to 200 μL of phosphate-buffered saline solution (PBS) and sonicated. This primary *w*/*o* emulsion was emulsified in PVA 1% *w*/*v* aqueous solution by sonication. Subsequently, this *w*/*o*/*w* emulsion was first diluted with PVA 1%, then heated for dichloromethane evaporation and finally the obtained NP were dialyzed and lyophilized. The NP showed a diameter of 175 nm with PDI of 0.14. In vitro biological studies on MCF-7 and Hs578T breast cancer cell lines proved a significant activity enhancement of EA in the encapsulated form, being its IC50 values more than 2-fold lower than those of the free form.

In a further attempt to curb the phagocytic activity, a combination of CS and PEG was considered to be surface coating material for EA-PLGA NPs [74]. The NPs were prepared by o/w single emulsion-solvent evaporation method as follows. EA and PLGA were separately dissolved in chloroform and emulsified with PVA 2% *w/v* aqueous solution containing 12% *w/w* CS and 5% *w/w* PEG 2 kDa through sonication. The emulsion was stirred overnight up to complete evaporation of the organic solvent. The coated CS-PEG-PLGA NPs were compared to PLGA NPs and PEG-PLGA NPs prepared in the same way. EE was always about 65%, while the mean hydrodynamic diameter was 220 nm for PLGA NPs and CS-PLGA NPs, and 255 nm for CS-PEG-PLGA NPs. As expected, positive charges were present on the surface of CS-PLGA NPs and CS-PEG-PLGA NPs (ζ = +27 and ζ = +38 mV, respectively); on the contrary, a negative zeta potential characterized PLGA NPs (ζ = −10 mV). Release studies, carried out at pH 7.4, showed an initial faster release of about 35% during the first 10 h, followed by a more controlled release phase, with further 55% of drug released in 24 h. In vitro anticancer activity against HepG2 hepatocellular carcinoma cells and HCT 116 colorectal cancer cells revealed a significant cytotoxic effect of EA loaded in CS-PEG-PLGA NP vs. free EA at every tested dosage (up to 100 μM), suggesting an efficient NPs uptake by the cells. Also Mady et al. used PCL for successful entrapment of EA through the emulsion-evaporation method [75]. In this case, EA, dissolved in PEG 200, was mixed with PCL, solubilized in ethyl acetate, and the mixture was emulsified by homogenization with an aqueous solution containing a stabilizer (PVA, DMAB or poloxamer 407 ranging from 0.1% to 1% *w/v*). The resulting *o/w* emulsion was sonicated for 1 min, then diluted in water and kept under stirring for 6 h up to complete evaporation of the organic solvent. The obtained NPs were centrifuged, washed with distilled water to remove unentrapped EA, and freeze-dried. As previously observed, 1% DMAB yielded the smallest mean NP size (193 nm). In fact, by creating a positive charge layer around the internal phase, DMAB provided electrostatic repulsion, while PVA and poloxamer, being uncharged, induced only a steric stabilizing effect. The type of stabilizer affected also EE and DL. DMAB gave the lowest EE (66.4%–73.5%) and DL (56.8%–63.9%), whereas PVA provided the highest EE (78.3%–90.3%) and DL (68.1%–78.6%). These differences in EA entrapment were probably linked to the unequal EA aqueous dissolution granted by the stabilizer. Release studies at pH 7.4 illustrated the typical two-step profile, with an initial fast release driven by diffusion for the first 12 h, and a second slow release due to the retarded diffusion of EA from the NPs inner layers. Finally, the release of EA from DMAB-PCL NPs reached up to 48% of the loaded amount in 8 days. The anticancer efficacy of EA-PCL NPs tested on HCT-116 colon adenocarcinoma cells was 6.9-fold enhanced in comparison to free EA, meaning that encapsulated EA was significantly superior in reducing HCT-116 cell survival. Moreover, a pharmacokinetic study by oral administration in rabbits showed that the nano-sized formulation improved the relative EA bioavailability by 3.6 times.

4.4.3. Chitosan Micro/Nanospheres

CS is a polysaccharide obtained by partial deacetylation of chitin, endowed by important features from the biomedical point of view. It is mucoadhesive, non-toxic, biocompatible, biodegradable and exerts slight antimicrobial properties. CS is a weak base (pKa value ~6.5) positively charged at physiologic pH. In a study by Arulmozhi et al., EA-CS NP were prepared by ionic gelation method using sodium tripolyphosphate (TPP) as gelating agent, with CS to TPP ratio of 4:1. CS was dissolved in 1% *v/v* acetic acid under magnetic stirring overnight and the final pH was adjusted to 5.0 [76]. Different EA amounts (25, 50, 100 mg) dissolved in DMSO (0.5% *v/v*) were added to the CS solution, and finally an equal volume of 1 mg/mL TPP solution was added dropwise under mild stirring. The mixture was kept under stirring till NPs formation. The lowest EA amount added led to the highest EE and DL, of 94% and 33% respectively. Spherical NP were obtained with a mean diameter of 176 nm and a slightly positive zeta potential (ζ = +4 mV), which could be due to the adsorption of EA on the particle surface, thus masking CS positive groups. As usually, the EA release showed a two-step profile, where 55% of loaded EA was rapidly released during the first 8 h and the remaining 20% was released more slowly until 48 h. Finally, EA-CS NPs were investigated as anticancer agents and proved higher cytotoxicity than free EA on KB human oral cancer cell line at almost all the tested doses. Successively, in another study by Gopalakrishnan et al., EA-CS NPs were been investigated as anti-hemorrhagic agents [77]. Also in this case, the NPs were prepared by ionic gelation procedure with 1:12 EA:CS ratio. They sized around 80 nm, being 50% their maximum EE. Release studies showed an EA fast dissolution (84% in 12 h), suitable for clotting purposes. In fact, EA-CS NPs yielded a significantly faster clotting time when compared to free EA, void CS NPs, and an EA:CS physical mixture.

A recent study by Ding et al. focused on the preparation of EA microspheres based on CS and sodium alginate as coating materials [78]. CS-alginate microparticles (MPs) were prepared by ionotropic gelation. The polycationic CS and Ca^{2+} were added to the EA alginate solution, thus a polyelectrolyte complex coating formed; MPs were further stabilized with 2% glutaraldehyde solution. SEM images revealed a mean size of 4.36 μm, with some EA crystals on the surface, while EE was around 30%. Regarding dissolution profiles, they reflected the structure of the MPs, because EA was quickly released at 0–3 h and 6–24 h, while it was slowly released from 3 to 6 h because of the necessary deconstruction of the strong coating, suggesting the effective dispersion of EA inside the MPs. Therefore, this formulation seems to be more suitable if a sustained release is desired. Finally, in vitro experiments on 3T3-L1 adipocytes showed a consistent inhibition of adipogenic differentiation by entrapped EA vs. EA alone, suggesting its possible use in obesity treatment.

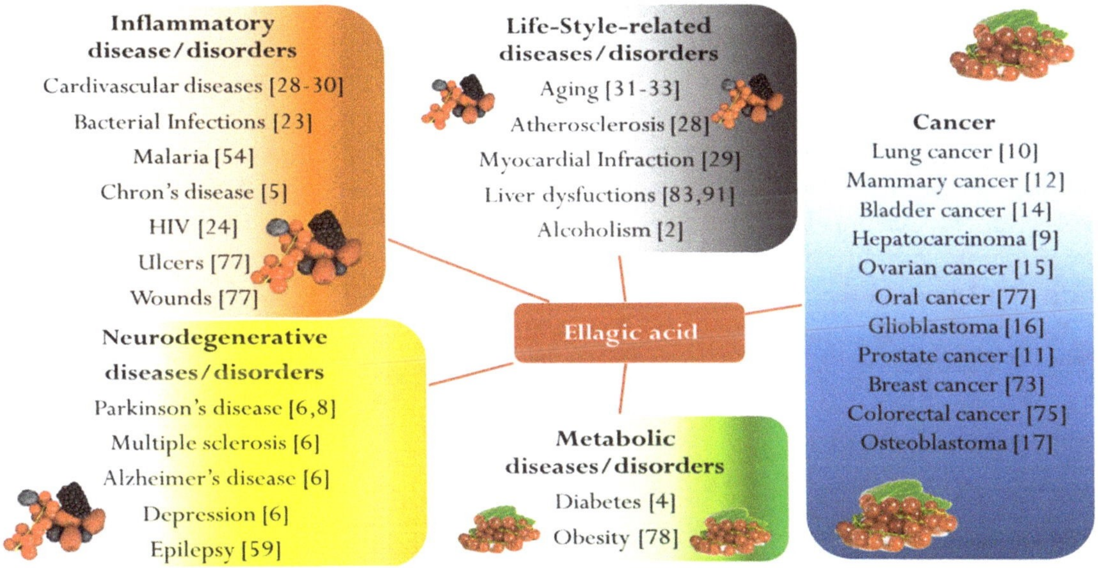

Figure 2. An overview of different ellagic acid's activities versus human diseases.

4.4.4. Zein Nanocapsules

Among the various formulations that have been designed to ameliorate EA bioavailability, only one attempt concerns nanocapsules (NCs). NCs, because of their hollow structure, display large surface-to-volume ratio, low density, short solid-state drug diffusion length, and good surface permeability. On the other hand, NCs present some disadvantages, such as weak mechanical properties and complex production procedures. Recently, EA has been successfully encapsulated into NCs made of zein, a group of water insoluble proteins (prolamins) extracted from corn gluten meal [79]. Ruan et al. developed a system, characterized by EA and a sacrifice template to form the core and by an outer film of zein mixed with a plasticizer to increase film flexibility. NCs were prepared by antisolvent coprecipitation in water using Na_2CO_3 as core-forming template. Firstly, EA was dissolved in 0.1 M NaOH solution and mixed with Na_2CO_3 aqueous solution (1% *w*/*w*). EA-Na_2CO_3 cores were formed by coprecipitation in 70% ethanol, then an ethanolic solution of triethyl citrate and zein was added to the core suspension, and finally the mixture was poured in distilled water to induce NCs precipitation and Na_2CO_3 diffusion outwards. Spherical NCs with an average diameter of 72 nm were obtained. EA content (326 mg/g) resulted much higher than that of NPs prepared without Na_2CO_3. Surprisingly, not remarkable differences were observed in the release behavior between solid and hollow NPs. Both formulations did not show a burst effect, achieving a well-controlled release. An in vitro permeability study on Caco-2 cells showed improved transporting ability of EA NCs compared to pure EA or solid zein NPs, because EA, either when free or present on NPs surface, tended to bind DNA and proteins, causing accumulation inside the cells. In addition, the superior anti-inflammatory activity of orally administered EA NCs was confirmed in a rat model and explained by pharmacokinetic experiments showing AUC 2.5 and 8.7 times higher than the ones of EA solid NPs and pure EA, respectively.

4.5. Dendrimers

Dendrimers are branched polymers characterized by a tree-like structure of globular shape of nanometric dimension endowed with inner cavities, able to host lipophilic drugs, and a peripheral shell rich in functionalized groups [80,81]. Among various typologies of dendrimers, the well-known polyamidoamine dendrimers (PAMAM) and branched polyethyleneimine polymers (b-PEI) are in vitro well-performant, but mainly because of their extremely cationic inner framework and poor biodegradability, they can exert hemolytic effect, which hindered their clinical translation. To reduce dendrimers cytotoxicity in the study by Alfei et al., PAMAM dendrimers were avoided and EA has been physically encapsulated into cationic dendrimers characterized by an uncharged polyester-based hydrolysable inner core peripherally esterified with a selection of four different amino acids [58]. Histidine, lysine, N-methyl-glycine and N, N-dimethylglycine were chosen to provide the carrier with primary, secondary, tertiary protonable amino groups and with the guanidine residue that is known to promote cellular up-take. Two dendrimers, one hydrophilic and one encompassing in the structure a C-18 chain that provides an amphiphilic character, were employed to encapsulate EA. Dendrimers were dissolved in MeOH and EA was added obtaining a conspicuous suspension maintained at acidic pH under magnetic stirring at room temperature for 48 h. The non-complexed EA was removed by filtration and the final EA dendrimer nanodispersions were brought to a constant weight under vacuum. The values of DL were of 46% (hydrophilic) and 53% (amphiphilic). NPs mean dimension was of 70 nm for both compounds while EA water solubility increased up to 1.7 mg/mL in the case of the amphiphilic dendrimer and up to 4.8 mg/mL in the case of the hydrophilic one.

4.6. Peptide Microtubes

In the last decade, there has been an increased focus on biomaterial fabrication, of which peptide micro and nanotubes provide a good example. These ordered structures origin from a dipeptide, usually L-diphenylalanine (FF), by self-assembling. Six FF units form cyclic hexamers, which can further be stacked to produce narrow channels with a diameter of approximately 10 Å. Various peptides can be used as building blocks, thereby these vehicles can be tailored according to the desired application [82]. In a study by Barnaby et al., EA was encapsulated by the self-assembling of the synthetic precursor bolaamphiphile bis (N-amido threonine)-1, 5-pentane dicarboxylate, with a pentyl chain between the head groups of the two aminoacids, according to the following procedure [83]. First, the bolaamphilile solution was allowed to assemble for 2–3 weeks with a higher yield at pH 6, then EA was added at a concentration of 0.06 mM, which maximizes EE, as at elevated concentrations EA forms discotic liquid crystal assemblies upon aggregation, while lower EA amounts efficiently insert into the nanotubes by capillarity. The self-assembled EA-loaded nanostructure had an average diameter ranging from 0.5 to 1 μm with an EE of about 80%. EA release was affected by pH, as expected, with about 50% of loaded acid released within 2 h at pH 6 and 7. EA antibacterial property was assessed in vitro against Gram-positive S. aureus and Gram-negative E. coli, and in both cases EA-loaded microtubes were significantly more efficacious than free EA. That was an unexpected result, since EA alone did not exert any action against S. aureus, but probably the explanation relies on the antibacterial activity of threonine itself.

4.7. Functionalized Graphene Oxide (GO) Carriers

GO is prepared by chemical oxidation of graphite and represent a promising pharmaceutical material due to its small size, biocompatibility, possible functionalization, and low cost. GO offers interesting opportunities for loading and delivering aromatic molecules such as flavonoids via simple physisorption [84]. To further improve GO aqueous solubility, it was covalently functionalized with hydrophilic excipients such as poloxamer F38, Tween 80 and maltodextrin through an esterification reaction. In a study by Kakran et al., EA loading was carried out by mixing 0.5 mg/mL functionalized GO aqueous solution with 50 mg/mL EA in 0.01 M NaOH solution [85]. After stirring overnight at rt, undissolved EA was removed by centrifugation, while the small amount of free dissolved EA was separated by dialysis. Therefore, EA was loaded by simple mixing, due to adsorption supported by hydrogen bonding, π-π stacking and hydrophobic interactions between the acid and the aromatic regions of graphene sheets [85]. Tween 80-GO exhibited the highest DL, with about 1.22 g of EA per g of excipient, as probably the poloxamer hindered GO surface with its higher molecular dimensions, differently Tween 80-GO exhibited a larger area available for the drug attachment. Release studies showed not differences among the three GO derivatives, probably due to the stronger hydrophobic interactions and hydrogen bonding between EA and the carriers, in any case an increasing release was observed raising pH values, which was attributed to the increased hydrophilicity and solubility of EA at higher pH. In vitro cytotoxic activity against MCF7 human breast cancer cells and HT29 human adenocarcinoma cells was found to be higher than the one of free EA, while the antioxidant property of EA-GO formulations was similar to that of EA alone, proving no interference of the carriers on EA scavenging activity as confirmed by DPPH assay.

4.8. Lipid-Based Carriers

4.8.1. Solid Lipid Nanoparticles (SLNs)

SLNs are colloidal delivery systems based on a high melting point lipid core coated by surfactants. In recent years, SLNs have been considered to be promising delivery systems due to the ease of manufacturing processes, scale up capability, biocompatibility and also biodegradability of formulation constituents [86]. SLNs also have some disadvantages, such as low drug loading efficiency and the possibility of drug expulsion due to its crystallization during storage [87]. Besides the initial burst release of drug which usually occurs represent an additional concern with these formulations [88]. These systems were proposed as carriers for improving the anticancer activity of EA against prostate cancer by Hajipour et al. [89]. EA-loaded SLNs were prepared by the homogenization method as follows. EA was added after dissolution in DMSO to the melted lipid phase, consisting of Precirol® and Tween 80, then the aqueous phase with poloxamer 407 was added dropwise at the same temperature under high speed homogenization. Finally, the obtained nanoemulsion was cooled for NP solidification. Tween 80 seemed to increase EA encapsulation, while the poloxamer at higher concentrations yielded unsuitable sizes. The optimal formulation showed an average diameter around 100 nm with a narrow size distribution (PDI = 0.28) and a negative zeta potential ($\zeta = -20$ mV). The EE was about 89% and DL 36%. Release studies performed at pH 7.4 demonstrated a noteworthy initial burst effect due to the drug present on or close to the surface, followed by a sustained release phase. Like polymer-based particulate systems, SLNs often lack uniformity of distribution of the drug in the nanostructure, which can explain the initial burst effect. In vitro biological studies revealed that EA loaded in SLNs was more efficacious than free EA on PC3 human prostate cancer cells, being the IC50 values of 61 and 82 μM, respectively.

4.8.2. Liposomes (LPs)

With the aim of producing an effective EA dietary supplement, a formulation based on phospholipids was developed by Murugan et al. [90]. EA and hydrogenated soy phosphatidylcholine (HSPC) in 1 to 4 molar ratio were dissolved in dichloromethane and refluxed at a temperature not exceeding 60 °C for 2 h. The solution was concentrated and then n-hexane was added for inducing the precipitation of the EA-LPs by anti-solvent method with a yield of encapsulation of 89% *w/w*. The resulting EE was around 29% and SEM images showed that EA was intercalated in the spherical lipid layer and that EA-LPs had a mean diameter ranging from 1 to 3 µm. In an in vivo CCl4-induced hepatic damage model, rats orally treated with EA-LPs exhibited a remarkably reduced antioxidant liver damage from oxidative stress. The same effect was obtained only with a double amount of free EA. Moreover, a pharmacokinetic study on the rats confirmed the enhancement of bioavailability exerted by the complexation as the AUC value resulted increased by 2.8-fold if compared to free EA administration.

With the aim of developing a nutritional support during chemotherapy with cyclophosphamide, a recent study by Stojiljković et al. evaluated the protective effect of EA encapsulated into nanoliposomes, in a cyclophosphamide-induced rat liver-damage model [91]. EA was incubated overnight with a suspension of LPs in 1:10 ratio, obtaining an EE equal to 60%. Stability studies were performed at 37 °C at different pH (from 4.5 to 9.9) or in the presence of metal ions. During the 3-h study, EA in the encapsulated form always resulted less degraded, whereas free EA showed higher chelating ability, thus indicating the effectiveness of encapsulation. Subsequently, the loaded liposomes were essayed in a cyclophosphamide-induced rat liver-damage model. The animals were treated for 5 days either with free or encapsulated EA, and only on the third day cyclophosphamide administration occurred. The authors determined serum liver-damage parameters, oxidative tissue damage parameters, and morphological changes of liver cells through histopathological observations. The results indicated that EA nanoliposome formulation could represent an efficacious tool in adjuvant cancer chemotherapy.

4.8.3. Self-Emulsifying Delivery Systems (SNEDDS)

Among the several approaches that were suggested to achieve better EA oral bioavailability, SNEDDS represent an attractive opportunity. SNEDDS are isotropic mixtures of active molecules, oils, surfactants, and coemulsifiers or solubilizers able to form an *o/w* nanoemulsion. Once in the gastrointestinal fluid, the fine droplet dispersion enhances water solubility of lipophilic molecules, thus providing more effective absorption. Though SNEDDS are not suitable for exerting controlled release, they demonstrated high potential in increasing oral bioavailability of several therapeutic agents, such as curcumin [92]. However, the poor palatability of the components and low compatibility with other excipients might be the major drawbacks in case of oral delivery. In this context, Avachat et al. developed a formulation containing EA starting from a mixture of EA and soy lecithin at 1:1 molar ratio [93]. This preliminary step was necessary to facilitate the incorporation of a larger amount of EA in the lipid phase and to increase its solubility. The EE was 95% and the water and n-octanol solubilities of complexed EA at 25 °C increased by about 3 and 6 times, respectively. Well-formulated SNEDDS should disperse in a few seconds under gentle stirring. Therefore, after a preliminary screening, the optimized composition was selected with the help of ternary phase diagrams. The final formulation included EA PL, glyceryl triacetate 40% *v/v* as oil, polyoxyl 40 hydrogenated castor oil 40% *v/v* as surfactant, PEG 400 20% *v/v* as co-surfactant. To prevent EA oxidation, tocopherol was added in the oil phase. This composition led to the smallest mean diameter (106 nm, PDI of 0.3388) and to a negative zeta potential ($\zeta = -13$ mV). As expected, EA release from SNEDDS was very fast at pH 6.8 (nearly 95% after 1 h), and a bit slower at pH 1.2, but this largest amount of dissolved EA may strongly increase gastrointestinal absorption. To support the hypothesis of a potential enhancement of oral bioavailability, an ex vivo permeability study was also carried out, which confirmed the good permeation of the SNEDDS through rat stomach and intestine.

In a more recent work by Wang et al., EA was entrapped in SNEDDS made of food-grade components to prepare a highly biocompatible formulation suitable for nutraceuticals, performing the procedure previously described [94]. Firstly, a preliminary study investigated the solubility of EA in different oils, surfactants, and co-surfactants, then ternary diagrams were constructed. The best formulation was selected on the basis of the weight of water added dropwise to the mixed ingredients without causing turbidity, and the best formula corresponded to EA 2.5 mg/mL, PEG 400 45% *v/v* as co-surfactant, Tween 80 45% *v/v* as surfactant, and caprylic/capric triacylglycerols 10% *v/v* as oil. This mixture was able to load EA in a concentration 250 times higher than its aqueous solubility and to release it completely within 1 h at pH 6.8. In addition, the authors developed a pharmacokinetic study on rats to evaluate in vivo oral bioavailability of EA in SNEDDS and the AUC value of the emulsified EA was 6.6 times higher than the one of the EA suspension.

An issue associated with SNEDDS is the possibility for the dissolved molecule to undergo precipitation if administered in high dose [95]. Therefore, a slight but important modification consists of adding a precipitation inhibitor, such as PVP or HPMC, capable of increasing drug loading and stability over time. On this purpose a supersaturable self-nanoemulsifying drug delivery system (S-SNEDDS) containing EA was developed by Zheng et al. [96]. As usual, according to the results of solubility studies, those vehicles highly mixable with EA were chosen for formulation optimization through ternary phase diagrams. The final formulation consisted of Tween 80, PEG 400 and ethyl oleate at the ratio of 67.5/22.5/10% *w/w*, which can be fully diluted with water without phase separation. In addition, to avoid EA precipitation during storage, 0.5% PVP K30 was added. DL was equal to 4 mg/g, while EA S-SNEDS droplet mean diameter was 45 nm and the zeta potential was negative ($\zeta = -23$ mV). The dissolution profiles were characterized by a slightly less rapid release, compared to EA-SNEDDS, since the complete delivery at pH 6.8 was reached after 4 h. Finally, in vitro and in vivo antioxidant activity was studied by DPPH assay or by detection of malondialdehyde, superoxide dismutase and glutathione in mice liver. The results indicated that the antioxidant ability of EA was noticeably improved by the S-SNEDDS vs. EA suspension, but it was of a lesser extent compared to vitamin C.

4.9. EA Formulations in Fixed Combination with Other Bioactive Molecules

With the aim to prevent or treat diseases associated with increased oxidative stress such as hyperglycemia, obesity, atherosclerosis, the industry of nutritional supplement has rapidly and greatly expanded over recent decades [97]. In a study by Ratnam et al., EA was combined with Coenzyme Q10 (CoQ10) in a PLGA nanoparticulate formulation to prevent hyperlipidemia [98]. The NP were prepared by emulsion-diffusion-evaporation method, dissolving PLGA and CoQ10 in ethyl acetate, and EA in PEG 400. The two solutions were mixed and emulsified in 1% PVA aqueous solution. The mean particle size obtained was around 259 nm with EE of 70% for EA and of 72% for CoQ10. In an in vivo experiment, rats were fed with a high fat diet and daily administered with oral suspension of free drugs or once in three days with EA-CoQ10 NP. The effects on reducing glucose and triglyceride levels were similar, but only EA-CoQ10 NP exerted a prolonged control on cholesterol levels for up to 2 weeks after treatment suspension.

With the aim at decreasing the risk of chemotherapy complications, further investigation concerning co-delivery systems involved EA and chemotherapy drugs, such as paclitaxel (PTX), for a combined anticancer therapy [99]. The idea of combining these actives was based on the evidence that PTX resistance relies on the NF-kB-dependent pathway, while EA hinders NF-kB. The two molecules were formulated with the temperature-sensitive amphiphilic copolymer poly (N-isopropylacrylamide-PEG acrylate), stable under physiological conditions, being its lower critical solution temperature higher than 37 °C. The NP were loaded directly by using the dialysis method at different temperatures. Several formulations were prepared, but the best one, in terms of EE and efficacy, contained the copolymer, PTX and EA in 20:1:1 weight ratio. The mixture was solubilized in DMF and dialyzed against deionized water, in which the copolymer self-assembled, developing core-shell nanoparticles. Since the drugs molecular weight is lower than the dialysis membrane cut-off

(12 kDa), a slight loss of EA and PTX was unavoidable. To limit this phenomenon and to achieve a high EE, the loading reaction was performed at 4 °C and an EE of 92% for PTX and of 98% for EA were achieved. After completion of the dialysis, the solution was filtered and lyophilized. NP size was below 200 nm and the release was well-controlled, as only the 8% of both drugs was released after 2 h, while the 61% of PTX and the 88% of EA were released after 48 h. In vitro cytotoxicity tests were performed against MCF-7 breast cell line. After 48 h PTX/EA-loaded NP showed slightly higher cytotoxicity compared to free PTX, deriving from an improved cellular uptake. However, further studies would be needed to assess an eventual synergism between the two loaded drugs.

Table 1. Solubility of ellagic acid in various vehicles.

	Vehicles	Solubility (mg/mL)	Temperature	Ref.
Solvents	N-methyl-2-pyrrolidone	25	37 °C	[36]
	DMSO	2.5	37 °C	[36]
	Pyridine	2.0	37 °C	[36]
	Methanol	$(671 \pm 17) \times 10^{-3}$	37 °C	[36]
	Ethanol	1.02 ± 0.04	25 °C	[96]
Cosolvents	PEG 200	4.178	25 °C	[94]
	PEG 400	11.0 ± 0.5	25 °C	[96]
	Propylene glycol	2.1 ± 0.1	25 °C	[96]
Oils	Palmester 3575 [1]	0.030	25 °C	[94]
	Cottonseed oil	0.005	25 °C	[94]
	Soybean oil	0.29 ± 0.01	25 °C	[95]
	Castor oil	1.63 ± 0.07	25 °C	[96]
	Oleic acid	0.29 ± 0.01	25 °C	[96]
	Ethyl oleate	2.34 ± 0.06	25 °C	[96]
Surfactants	Tween 20	1.605	25 °C	[94]
	Sucrose esters	0.115	25 °C	[94]
	Isopropyl myristate	1.94 ± 0.07	25 °C	[96]
	Cremophor RH40 [2]	2.5 ± 0.1	25 °C	[96]
	Tween 80	3.5 ± 0.1	25 °C	[96]
	Lecithin	0.085 ± 0.004	25 °C	[96]
	Poloxamer F68	0.036 ± 0.002	25 °C	[96]
Aqueous Solutions	Phosphate buffer pH 7.4	$(33 \pm 16) \times 10^{-3}$	37 °C	[36]
	Phosphate buffer pH 6.8	$(11.1 \pm 0.4) \times 10^{-3}$	25 °C	[96]
	Acetate buffer pH 4.5	$(6.9 \pm 0.3) \times 10^{-3}$	25 °C	[96]
	Distilled water	$(8.2 \pm 0.4) \times 10^{-3}$	25 °C	[96]
	HCl 0.1 M in water	$(1.03 \pm 0.06) \times 10^{-3}$	25 °C	[96]

[1] Caprylic/capric triacylglycerols [2] Polyoxyl 40 hydrogenated castor oil.

In a multiple drug co-delivery study by Fahmy et al., fluvastatin (FLV), alpha lipoic acid (ALA) and EA were chosen for their anticancer properties [100]. As dosage form, nanostructured lipid carriers (NLCs) were taken into consideration. NLCs are a relatively new generation delivery system, developed to overcome SLNs drawbacks such as low payload, crystallization of the lipid matrix, and drug expulsion during storage. In fact, NLCs, being composed of both solid and liquid lipids, do not undergo crystallization, allowing higher drug loading and consequent better bioavailability of low soluble drugs. Furthermore, NLCs are composed of highly biocompatible and biodegradable lipids, so they have a wider range of applications. As an example, NLCs are useful nutraceutical delivery systems with high drug loading, stability, capability in increasing bioavailability of bioactive compounds and consumer acceptability. In addition, they may provide controlled release of the encapsulated materials [101]. In this work, NLCs were prepared by hot emulsification–ultrasonication method starting from 1% almond oil, 3% glyceryl dibehenate, 0.5% L-α-phosphatidylcholine phospholipid,

0.25% FLV, 0.02% EA and 0.3% ALA. The mixture was melted heating up to 50 °C in chloroform:ethyl acetate 1:1. To this lipid phase 1% Gelucire® 44/14 aqueous solution was added and the resultant emulsion was sonicated, cooled down and collected by ultracentrifugation. The NPs had a mean particle size of 85 nm (PDI = 0.58) and a negative zeta potential ($\zeta = -25$ mV). The EE was 98% for FLV, 92% for ALA, and 96% for EA. The release rate was rather slow after an initial burst effect. The formulation was evaluated for its in vitro cytoxicity against PC3 prostate carcinoma cells. The co-delivery of FLV, ALA and EA from NLCs always provided better results in comparison with free drugs both when administered individually and mixed together, with significant differences in terms of cell survival, caspase-3 expression and incidence of apoptosis.

In another interesting study, Abd Elwakil et al. focused on the preparation of an inhalable spray dried powder for targeted co-delivery of EA and doxorubicin (DOX) to lung carcinoma [102]. This system consisted of nanocomposites comprised of drug-loaded NP and excipients like sugars just to reach the micro-range size necessary to ensure deposition in deep lung tissue. Once at the alveolar surface, the carbohydrate fraction rapidly dissolves, releasing the NP components apt to be internalized by the cancer cells. NP matrix was composed of lactoferrin (Lf), a cationic glycoprotein chosen for its ability to bind transferrin receptors overexpressed on cancer cells, and chondroitin sulfate (ChS), a polyanionic glycosaminoglycan able to bind hyaluronic acid CD44 receptors. The first step of this procedure was the nanocrystallization of raw EA via antisolvent precipitation in order to increase EA incorporation in the hydrophilic matrix. A methanolic EA solution was added in a 1:10 volume ratio to an aqueous phase containing 0.5% *w/v* poloxamer F188 as a stabilizer at 4 °C and the mixture was stirred for 15 min. The resulting EA nanocrystals had an average size of 148 nm (PDI of 0.185) and an aqueous solubility 33.3-fold higher than raw EA. The loaded Lf-ChS NPs exploited the polyelectrolyte electrostatic complexation. DOX dissolved in distilled water was dropped gradually into 2% *w/v* ChS solution containing lyophilized nano-sized EA; this dispersion was added by controlled dripping to 2% *w/v* Lf solution, at a suitable pH to allow formation and stabilization of NPs. The resulting product was harvested by centrifugation. The loaded NPs showed a size of around 192 nm and a negative zeta potential ($\zeta = -27$ mV). The EE was 91% for DOX and 96% for EA. The in vitro anticancer efficacy was tested against A495 human lung cancer cell line. Co-encapsulated DOX and EA Lf–ChS NPs enhanced the potency of the drug co-administrated in mixture, as demonstrated by the significant reduction of IC50 value by 3.8-fold compared with combined free drug solution. This system was not expensive, scalable, and made of natural and highly biocompatible components, characteristics that make it potentially useful for preparation of EA-enriched foods.

Table 2. EA micro-sized formulations and their distinctive characteristics.

Formulation Type	Fabrication Method	Excipients	Mean Size	Remarkable Features	Highlights	Ref.
Micro-sized EA	Anti-solvent precipitation	-	n.a.	Use of a syringe pump Good dispersion	In vitro and in vivo inhibition of blood parasites	[54]
Micro-sized EA	Supercritical anti-solvent process	Eudragit® L 100	3.73 µm	Co-precipitate product EA content 49% Residual NMP 148 ppm	Increased EA dissolution rate	[55]
Amorphous solid dispersion	Freeze drying	Maltodextrin	n.a.	Use of cloudberry extract	Higher storage stability up to 32 days Food supplement formulation	[56]
Amorphous solid dispersion	Spray drying	Hydroxypropyl-methyl cellulose acetate succinate	n.a.	EA solubility 280 µg/mL EA content 25%Stable supersaturated EA solution at pH 6.8	pH-sensitive polymer Minimal release in the stomach, quite fast at pH 6.8 (35% after 0.5 h)	[57]
Amorphous solid dispersion	Spray drying	Pectin	10 µm	EA solubility 63 µg/mL EA content 21% No organic solvent used	High biocompatibility Suitable to formulate antioxidant-rich functional food	[58]
Amorphous solid dispersion	Spray drying	Alginic acid	670 nm	EA solubilized in basic solution Crosslinking with $CaCl_2$ Complete release after 8 h	Highly biocompatible formulation Improved in vivo neuroprotective and anticonvulsant effect in orally treated mice	[60]
Polymeric microspheres	Emulsion-evaporation technique in oil phase (acetone/light liquid paraffin)	Eudragit® P-4135F	113 µm	EA content 35% EE 81% Total release after 6 h	pH responsive release Ileocaecal targeting	[70]
Polymeric microspheres	Ionotropic gelation by sodium alginate	Chitosan	4.36 µm	EE 29% Sustained release	Obesity prevention and treatment	[78]
Peptide microtubes	Self-assembling	bis(N-α-amido threonine)-1, 5-pentane dicarboxylate	0.5–1 µm	EE 80% Rate release dependent on the EA deprotonation process at different pH	High biocompatibility Enhanced antibacterial activity	[83]
Phospholipidvesicles	Anti-solvent precipitation	Hydrogenated soy phosphatidyl-choline	1–3 µm	EE 29%	High biocompatibility Liver protection Relative AUC increase by2.8-fold	[83]

Table 3. EA nano-sized formulations and their distinctive characteristics.

Formulation Type	Fabrication Method	Excipients	Mean Size	Remarkable Features	Highlights	Ref.
Nano-sized EA	Anti-solvent precipitation	-	428 nm	EA water solubility 11.67 μg/mL Lyophilized product with maltodextrin as diluent Residual NMP 405 ppm	Higher radical scavenging activity Enhanced relative AUC by 2 times	[52]
Polymer nanospheres	Emulsion-diffusion-evaporation	PLGA or PCL	125 nm	EA content 62% Slow EA release (about 24% after 6 days)	Sustained release for 20 days Good stability Potential prophylaxis system Higher in situ uptake and greater in vivo nephron-protection in CyA-treated rats	[22,72]
Dendrimer	Self-assembling	Aminoacid-modifed hetero dendrimer	70 nm	EA solubility 9 mg/mL EA content 53%	EA solubility increase	[58]
Inclusion complex	Freeze drying	HP-β-CD	n.a.	Formation of 1:2 EA:HP-β-CD complex Increased total EA solubility up to 54.40 μg/mL 60% EA released after 0.5 h	Enhanced in vivo anti-inflammatory effect	[61]
Inclusion complex	Freeze drying	β-CD	n.a.	Formation of 1:2 EA:β-CD complex Increased EA solubility up to 39.14 μg/mL Less than 30% EA released after 0.5 h	Enhanced in vivo anti-inflammatory effect	[62,63]
Inclusion complex	Overnight shaking	β-CD nanosponge	423 nm	EA solubility up to 49.79 μg/mL EA content 69% Prolonged release	High biocompatibility Increased relative AUC by 2.2-fold	[64]
Inclusion complex	Stirring-ultrasonic and final freeze drying	HP-β-CD	n.a.	Optimized production process EE 84%	Antibacterial activity	[67]
Inclusion complex	Precipitation	Arene-Ru metalla-prisms	n.a.	Yield 92% High complex stability	Enhanced antitumor activity against A549 cells	[69]
Polymeric nanospheres	Double emulsion-evaporation (*w/o/w*)	PLGA-PEG	175 nm	Opsonization avoided Prolonged circulation time in blood Suitable for i.v. administration	Inhibition of breast cancer cell growth More than 2-fold IC_{50} reduction in MCF-7 cells	[73]
Polymeric nanospheres	Emulsion-evaporation in aqueous phase	PLGA coated with chitosan and PEG	255 nm	Opsonization avoided Sustained release Suitable for i.v. administration	3-fold IC_{50} reduction in HepG2 and HCT 116 cells	[74]
Polymeric nanospheres	Emulsion-diffusion-evaporation	PCL	193 nm	EA content 58% EE 66% Slow EA release: approx. 48% after 8 days	Long-term release 6.9-fold cytotoxicity increase against HCT 116 cells Improved relative AUC by 3.6 times	[75]

Table 3. *Cont.*

Formulation Type	Fabrication Method	Excipients	Mean Size	Remarkable Features	Highlights	Ref.
Polymeric nanospheres	Ionic gelation by sodium tripolyphosphate	Chitosan	176 nm	EA content 33% Rapid release up to 8 h, then more controlled up to 48 h	More than 3-fold IC_{50} reduction in KB cells Faster clotting time	[76,77]
Polymeric nanocapsules	Anti-solvent coprecipitation	Zein	72 nm	Shell thickness of 20 nm 326 mg EA loaded per 1 g of excipient Sustained release up to 6 days	High biocompatibility Enhanced in vivo anti-inflammatory effect Relative AUC increased by 8.7-fold	[79]
Adsorption complex	Overnight shaking	Functionalized graphene oxide	Sheets ranged from 20 to 120 nm	Easy EA loading by physisorption EA solubility up to 610 µg/mL 1.22 g EA loaded per 1 g of excipient 23% EA released at pH 4 38% at pH 10 after 72 h	Enhanced in vitro cytotoxicity against MCF7 and HT29 cells	[85]
Solid lipid nanoparticle	Hot homogenization method	Precirol® Poloxamer 407 Tween 80	100 nm	EE 89% EA content 36% Initial burst effect (>40%) followed by a sustained release	Enhanced antitumor activity against PC3 cells	[89]
Liposome	Overnight mixing	Phospholipid nanoparticles solution (10%) in form of nanospheres	n.a.	EE 60% Good EA protection in different pH buffers and metal ion containing solutions	For nutritional supplements as adjuvant therapy in cancer	[91]
Self-nanoemulsifying delivery systems	Preliminary EA and soy lecithin complex obtained by anti-solvent precipitation	Soy lecithin Captex® 500 Cremophor® RH40 PEG 400 Tocopherol	106 nm	EE 95% Fast release of nearly 95% after 1 h	Improved ex vivo intestinal permeability	[93]
Self-nanoemulsifying delivery systems	Vortex mixing	Palmester® 3575 Tween 80 PEG 400	120 nm	2.5 mg/mL EA loading into SNEDDS Fast release	Food-grade components Increased relative AUC by 6.6-fold	[94]
Self-nanoemulsifying delivery systems	Vortex mixing	Ethyl oleate Tween 80 PEG 400	45 nm	4 mg/g EA loading into SNEDDS Adjunct of PVP 0.5% as stabilizer Less fast release	Enhanced in vitro and in vivo radical scavenging activity	[96]
Polymeric nanospheres	Emulsion-diffusion-evaporation	PLGA	259 nm	Fixed formulation with CoQ10 EE of 70% for EA and of 72% for CoQ10	Prolonged control on cholesterol levels in rats	[98]
Polymeric nanospheres	Self-assembling and dialysis method for drug loading	Poly (N-iso-propylacrylamide-PEG acrylate)	200 nm	Combined formulation with paclitaxel Controlled release (only 8% after 2 h) EE 98% for EA and 92% for paclitaxel	Enhanced in vitro cytotoxicity against MCF-7 cells	[99]
Nanostructured lipid carrier	Hot emulsification-ultrasonication	Almond oil Compritol® ATO Phosphatidylcholine Gelucire®	85 nm	Co-delivery of EA, fluvastatin, alpha lipoic acid Total drug released within 3 h	Enhanced in vitro cytotoxicity against PC3 cells	[100]
Polymeric nanoparticles	EA nanocrystallization by anti-solvent precipitation + polyelectrolyte electrostatic complexation	Lactoferrin Chondroitin sulfate	192 nm	Inhalable combined formulation with doxorubicin	Low cost of production Easy scalability Excipients usable in food products	[102]

5. Conclusions

In recent decades, a growing interest in the administration of polyphenolic compounds for prevention of several diseases has arisen, since epidemiological studies have revealed a correlation between dietary habits and disease risks. In particular, EA exerts various health-promoting activities, suggesting that it may play an important role in dietary supplements. Furthermore, a few research studies proved that EA is endowed with a wide spectrum of therapeutic effects against oxidation-linked chronic illnesses such as, above all, diabetes, cancer, neurodegenerative disorders, and cardiovascular diseases. Unfortunately, EA presents unsuitable biopharmaceutical features, including poor bioavailability and interindividual variability that hamper its successful employment in prophylaxis and disease treatment. To date, on the market, EA is present in beverages, capsules, and tablets, which obviously do not overcome the problems associated with low oral EA intake; furthermore liquid formulation submits it to fast degradation. From this background, in order to address the many drawbacks associated with EA in vivo absorption, strategies mainly consisting of micro and nanotechnology approaches were designed and performed. The obtained EA formulations demonstrated modifying its release and improving its solubility, stability during storage, and bioavailability in animal models. However, from the evaluation of the various developed formulations, some considerations may be made. For example, approaches starting from basic EA solutions lead to higher EA content, but the preparation timing may represent a crucial factor as undesirable reactions such as oxidation and hydrolysis may occur. As a matter of fact, the choice of a proper vehicle for dissolving EA is challenging, because EA results rather insoluble in most common solvents. The attempt of reducing the size of EA powder through anti-solvent precipitation could be a recommended preliminary step as reported by different authors. Regarding micro and nanosystems preparative methods, encapsulation in biodegradable PLGA or PCL micro and nanospheres represents a valid route when effective EA protection, long circulation and controlled release are required, as, despite an initial burst effect, these systems provided a sustained release over one week. Thanks to its biocompatibility, chitosan was also extensively used, providing a rather fast EA release (50% within 8 h). Concerning lipid carriers, self-emulsifying systems are the most investigated ones, since they were usually endowed with high EA loading capacity and gastrointestinal release within 1 h. Although in the work of Wang et al. food-grade excipients were used, the effects of surfactants concentration on intestinal epithelial integrity has to be taken into consideration. In this regard, it is of great importance to develop formulations with residual organic solvents or surfactants below the recommended maximum levels indicated by regulatory agencies. The most recent, innovative, and highly biocompatible EA formulations consisted of pectin spray dried dispersion, cyclodextrin-based nanosponges, zein nanocapsules, chitosan/alginate microspheres, lactoferrin/chondroitin sulfate nanoparticles, and supersaturatable self-microemulsifying delivery systems. With these promising advances, novel and more effective strategies could be applied for allowing extensive investigations on EA in vivo beneficial effects. In this regard, in the last pharmacokinetic study in humans, it was reported that after pomegranate extracts consumption, the key factors hampering EA effectiveness are: its low solubility at the gastric pH, its bounding to intestinal epithelium, the saturable transcellular transport and the interindividual variability to produce urolithins. All these drawbacks may be overcome at least to a large extent by applying micro or nanocarrier-based approaches, suggesting that future pharmacokinetic studies will provide more encouraging results if they are performed by using an optimized pomegranate acid delivery system.

Author Contributions: Conceptualization, G.Z., S.B. and G.C.; resources, G.Z., F.T., S.A. and S.B.; writing—original draft preparation, G.Z.; writing—review and editing, G.Z., S.B., G.C., G.A., S.A. and F.T. All authors have read and agreed to the published version of the manuscript.

References

1. Miguel, M.G.; Neves, M.A.; Antunes, M.D. Pomegranate (*Punica granatum* L.): A medicinal plant with myriad biological properties—A short review. *J. Med. Plants Res.* **2010**, *4*, 2836–2847.
2. Ríos, J.L.; Giner, R.M.; Marín, M.; Recio, M.C. A Pharmacological Update of Ellagic Acid. *Planta Med.* **2018**, *84*, 1068–1093. [CrossRef] [PubMed]
3. Cai, Y.; Zhang, J.; Chen, N.G.; Shi, Z.; Qiu, J.; He, C.; Chen, M. Recent Advances in Anticancer Activities and Drug Delivery Systems of Tannins. *Med. Res. Rev.* **2017**, *37*, 665–701. [CrossRef] [PubMed]
4. Ahangarpour, A.; Sayahi, M.; Sayahi, M. The antidiabetic and antioxidant properties of some phenolic phytochemicals: A review study. *Diabetes Metab. Syndr. Clin. Res.* **2019**, *13*, 854–857. [CrossRef]
5. Baradaran Rahimi, V.; Ghadiri, M.; Ramezani, M.; Askari, V.R. Anti-inflammatory and anti-cancer activities of pomegranate and its constituent, ellagic acid: Evidence from cellular, animal, and clinical studies. *Phytother. Res.* **2020**, in press. [CrossRef]
6. Alfei, S.; Turrini, F.; Catena, S.; Zunin, P.; Grilli, M.; Pittaluga, A.M.; Boggia, R. Ellagic acid a multi-target bioactive compound for drug discovery in CNS? A narrative review. *Eur. J. Med. Chem.* **2019**, *183*, 111724. [CrossRef]
7. Kang, I.; Buckner, T.; Shay, N.F.; Gu, L.; Chung, S. Improvements in Metabolic Health with Consumption of Ellagic Acid and Subsequent Conversion into Urolithins: Evidence and Mechanisms. *Adv. Nutr.* **2016**, *7*, 961–972. [CrossRef]
8. Sarkaki, A.; Farbood, Y.; Dolatshahi, M.; Mansouri, S.M.; Khodadadi, A. Neuroprotective Effects of Ellagic Acid in a Rat Model of Parkinson's Disease. *Acta Med. Iran.* **2016**, *54*, 494–502.
9. Das, U.; Biswas, S.; Chattopadhyay, S.; Chakraborty, A.; Dey Sharma, R.; Banerji, A.; Dey, S. Radiosensitizing effect of ellagic acid on growth of Hepatocellular carcinoma cells: An in vitro study. *Sci. Rep.* **2017**, *7*, 14043. [CrossRef]
10. Jeong, H.; Phan, A.N.H.; Choi, J.W. Anti-cancer Effects of Polyphenolic Compounds in Epidermal Growth Factor Receptor Tyrosine Kinase Inhibitor-resistant Non-small Cell Lung Cancer. *Pharmacogn. Mag.* **2017**, *13*, 595–599. [CrossRef]
11. Vanella, L.; Di Giacomo, C.; Acquaviva, R.; Barbagallo, I.; Li Volti, G.; Cardile, V.; Abraham, N.; Sorrenti, V. Effects of Ellagic Acid on Angiogenic Factors in Prostate Cancer Cells. *Cancers* **2013**, *5*, 726–738. [CrossRef] [PubMed]
12. Dai, Z.; Nair, V.; Khan, M.; Ciolino, H.P. Pomegranate extract inhibits the proliferation and viability of MMTV-Wnt-1 mouse mammary cancer stem cells in vitro. *Oncol. Rep.* **2010**, *24*, 1087–1091. [CrossRef] [PubMed]
13. Kowshik, J.; Giri, H.; Kishore, T.; Kesavan, R.; Vankudavath, R.; Reddy, G.; Dixit, M.; Nagini, S. Ellagic Acid Inhibits VEGF/VEGFR2, PI3K/Akt and MAPK Signaling Cascades in the Hamster Cheek Pouch Carcinogenesis Model. *Anticancer Agents Med. Chem.* **2014**, *14*, 1249–1260. [CrossRef] [PubMed]
14. Ceci, C.; Tentori, L.; Atzori, M.; Lacal, P.; Bonanno, E.; Scimeca, M.; Cicconi, R.; Mattei, M.; de Martino, M.; Vespasiani, G.; et al. Ellagic Acid Inhibits Bladder Cancer Invasiveness and In Vivo Tumor Growth. *Nutrients* **2016**, *8*, 744. [CrossRef]
15. Liu, H.; Zeng, Z.; Wang, S.; Li, T.; Mastriani, E.; Li, Q.H.; Bao, H.X.; Zhou, Y.J.; Wang, X.; Liu, Y.; et al. Main components of pomegranate, ellagic acid and luteolin, inhibit metastasis of ovarian cancer by down-regulating MMP2 and MMP9. *Cancer Biol. Ther.* **2017**, *18*, 990–999. [CrossRef]
16. Wang, D.; Chen, Q.; Tan, Y.; Liu, B.; Liu, C. Ellagic acid inhibits human glioblastoma growth in vitro and in vivo. *Oncol. Rep.* **2017**, *37*, 1084–1092. [CrossRef]
17. Xu, W.; Xu, J.; Wang, T.; Liu, W.; Wei, H.; Yang, X.; Yan, W.; Zhou, W.; Xiao, J. Ellagic acid and Sennoside B inhibit osteosarcoma cell migration, invasion and growth by repressing the expression of c-Jun. *Oncol. Lett.* **2018**, *16*, 898–904. [CrossRef]
18. Ceci, C.; Lacal, P.; Tentori, L.; De Martino, M.; Miano, R.; Graziani, G. Experimental Evidence of the Antitumor, Antimetastatic and Antiangiogenic Activity of Ellagic Acid. *Nutrients* **2018**, *10*, 1756. [CrossRef]
19. Umesalma, S.; Nagendraprabhu, P.; Sudhandiran, G. Ellagic acid inhibits proliferation and induced apoptosis via the Akt signaling pathway in HCT-15 colon adenocarcinoma cells. *Mol. Cell. Biochem.* **2015**, *399*, 303–313. [CrossRef]

20. Goyal, Y.; Koul, A.; Ranawat, P. Ellagic acid ameliorates cisplatin induced hepatotoxicity in colon carcinogenesis. *Environ. Toxicol.* **2019**, *34*, 804–813. [CrossRef]
21. Lin, M.; Yin, M. Preventive Effects of Ellagic Acid Against Doxorubicin-Induced Cardio-Toxicity in Mice. *Cardiovasc. Toxicol.* **2013**, *13*, 185–193. [CrossRef] [PubMed]
22. Sonaje, K.; Italia, J.L.; Sharma, G.; Bhardwaj, V.; Tikoo, K.; Kumar, M.N.V.R. Development of Biodegradable Nanoparticles for Oral Delivery of Ellagic Acid and Evaluation of Their Antioxidant Efficacy Against Cyclosporine A-Induced Nephrotoxicity in Rats. *Pharm. Res.* **2007**, *24*, 899–908. [CrossRef] [PubMed]
23. Sepúlveda, L.; Ascacio, A.; Rodríguez-Herrera, R.; Aguilera-Carbó, A.; Aguilar, C.N. Ellagic acid biological properties and biotechnological development. *Afr. J. Biotechnol.* **2011**, *10*, 4518–4523. [CrossRef]
24. Notka, F.; Meier, G.; Wagner, R. Concerted inhibitory activities of Phyllanthus amarus on HIV replication in vitro and ex vivo. *Antivir. Res.* **2004**, *64*, 93–102. [CrossRef]
25. Govindarajan, R.; Vijayakumar, M.; Rao, C.V.; Shirwaikar, A.; Mehrotra, S.; Pushpangadan, P. Healing potential of Anogeissus latifolia for dermal wounds in rats. *Acta Pharm.* **2004**, *54*, 331–338.
26. Giménez-Bastida, J.A.; González-Sarrías, A.; Larrosa, M.; Tomás-Barberán, F.; Espín, J.C.; García-Conesa, M.T. Intestinal ellagitannin metabolites ameliorate cytokine-induced inflammation and associated molecular markers in human colon fibroblasts. *J. Agric. Food Chem.* **2012**, *60*, 8866–8876. [CrossRef]
27. Prabha, B.; Sini, S.; Priyadarshini, T.S.; Sasikumar, P.; Gopalan, G.; Jayesh, P.J.; Jithin, M.M.; Sivan, V.V.; Jayamurthy, P.; Radhakrishnan, K.V. Anti-inflammatory effect and mechanism of action of ellagic acid-3,3′,4-trimethoxy-4′-O-α-L-rhamnopyranoside isolated from Hopea parviflora in lipopolysaccharide-stimulated RAW 264.7 macrophages. *Nat. Prod. Res.* **2019**, *12*, 1–5. [CrossRef]
28. Mele, L.; Mena, P.; Piemontese, A.; Marino, V.; López-Gutiérrez, N.; Bernini, F.; Brighenti, F.; Zanotti, I.; Del Rio, D. Antiatherogenic effects of ellagic acid and urolithins in vitro. *Arch. Biochem. Biophys.* **2016**, *599*, 42–50. [CrossRef]
29. Jordão, J.B.R.; Porto, H.K.P.; Lopes, F.M.; Batista, A.C.; Rocha, M.L. Protective Effects of Ellagic Acid on Cardiovascular Injuries Caused by Hypertension in Rats. *Planta Med.* **2017**, *83*, 830–836. [CrossRef]
30. Turrini, F.; Boggia, R.; Donno, D.; Parodi, B.; Beccaro, G.; Baldassari, S.; Signorello, M.G.; Catena, S.; Alfei, S.; Zunin, P. From pomegranate marcs to a potential bioactive ingredient: A recycling proposal for pomegranate squeezed-marcs. *Eur. Food Res. Technol.* **2019**, *246*, 273–285. [CrossRef]
31. Kim, Y.H.; Kim, K.H.; Han, C.S.; Yang, H.C.; Park, S.H.; Jang, H.-I.; Kim, J.-W.; Choi, Y.-S.; Lee, N.H. Anti-wrinkle activity of Platycarya strobilacea extract and its application as a cosmeceutical ingredient. *J. Cosmet. Sci.* **2018**, *14*, 211–223.
32. Liu, R.; Li, J.; Cheng, Y.; Huo, T.; Xue, J.; Liu, Y.; Liu, J.; Chen, X. Effects of ellagic acid-rich extract of pomegranates peel on regulation of cholesterol metabolism and its molecular mechanism in hamsters. *Food Funct.* **2015**, *6*, 780–787. [CrossRef]
33. Boggia, R.; Turrini, F.; Villa, C.; Lacapra, C.; Zunin, P.; Parodi, B. Green extraction from pomegranate marcs for the production of functional foods and cosmetics. *Pharmaceuticals* **2016**, *9*, 63. [CrossRef] [PubMed]
34. Núñez-Sánchez, M.A.; García-Villalba, R.; Monedero-Saiz, T.; GarcíaTalavera, N.V.; Gómez-Sánchez, M.B.; Sánchez-Álvarez, C.; García-Albert, A.M.; Rodríguez-Gil, F.J.; Ruiz-Marín, M.; Pastor-Quirante, F.A.; et al. Targeted metabolic profiling of pomegranate polyphenols and urolithins in plasma, urine and colon tissues from colorectal cancer patients. *Mol. Nutr. Food Res.* **2014**, *58*, 1199–1211. [CrossRef] [PubMed]
35. Bellone, J.A.; Murray, J.R.; Jorge, P.; Fogel, T.G.; Kim, M.; Wallace, D.R.; Hartman, R.E. Pomegranate supplementation improves cognitive and functional recovery following ischemic stroke: A randomized trial. *Nutr. Neurosci.* **2019**, *22*, 738–743. [CrossRef] [PubMed]
36. Bala, I.; Bhardwaj, V.; Hariharan, S.; Kumar, M.N. Analytical methods for assay of ellagic acid and its solubility studies. *J. Pharm. Biomed. Anal.* **2006**, *40*, 206–210. [CrossRef]
37. Muzolf, M.; Szymusiak, H.; Gliszczynska-Swiglo, A.; Rietjens, I.M.C.M.; Tyrakowska, B. pH-Dependent radical scavenging capacity of green tea catechins. *J. Agric. Food Chem.* **2008**, *56*, 816–823. [CrossRef]
38. Panichayupakaranant, P.; Itsuriya, A.; Sirikatitham, A. Preparation method and stability of ellagic acid-rich pomegranate fruit peel extract. *Pharm. Biol.* **2010**, *48*, 201–205. [CrossRef]
39. Mao, X.; Wu, L.-F.; Zhao, H.; Liang, W.-Y.; Chen, W.-J.; Han, S.-X.; Qi, Q.; Cui, Y.-P.; Li, S.; Yang, G.-H.; et al. Transport of Corilagin, Gallic Acid, and Ellagic Acid from Fructus Phyllanthi Tannin Fraction in Caco-2 Cell Monolayers. *Evid. Based Complementary Altern. Med.* **2016**, *2016*, 9205379. [CrossRef] [PubMed]

40. Mertens-talcot, S.U.; Jilma-Stohlawetz, P.; Rios, J.; Hingorani, L.; Derendorf, H. Absorption metabolism and antioxidant effects of pomegranate. *J. Agric. Food Chem.* **2006**, *54*, 8956–8961. [CrossRef]
41. Seeram, N.P.; Henning, S.M.; Zhang, Y.; Suchard, M.; Li, Z.; Heber, D. Pomegranate juice ellagitannin metabolites are present in human plasma and some persist in urine for up to 48 hours. *J. Nutr.* **2006**, *136*, 2481–2485. [CrossRef] [PubMed]
42. Tomás-Barberán, F.A.; García-Villalba, R.; González-Sarrías, A.; Selma, M.V.; Espín, J.C. Ellagic acid metabolism by human gut microbiota: Consistent observation of three urolithin phenotypes in intervention trials, independent of food source, age, and health status. *J. Agric. Food Chem.* **2014**, *62*, 6535–6538. [CrossRef] [PubMed]
43. Tomás-Barberán, F.A.; González-Sarrias, A.; Garcıa-Villalba, R.; Nunez-Sanchez, M.A.; Selma, M.V.; Garcıa-Conesa, M.T.; Espın, J.C. Urolithins, the rescue of "old" metabolites to understand a "new" concept: Metabotypes as a nexus among phenolic metabolism, microbiota dysbiosis, and host health status. *Mol. Nutr. Food Res.* **2017**, *61*, 1500901. [CrossRef] [PubMed]
44. Cortés-Martín, A.; García-Villalba, R.; González-Sarrías, A.; Romo-Vaquero, M.; Loria-Kohen, V.; Ramírez-de-Molina, A.; Tomás-Barberán, F.A.; Selma, M.V.; Espín, J.C. The gut microbiota urolithin metabotypes revisited: The human metabolism of ellagicacid is mainly determined by aging. *Food Funct.* **2018**, *9*, 4100–4106. [CrossRef] [PubMed]
45. González-Sarrías, A.; García-Villalba, R.; Núñez-Sánchez, M.Á.; Tomé-Carneiro, J.; Zafrilla, P.; Mulero, J.; Tomás-Barberán, F.A.; Espín, J.C. Identifying the limits for ellagic acid bioavailability: A crossover pharmacokinetic study in healthy volunteers after consumption of pomegranate extracts. *J. Funct. Foods* **2015**, *19*, 225–235. [CrossRef]
46. Tennant, D.R.; Davidson, J.; Day, A.J. Phytonutrient intakes in relation to European fruit and vegetable consumption patterns observed in different food surveys. *Br. J. Nutr.* **2014**, *112*, 1214–1225. [CrossRef]
47. Whitley, A.C.; Stoner, G.D.; Darby, M.V.; Walle, T. Intestinal epithelial cell accumulation of the cancer preventive polyphenol ellagic acid—Extensive binding to protein and DNA. *Biochem. Pharmacol.* **2003**, *66*, 907–915. [CrossRef]
48. Srivastava, A.K.; Bhatnagar, P.; Singh, M.; Mishra, S.; Kumar, P.; Shukla, Y.; Gupta, K.C. Synthesis of PLGA nanoparticles of tea polyphenols and their strong in vivo protective effect against chemically induced DNA damage. *Int. J. Nanomed.* **2019**, *14*, 7001–7002. [CrossRef]
49. Xie, X.; Tao, Q.; Zou, Y.; Zhang, F.; Guo, M.; Wang, Y.; Wang, H.; Zhou, Q.; Yu, S. PLGA Nanoparticles Improve the Oral Bioavailability of Curcumin in Rats: Characterizations and Mechanisms. *J. Agric. Food Chem.* **2011**, *59*, 9280–9289. [CrossRef]
50. Sanna, V.; Siddiqui, I.A.; Sechi, M.; Mukhtar, H. Resveratrol-Loaded Nanoparticles Based on Poly (epsilon-caprolactone) and Poly (d l-lactic-*co*-glycolic acid)–Poly (ethylene glycol) Blend for Prostate Cancer Treatment. *Mol. Pharmaceut.* **2013**, *10*, 3871–3881. [CrossRef]
51. Noyes, A.A.; Whitney, W.R. The rate of solution of solid substances in their own solutions. *J. Am. Chem. Soc.* **1987**, *19*, 930–934. [CrossRef]
52. Li, Y.; Zhao, X.; Zu, Y.; Zhang, Y.; Ge, Y.; Zhong, C.; Wu, W. Preparation and characterization of micronized ellagic acid using antisolvent precipitation for oral delivery. *Int. J. Pharmaceut.* **2015**, *486*, 207–216. [CrossRef] [PubMed]
53. Committee for Human Medicinal Products ICH guideline Q3C (R6) on impurities: Guideline for residual solvents. *EMA/CHMP/ICH/82260/* **2006**, *2006*, 1–39.
54. Beshbishy, A.M.; Batiha, G.E.-S.; Yokoyama, N.; Igarashi, I. Ellagic acid microspheres restrict the growth of Babesia and Theileria in vitro and Babesia microti in vivo. *Parasites Vectors* **2019**, *12*, 269. [CrossRef] [PubMed]
55. Montes, A.; Wehner, L.; Pereyra, C.; Martínez de la Ossa, E.J. Generation of microparticles of ellagic acid by supercritical antisolvent process. *J. Supercrit. Fluids* **2016**, *116*, 101–110. [CrossRef]
56. Laine, P.; Kylli, P.; Heinonen, M.; Jouppila, K. Storage Stability of Microencapsulated Cloudberry (*Rubus chamaemorus*) Phenolics. *J. Agric. Food Chem.* **2008**, *56*, 11251–11261. [CrossRef]
57. Li, B.; Harich, K.; Wegiel, L.; Taylor, L.S.; Edgar, K.J. Stability and solubility enhancement of ellagic acid in cellulose ester solid dispersions. *Carbohyd. Polym.* **2013**, *92*, 1443–1450. [CrossRef]

58. Alfei, S.; Turrini, F.; Catena, S.; Zunin, P.; Parodi, B.; Zuccari, G.; Pittaluga, A.M.; Boggia, R. Preparation of ellagic acid micro and nano formulations with amazingly increased water solubility by its entrapment in pectin or non-PAMAM dendrimers suitable for clinical applications. *New J. Chem.* **2019**, *43*, 2438–2448. [CrossRef]
59. Food Additive Database. Available online: https://webgate.ec.europa.eu/foods_system/main/?sector=FAD&auth=SANCAS (accessed on 2 February 2017).
60. El-Missiry, M.A.; Othman, A.I.; Amer, M.A.; Sedki, M.; Ali, S.M.; El-Sherbiny, I.M. Nanoformulated ellagic acid ameliorates pentylenetetrazol-induced experimental epileptic seizures by modulating oxidative stress, inflammatory cytokines and apoptosis in the brains of male mice. *Metab. Brain Dis.* **2020**, *35*, 385–399. [CrossRef]
61. Bulani, V.D.; Kothavade, P.S.; Nagmoti, D.M.; Kundaikar, H.S.; Degani, M.S.; Juvekar, A.R. Characterisation and anti-inflammatory evaluation of the inclusion complex of ellagic acid with hydroxypropyl-β-cyclodextrin. *J. Incl. Phenom. Macrocycl. Chem.* **2015**, *82*, 361–372. [CrossRef]
62. Bulani, V.D.; Kothavade, P.S.; Kundaikar, H.S.; Gawali, N.B.; Chowdhury, A.A.; Degani, M.S.; Juvekar, A.R. Inclusion complex of ellagic acid with β-cyclodextrin: Characterization and in vitro anti-inflammatory evaluation. *J. Mol. Struct.* **2016**, *1105*, 308–315. [CrossRef]
63. Wang, H.; Zhang, Y.; Tian, Z.; Ma, J.; Kang, M.; Ding, C.; Ming, D. Preparation of β-CD-Ellagic Acid Microspheres and Their Effects on HepG2 Cell Proliferation. *Molecules* **2017**, *22*, 2175. [CrossRef] [PubMed]
64. Mady, F.M.; Ibrahim, S.R.M. Cyclodextrin-based nanosponge for improvement of solubility and oral bioavailability of Ellagic acid. *Pak. J. Pharm. Sci.* **2018**, *31*, 2069–2076. [PubMed]
65. Joseph, E.; Singhvi, G. *Nanomaterials for Drug Delivery and Therapy*; Elsevier: Amsterdam, The Netherlands, 2019; pp. 91–111.
66. Lu, G.W.; Gao, P. *Handbook of Non-Invasive Drug Delivery Systems*; Elsevier: Amsterdam, The Netherlands, 2010; pp. 59–94.
67. Fan, G.; Cai, Y.; Fu, E.; Yuan, X.; Tang, J.; Sheng, H.; Gong, J. Preparation and process optimization of pomegranate ellagic acid-hydroxypropyl-β-cyclodextrin inclusion complex and its antibacterial activity in vitro. *Acta Medica. Mediterr.* **2019**, *35*, 383–389. [CrossRef]
68. Gontijo, A.V.G.; Sampaio, A.; Da, G.; Koga-Ito, C.Y.; Salvador, M.J. Biopharmaceutical and antifungal properties of ellagic acid-cyclodextrin using an *in vitro* model of invasive candidiasis. *Future Microbiol.* **2019**, *14*, 957–967. [CrossRef]
69. An, S.S.; Chi, K.-W.; Kang, S.C.; Dubey, A.; Park, D.W.; Kwon, J.E.; Jeong, Y.J.; Kim, T.; Kim, I. Investigation of the biological and anti-cancer properties of ellagic acid-encapsulated nano-sized metalla-cages. *Int. J. Nanomed.* **2015**, *10*, 227–240. [CrossRef]
70. Jeong, Y.-I.; Yv, R.P.; Ohno, T.; Yoshikawa, Y.; Shibata, N.; Kato, S.; Takeuchi, K.; Takada, K. Application of Eudragit P-4135F for the delivery of ellagic acid to the rat lower small intestine. *J. Phar. Pharmacol.* **2001**, *53*, 1079–1085. [CrossRef]
71. Danhier, F.; Ansorena, E.; Silva, J.M.; Coco, R.; Le Breton, A.; Préat, V. PLGA-based nanoparticles: An overview of biomedical applications. *J. Control. Release* **2012**, *161*, 505–522. [CrossRef]
72. Bala, I.; Bhardwaj, V.; Hariharan, S.; Kharade, S.V.; Roy, N.; Ravi Kumar, M.N.V. Sustained release nanoparticulate formulation containing antioxidant-ellagic acid as potential prophylaxis system for oral administration. *J. Drug Target.* **2006**, *14*, 27–34. [CrossRef]
73. Reliene, R.; Shirode, A.; Coon, J.; Nallanthighal, S.; Bharali, D.; Mousa, S. Nanoencapsulation of pomegranate bioactive compounds for breast cancer chemoprevention. *Int. J. Nanomed.* **2015**, *10*, 475–484. [CrossRef]
74. Abd-Rabou, A.A.; Ahmed, H.H. CS-PEG decorated PLGA nano-prototype for delivery of bioactive compounds: A novel approach for induction of apoptosis in HepG2 cell line. *Adv. Med. Sci.* **2017**, *62*, 357–367. [CrossRef] [PubMed]
75. Mady, F.; Shaker, M. Enhanced anticancer activity and oral bioavailability of ellagic acid through encapsulation in biodegradable polymeric nanoparticles. *Int. J. Nanomed.* **2017**, *12*, 7405–7417. [CrossRef]
76. Arulmozhi, V.; Pandian, K.; Mirunalini, S. Ellagic acid encapsulated chitosan nanoparticles for drug delivery system in human oral cancer cell line (KB). *Colloids Surf. B* **2013**, *110*, 313–320. [CrossRef] [PubMed]
77. Gopalakrishnan, L.; Ramana, L.N.; Sethuraman, S.; Krishnan, U.M. Ellagic acid encapsulated chitosan nanoparticles as anti-hemorrhagic agent. *Carbohydr. Polym.* **2014**, *111*, 215–221. [CrossRef] [PubMed]

78. Ding, C.; Bi, H.; Wang, D.; Kang, M.; Tian, Z.; Zhang, Y.; Wang, H.; Zhu, T.; Ma, J. Preparation of Chitosan/Alginate-ellagic acid sustained-release microspheres and their Inhibition of preadipocyte adipogenic differentiation. *Curr. Pharm. Biotechnol.* **2019**, *20*, 1213–1222. [CrossRef] [PubMed]
79. Ruan, J.; Yang, Y.; Yang, F.; Wan, K.; Fan, D.; Wang, D. Novel oral administrated ellagic acid nanoparticles for enhancing oral bioavailability and anti-inflammatory efficacy. *J. Drug Deliv. Sci. Technol.* **2018**, *46*, 215–222. [CrossRef]
80. Padilla De Jesus, O.L.; Ihre, H.R.; Gagne, L.; Frechet, J.M.J.; Szoka, F.C. Polyester dendritic systems for drug delivery applications: In vitro and in vivo evaluation. *Bioconjug. Chem.* **2002**, *13*, 453–461. [CrossRef]
81. Alfei, S.; Marengo, B.; Domenicotti, C. Polyester-Based Dendrimer Nanoparticles Combined with Etoposide Have an Improved Cytotoxic andmPro-Oxidant Effect on Human Neuroblastoma Cells. *Antioxidants* **2020**, *9*, 50. [CrossRef]
82. Tesauro, D.; Accardo, A.; Diaferia, C.; Milano, V.; Guillon, J.; Ronga, L.; Rossi, F. Peptide based drug delivery systems in biotechnological applications. *Molecules* **2019**, *24*, 351. [CrossRef]
83. Barnaby, S.N.; Fath, K.R.; Tsiola, A.; Banerjee, I.A. Fabrication of ellagic acid incorporated self-assembled peptide microtubes and their applications. *Colloid Surf. B* **2012**, *95*, 154–161. [CrossRef]
84. Rahmanian, N.; Hamishehkar, H.; Dolatabadi, J.E.; Arsalani, N. Nano graphene oxide: A novel carrier for oral delivery of flavonoids. *Colloids Surf. B* **2014**, *123*, 331–338. [CrossRef] [PubMed]
85. Kakran, M.G.; Sahoo, N.; Bao, H.; Pan, Y.; Li, L. Functionalized graphene oxide as nanocarrier for loading and delivery of ellagic acid. *Curr. Med. Chem.* **2011**, *18*, 4503–4512. [CrossRef]
86. Ghasemiyeh, P.; Mohammadi-Samani, S. Solid lipid nanoparticles and nanostructured lipid carriers as novel drug delivery systems: Applications, advantages and disadvantages. *Res. Pharm. Sci.* **2018**, *13*, 288–303. [PubMed]
87. Yoon, G.; Park, J.W.; Yoon, I.S. Solid lipid nanoparticles (SLNs) and nanostructured lipid carriers (NLCs): Recent advances in drug delivery. *J. Pharm. Investig.* **2013**, *43*, 353–362. [CrossRef]
88. Makwana, V.; Jain, R.; Patel, K.; Nivsarkar, M.; Joshi, A. Solid lipid nanoparticles (SLN) of Efavirenz as lymph targeting drug delivery system: Elucidation of mechanism of uptake using chylomicron flow blocking approach. *Int. J. Pharm.* **2015**, *495*, 439–446. [CrossRef] [PubMed]
89. Hajipour, H.; Hamishehkar, H.; Rahmati-yamchi, M.; Shanehbandi, D.; Nazari Soltan Ahmad, S.; Hasani, A. Enhanced anti-cancer capability of ellagic acid using solid lipid nanoparticles (SLNs). *Int. J. Cancer Manag.* **2018**, *11*, e9402. [CrossRef]
90. Murugan, V.; Mukherjee, K.; Maiti, K.; Mukherjee, P.K. Enhanced oral bioavailability and antioxidant profile of ellagic acid by phospholipids. *J. Agric. Food Chem.* **2009**, *57*, 4559–4565. [CrossRef]
91. Stojiljković, N.; Ilić, S.; Stojanović, N.; Janković-Veličković, L.; Stojnev, S.; Kocić, G.; Radenković, G.; Arsić, I.; Stojanović, M.; Petković, M. Nanoliposome-encapsulated ellagic acid prevents cyclophosphamide-induced rat liver damage. *Mol. Cell. Biochem.* **2019**, *458*, 185–195. [CrossRef]
92. Wang, X.; Jiang, Y.; Wang, Y.-W.; Huang, M.-T.; Ho, C.-T.; Huang, Q. Enhancing anti-inflammation activity of curcumin through O/W nanoemulsions. *Food Chem.* **2008**, *108*, 419–424. [CrossRef]
93. Avachat, A.M.; Patel, V.G. Self nanoemulsifying drug delivery system of stabilized ellagic acid–phospholipid complex with improved dissolution and permeability. *Saudi Pharm. J.* **2015**, *23*, 276–289. [CrossRef]
94. Wang, S.-T.; Chou, C.-T.; Su, N.-W. A food-grade self-nanoemulsifying delivery system for enhancing oral bioavailability of ellagic acid. *J. Funct. Foods* **2017**, *34*, 207–215. [CrossRef]
95. Dokania, S.; Joshi, A.K. Self-microemulsifying drug delivery system (SMEDDS)—Challenges and road ahead. *Drug Deliv.* **2015**, *22*, 675–690. [CrossRef] [PubMed]
96. Zheng, D.; Lv, C.; Sun, X.; Wang, J.; Zhao, Z. Preparation of a supersaturatable self-microemulsion as drug delivery system for ellagic acid and evaluation of its antioxidant activities. *J. Drug Deliv. Sci. Technol.* **2019**, *53*, 101209. [CrossRef]
97. Tavano, L.; Muzzalupo, R.; Picci, N.; de Cindio, B. Co-encapsulation of antioxidants into niosomal carriers: Gastrointestinal release studies for nutraceutical applications. *Colloid Surf. B* **2014**, *114*, 82–88. [CrossRef] [PubMed]
98. Ratnam, D.V.; Chandraiah, G.; Meena, A.K.; Ramarao, P.; Kumar, M.N. The co-encapsulated antioxidant nanoparticles of ellagic acid and coenzyme Q10 ameliorates hyperlipidemia in high fat diet fed rats. *Nanosci. Nanotechnol.* **2009**, *9*, 6741–6746. [CrossRef] [PubMed]

99. Suri, S.; Mirza Mohd, A.; Anwer, M.K.; Alshetaili, A.S.; Alshahrani, S.M.; Ahmed, F.J.; Iqbal, Z. Development of NIPAAm-PEG acrylate polymeric nanoparticles for co-delivery of paclitaxel with ellagic acid for the treatment of breast cancer. *J. Polym. Eng.* **2019**, *39*, 271–278. [CrossRef]
100. Fahmy, U.A. Augmentation of fluvastatin cytotoxicity against prostate carcinoma PC3 cell line utilizing alpha lipoic–ellagic acid nanostructured lipid carrier formula. *AAPS PharmSciTech* **2018**, *19*, 3454–3461. [CrossRef]
101. Tamjidi, F.; Shahedi, M.; Varshosaz, J.; Nasirpour, A. Nanostructured lipid carriers (NLC): A potential delivery system for bioactive food molecules. *Innov. Food Sci. Emerg. Technol.* **2013**, *19*, 23–43. [CrossRef]
102. Abd Elwakil, M.M.; Mabrouk, M.T.; Helmy, M.W.; Abdelfattah, E.-Z.A.; Khiste, S.K.; Elkhodairy, K.A.; Elzoghby, A.O. Inhalable lactoferrin–chondroitin nanocomposites for combined delivery of doxorubicin and ellagic acid to lung carcinoma. *Nanomedicine* **2018**, *13*, 2015–2035. [CrossRef]

12

Phytochemical Characterization and Bioactivity Evaluation of Autumn Olive (*Elaeagnus umbellata* Thunb.) Pseudodrupes as Potential Sources of Health-Promoting Compounds

Giovanni Gamba [1,*], Dario Donno [1], Maria Gabriella Mellano [1], Isidoro Riondato [1], Marta De Biaggi [1], Denis Randriamampionona [2] and Gabriele Loris Beccaro [1]

1 Dipartimento di Scienze Agrarie, Forestali e Alimentari, Università degli Studi di Torino, 10095 Grugliasco (TO), Italy; dario.donno@unito.it (D.D.); gabriella.mellano@unito.it (M.G.M.); isidoro.riondato@unito.it (I.R.); marta.debiaggi@unito.it (M.D.B.); gabriele.beccaro@unito.it (G.L.B.)

2 Mention Agriculture Tropicale et Développement Durable—Ecole Supérieure des Sciences Agronomiques, Université d'Antananarivo, 101 Antananarivo, Madagascar; denisr07@yahoo.fr

* Correspondence: giovanni.gamba@unito.it

Abstract: Autumn olive (*Elaeagnus umbellata* Thunb.) is a deciduous shrub tree widely distributed in Asia and Southern Europe and grown as ornamental species. It is locally used for human consumption, as relevant medical value is attributed to the berries. Information about its composition, especially concerning the characterization of bioactive and health-promoting compounds, is limited. The aim of the present study is to evaluate the main bioactive compounds and nutraceutical proprieties of autumn olive fruits, via high-performance liquid chromatography (HPLC) fingerprint and spectrophotometric analysis, in order to strengthen the knowledge about this underrated species and promote potential applications as a food supplement. Concerning nutraceutical traits, total polyphenolic content (325.366 ± 13.019 mg of gallic acid equivalents (mg GAE)/100 of fresh weight (g FW)) and total anthocyanin content (194.992 ± 0.817 mg of cyanidin-3-O-glucoside (mg C3G)/100 g FW) recorded considerable values. The phytochemical fingerprint revealed the presence 23 bioactive compounds. Polyphenols (65.56%) were the largest class, followed by monoterpenes (27.40%) and vitamin C (7.04%). Anthocyanins were the most represented compounds among polyphenols (71.9%). The antioxidant capacity (20.031 ± 1.214 mmol Fe^{2+}/kg) was similar to that recorded for other small fruits with proven health-promoting properties. The present work underlined the potential of *E. umbellata* as a source of health-promoting bioactive compounds. Further studies should deepen the knowledge of nutraceutical aspects, which turned out to be interesting.

Keywords: berry fruit; antioxidant activity; anthocyanins; HPLC fingerprint; underrated species; multipurpose tree

---

1. Introduction

The genus *Elaeagnus* includes 98 species belonging to the Elaeagnaceae family [1]. This family includes shrubs and small trees that produce fruits with a nutritional and ornamental value. Japanese silverberry (*Elaeagnus umbellata* Thunb), also known as autumn olive or goumi, is a deciduous small tree widely used along highways, as the hedges provide a protective screen against wind, and to prevent soil erosion [2]. Due to its ornamental value, drought tolerance, adaptability to different environments, and compact structure, it is grown in urban areas as a hedge [3]. Locally, it is employed for making artefacts such as fencing, fodder, and baskets and as a fuel wood [4]. Originally from Southern Europe, Central and Meridional Asia, it grows wild in its native range as a shrub, where the topographic features of the area limit the cultivation of extensive crops [5]. The autumn olive produces almost spherical fruits called pseudodrupes: 7 mm long and deep-red at fully ripening stage, highly attractive to birds, and locally used for human consumption. The fruit is astringent until ripe, when it acquires a sweet-tart flavor. Pseudodrupes can be consumed fresh or processed for preserves, juices, fruit rolls, and condiments [6]. They are composed of 69.4% moisture, 14.5% total soluble solids, 8.34% total sugars, and 1.51% acids. The content of ash, expression of the total mineral content, is 1.045% [7]. The berries are rich in oil, 7.43–8.11 g/100 g and 5.84–6.11 g/100 g, respectively, in pulp and seed. The composition of these oils contains vitamin E (tocopherol) and phytosterols, which could have significant values in medicine [4].

In the native range of the species, relevant medical value is attributed to the berries. Inhabitants used to eat them, either raw or cooked, as a remedy to reduce blood pressure, against coughs, and for pulmonary infections [7]. Recent studies have shown the antibacterial activity of aqueous extracts from fruits of *E. umbellata* in inhibiting the growth of *Staphylococcus aureus* and *Escherichia coli* [8]. In some areas of China, Japan, and Korea the fruits of *E. umbellata* are incorporated into the local diet, due to their putative health benefits [9].

Little information is available regarding the cultivation of *E. umbellata*. It is considered an invasive exotic species in multiple American states [3]. Until the early 1990s, there were only four recognized cultivars in the US, that mainly differed due to their adaptations to different climatic regions [10]. In the last few years, new cultivars were selected based on the color of the berries.

In Italy, this species is mainly used for ornamental purposes, as it can easily grow over 2 m, has little white flowers with intense scent, and does not require specific plant care. Indeed, autumn olive is a very rustic tree, resistant to cold temperatures and drought, and highly tolerant to pruning. Cultivation areas also include coastal zones, since autumn olive can grow at high soil salt concentrations [11]. The berries are consumed fresh, a tradition derived from tropical and temperate Asia, the native area of the species [12]. Few cultivars are available on the market, mainly selected and registered in North European regions over the last years, which underlines the marginal role of the cultivation of *E. umbellata*.

Thus far, few studies have explored the antioxidant and bioactive compounds of autumn olive. Berries are a valuable source of carotenoids such as lycopene, α-cryptoxanthin, β-cryptoxanthin, β-carotene, lutein, phytoene, and phytofluene. Regarding lycopene (15–54 mg/100 g), the concentration is rather higher than in fresh tomato fruits [13]. Scientific research has reported on the anticancer efficacy of lycopene, represented by a high singlet oxygen quenching ability, twice that of β-carotene and 10 times that of α-tocopherol [5]. The total phenolic content, ranging from 190 to 275 mg of gallic acid equivalents (mg GAE)/100 g of fresh weight (g FW), falls within the range of many other berry fruits with proven health-promoting effects [14]. Furthermore, it is a source of vitamin C, whose content ranges between 14–17 mg/100 g FW [4].

However, at the European and national level little information is yet available on *E. umbellata*, due to the limited consumption of its berries. Several aspects of its composition and potential health benefits need to be further explored, in particular regarding the polyphenol composition.

The objective of the present work is to enhance the knowledge of the autumn olive (*Elaeagnus umbellata* Thunb.), evaluating its fruits as a potential source of bioactive and antioxidant compounds. The main phytochemical compounds, selected on the basis of their health-promoting demonstrated efficacy, were measured through the use of high-performance liquid chromatography (HPLC).

2. Materials and Methods

2.1. *Plant Material, Harvesting Site, and Sample Preparation*

E. umbellata fruits were collected in the germplasm collection of the Department of Agricultural, Forest and Food Sciences of the University of Turin (DISAFA), located in Chieri (45°02′26.3″ N,

7°50′16.8″ E, at 305 m a.s.l.), Piemonte (northwest Italy). Berries were harvested manually (500 g for each replication) at the beginning of November 2018 and randomized from three different trees, so that each tree represented one biological replication. The ripening evaluation was based on pericarp color and fruit development. This work is a preliminary research on the autumn olive; therefore, the investigation did not focus on a single genotype, but rather on the entire *E. umbellata* species. The climate of the area is temperate and for 2018 the average precipitation recorded a value of approximately 770 mm. The soil at the germplasm repository is loam-clay.

After the harvest, berries were immediately stored in refrigerated containers and sent to the laboratory at the DISAFA in Grugliasco (Province of Turin). Then, selection was performed in order to discard any defective fruits from analysis. Finally, the samples were separated into two equal portions. The same day of harvest, physio-chemical parameters were assessed using one portion. The other portion was stocked for one day at 4 °C and 95% relative humidity and further used to extract the bioactive compounds.

2.2. Chemicals

The solvents and chemicals used for extractions and analysis are described in more detail in the Supplementary Materials. All the references (Company, City, State Abbr. and Country) are reported.

2.3. Determination of Morphological and Quality Parameters

One portion of the samples (250 g each replication) was used for the measurement of the fruits' physio-chemical parameters. To assess width and length, a 0.01 mm sensitive digital caliper was used (Traceable Digital Caliper-6″, VWR International, Milan, Italy). Weight was measured to the nearest 0.01 g (Mettler-Toledo AG, Greifensee, Switzerland). For the assessment of pH, total soluble solids (TSS) and titratable acidity (TA), samples were firstly homogenized in a blender (Ultra-Turrax model T25, Ika, Staufen, Germany) and later centrifuged at 4000 rpm for 10 min. The remaining samples were stored at 4 °C and 95% relative humidity for further analysis.

The pH was determined on the fruit juice with the support of a potentiometric pH-meter (Crison, Alella, Spain). The TSS, expressed as °Brix, was quantified with the aid of a digital refractometer (Tsingtao Unicom-Optics Instruments, Laixi, China). Finally, the TA (meq L^{-1}) was measured by titration of a mixture of autumn olive juice (10 mL) diluted in Milli-Q water (90 mL) with the addition of 0.2 M NaOH solution using an automatic titrator (Crison, Alella, Spain) to an end-point of pH 8.2.

2.4. Spectrophotometric Analysis

A single-beam UV–Vis spectrophotometer (1600-PC, VWR International, Milan, Italy) was used to determine the total polyphenolic content (TPC), total anthocyanin content (TAC), and antioxidant capacity (AC). The Folin–Ciocalteu colorimetric method was performed to assess the TPC [15]. The results were expressed as mg of gallic acid equivalents (GAE) per 100 g of fresh weight (FW). Standard solution of gallic acid was prepared at 0.02–0.10 mg mL^{-1}. The pH-differential method was used for the evaluation of TAC [16,17], and results were reported as cyanidin-3-O-glucoside (C3G) per 100 g of FW (mg C3G/100 g FW). Anthocyanins demonstrate maximum absorbance at 515 nm at pH 1.0 and at 700 nm at pH 4.5. The colored oxonium form of anthocyanin predominates at pH 1.0, and the colorless hemiketal form at pH 4.5. The pH-differential method is based on the reaction producing oxonium forms. Finally, the AC was determined through the ferric reducing antioxidant power (FRAP) assay [18], expressing results as millimoles of ferrous iron (Fe^{2+}) equivalents per kilogram (solid food) of FW. The standard curve was plotted using FeSO4·7H2O at 100–1000 μmol/L.

2.5. HPLC Fingerprint: Bioactive Compound Extraction

Polyphenolic compounds, organic acids, monoterpenes, and vitamin C were extracted following effective protocols used in previous works [19,20]. The full description of the protocols used to extract each compound class is fully explained in the Supplementary Materials.

2.6. *Chromatographic Analysis*

2.6.1. Sample Preparation and Chromatographic Analysis

Before the HPLC-DAD (diode array detector) analysis, circular pre-injection filters were used to filter methanolic extracts (0.45 μm, polytetrafluoroethylene membrane, PTFE). For the absorption of the polyphenolic fraction for the vitamin C analysis, a C_{18} cartridge was applied for solid phase extraction (Waters, Milford, MA, USA). Then, for dehydroascorbic acid (DHAA) derivatization into the fluorophore 3-(1,2-dihydroxyethyl)furo(3,4-b)quinoxaline-1-one (DFQ), 750 μL of each sample were diluted with *o*-phenylenediamine (OPDA) solution (18.8 mmol L^{-1}). After 37 min in the dark, samples were ready to be analyzed using HPLC-DAD [21].

Concerning the chromatographic analysis, an Agilent 1200 High-Performance Liquid Chromatograph combined to an Agilent UV–Vis diode array detector (Agilent Technologies, Santa Clara, CA, USA) was used. To separate the bioactive substances, a Kinetex C18 column (4.6 × 150 mm, 5 μm; Phenomenex, Torrance, CA, USA) was used. The samples were analyzed using five chromatographic methods and different mobile phases were used in order to separate and identify the compounds, while UV spectra were recorded at different wavelengths [22] (the mobile phases are listed in Table S1).

In order to obtain a phytochemical fingerprint with all the relevant information on the chemical composition, with a proper resolution and a reasonable analysis time, the chromatographic conditions were set. To optimize the molecule separation, different linear gradients in different slopes were used. Indeed, the same chemical class had similar compounds in term of structure. Since most of the compounds were also weakly acidic, we added formic and phosphoric acid to enhance the resolution and eliminate peak tailing. The selection of the wavelengths was essential to develop a reliable fingerprint. As a matter of fact, only the selected wavelengths achieved more specific peaks, as well as a smooth baseline after a full-scan on the chromatogram from 190 to 400 nm.

2.6.2. Identification and Quantification of Bioactive Compounds

For the quantitative determination of bioactive compounds, the external standard calibration method was used. This is an effective method already performed with success in previous studies [19,20]. A more detailed description is reported in the Supplementary Materials (Table S2).

2.7. *Statistical Analysis*

The results were subjected to variance analysis (ANOVA) for comparison of means, followed by Tukey's honest significant different (HSD) multiple range test ($p < 0.05$). The samples were prepared and analyzed in triplicate (three samples for three biological repetitions). Statistical analysis was performed with SPSS Statistics 22.0 (IBM, Armonk, NY, USA, 2013).

3. Results and Discussion

3.1. *Morphological and Quality Parameters*

Japanese silverberry produced almost spherical fruits (6.92 ± 0.11 mm in width and 6.46 ± 0.08 mm in length) with a mean weight of 0.32 ± 0.02 g for each berry at fully ripe stage (Table 1). Results are in accordance with previous research [6,7,11], except for the weight, which turned out to be slightly higher [4].

Analysis on quality traits revealed a TSS mean value of 16.23 ± 0.15° Brix (Table 1). These findings are partially confirmed in the literature: a study on *Elaeagnus umbellata* berries cultivated in five different localities showed lower values of TSS [23], while the results of six autumn olive genotypes grown in Cookeville (TN, USA) recorded TSS values ranging from 10.6 to 18.4° Brix [5].

Table 1. Morphological, quality, and antioxidant traits of autumn olive fruits.

Parameter	Unit of Measurement	Mean Value ± SD
Weight	(g)	0.32 ± 0.02
Width	(mm)	6.92 ± 0.11
Length	(mm)	6.46 ± 0.08
Total soluble solids	(°Brix)	16.23 ± 0.15
Titratable acidity	(meq/L)	342 ± 79.37
pH	(pH units)	3.53 ± 0.20
Total polyphenolic content (TPC)	(mgGAE/100 gFW)	325.366 ± 13.019
Total anthocyanin content (TAC)	(mgC3G/100 gFW)	194.992 ± 0.817
Antioxidant capacity (AC)	(mmol Fe^{2+}/kg)	20.031 ± 1.214

Mean value and standard deviation are given for each sample ($n = 3$).

Free sugars are among the principal constituents and are essential to determine the quality of fruits [24]. Within the sugar class, many studies have reported fructose and glucose as the major contributors of fruit flavor. As proof of this, fructose turned out to be 1.8 time sweeter than sucrose [25]. Many studies on oleaster fruits revealed fructose and glucose as the main sugars during ripening stage [5,26], highlighting the palatability of *Elaeagnus* fruits.

Autumn olive berries had a pH mean value of 3.53 ± 0.20, falling within the range found in a previous study (3.30–3.90) [23], although in contrast with the study of Khattak on the same species [27]. TA ranged from 252 to 402 meq/L, with a mean value of 342 ± 79.37 meq/L (Table 1). In order to make this value comparable, it was converted in percentage of malic acid equivalent. Therefore, titratable acidity was found to be 1.64% (equal to 1.64 g of malic acid/100 g), considerably lower than the findings of Hussain [23] and Khattak [27], which were 2.20–2.94% and 3.1 ± 0.1%, respectively. The differences in terms of TA could be due to many factors, among which locality, weather conditions, genotype (cultivar), and agronomic techniques play a key role. Considering the non-climacteric attitude of the berries, the time of the harvest is also essential in determining the TSS:TA ratio. All of these aspects have to be taken into account when comparing fruits grown in tropical or sub-tropical areas rather than in temperate regions [28].

The TSS:TA ratio of 9.90 observed in this study further emphasized the large intraspecific variability of the *E. umbellata* fruits, partially confirming previous studies [5,23,27].

3.2. Antioxidant Potential Properties

Berry fruits have considerable amounts of health-promoting compounds, such as phenolic compounds like phenolic acids, anthocyanins, tannins, and flavonoids [28]. Natural phenolic compounds exert healthy actions by reducing oxidative stress and inhibiting macromolecular oxidations, thus counteracting the risk of degenerative diseases [29].

Autumn olive is a multipurpose plant, whose fruits have been consumed over the centuries for many uses. Among these, especially in the native range of the species, the berries have a relevant medical value. To partially support the effectiveness of these local remedies, a study on *E. umbellata* conducted in 2007 reported the capacity of the plant extracts to inhibit the growth of *E. coli*, *S. aureus*, *P. aeruginosa*, and *B. subtilis* [8].

The TPC value is expressed in milligrams of gallic acid equivalents and recorded a considerable value (Table 1), higher than other studies on the same species [5,14]. These results make autumn olive berries comparable to other small fruits such as red raspberry (357.83 ± 7.06 mg GAE/100 g FW), blueberry (305.38 ± 5.09 mg GAE/100 g FW), and cherry (314.45 ± 5.95 mg GAE/100 g FW) [28]. Regarding TAC, no values have been reported so far in this species. The clear identification of the different Elaeagnaceae species and cultivars is often difficult; moreover, it is hard to find specific information on the different species. However, the observed value of total anthocyanins (Table 1), expressed as milligrams of cyanidin-3-O-glucoside (C3G) per 100 g of fresh weight, was higher than those found on other berry fruits such as blackberry, strawberry, blueberry, and red currant, but lower than the values detected in black currant and black chokeberry [28,30]. The present results are in accordance with previous research on different genotypes of Russian olive (*Elaeagnus angustifolia* L.), where values ranged from 115.45 to 260.52 mg C3G/100 g FW and from 116.84 to 630.1 mg C3G/100 g FW [31,32]. Genetic and environmental factors contribute to determining a large intraspecific variability on these parameters, as confirmed by the results in literature.

Ferric reducing antioxidant power (FRAP), a technique based on the ability of antioxidants to reduce ferric (III) ions to ferrous (II) ions, was performed to assess the antioxidant activity. There are several techniques to estimate this parameter. Among them, FRAP methodology represents a fast, low-cost, and comparable in vitro method widely used for screening. Despite the abundance of phenolic and antioxidant compounds, only a few studies report the antioxidant capacity of *Elaeagnus* berries. The value obtained in this study (Table 1) is very close to the ones observed for similar berries with demonstrated health-promoting properties, such as cornelian cherry (*Cornus mas* L.) and jostaberry (*Ribes* x *nidigrolaria* Rud. Bauer & A. Bauer) at 20.41 mmol $Fe2^{+}$/kg and 24.09 mmol $Fe2^{+}$/kg, respectively [33,34], but lower than other common berries such as blackberry (*Rubus ulmifolius* L.) 79.17 mmol $Fe2^{+}$/kg, highbush blueberry (*Vaccinium corymbosum* L.) 49.45 mmol $Fe2^{+}$/kg, black currant (*Ribes nigrum* L.) 58.43 mmol $Fe2^{+}$/kg, and white currant (*Ribes rubrum* L.) 85.97 mmol $Fe2^{+}$/kg [35]. The results of nutraceutical compounds are in accordance with a previous study on *Elaeagnus angustifolia* (L.), member of the Elaeagnaceae family with berries similar to the E. umbellata species [31]. The FRAP value was highly correlated with TAC (r = 0.929) and flavonols content (r = 0.962), pointing out the main role of these compounds in antioxidant activities.

3.3. Organic Acids

Organic acids are located in the fleshy parts of fruits and can affect sensory properties and consumer acceptability. A study conducted on juices of six cultivars of sea buckthorn (*Elaeagnus rhamnoides* L.), a berry tree of the Elaeagnaceae family, found that titratable acidity had a positive correlation with the intensity of sourness and astringency [35]. The quantity of organic acids can vary depending on many factors; for example, in a study on two blueberry species native to Turkey (*Vaccinium arctostaphylos* and *V. myrtillus*), the amount of malic, citric, and quinic acids changed significantly during different ripening stages [36]. Other factors include cultivar choice, soil, and climate conditions. Organic acids were the most represented secondary metabolites (1890 ± 182.02 mg/100 g FW) in *E. umbellata* berries. The compounds detected were citric, malic, oxalix, quinic, succinic, and tartaric acids (Table 2). Succinic was the primary organic acid (490.78 mg/100 g FW) accounting for about 25% of the total acid concentration, followed by quinic (468.83 mg/100 g FW) and citric (370.15 mg/100 g FW). Results are in accordance with previous studies on the autumn olive, where the main organic acids detected were malic, quinic, and citric acids, although in smaller quantities [5,6]. Among the acids, citric was the one with the higher correlation to titratable acidity (r = 0.932).

Table 2. Organic acids composition of autumn olive berries.

	Citric Acid	Malic Acid	Oxalic Acid	Quinic Acid	Succinic Acid	Tartaric Acid
Mean value	370.15	382.43	60.69	468.83	490.58	117.77
SD	14.28	15.65	6.34	39.76	18.20	22.48

The results are reported as mg/100 g FW (FW = fresh weight). Mean value and standard deviation are given for each sample ($n = 3$).

3.4. Phytochemical Composition

Phytochemicals are secondary metabolites produced by plants. These bioactive non-nutritive compounds may provide desirable health benefits to contrast the development of chronic diseases. Indeed, the regular consumption of phytochemicals (antioxidant compounds) help to prevent or slow oxidative stress caused by free radicals [37]. There is currently little available research on the phytochemical composition of *E. umbellata* species.

Several factors are relevant in determining the composition of bioactive compounds, such as genetic and environmental factors. Among the environmental ones, soil composition, agronomic management, and weather are the most influential variables. Nevertheless, the composition can change due to oxidative reactions during processing and storage [38]. In addition, the analytical method is discriminatory.

The phytochemical fingerprint of autumn olive berries was carried out via HPLC-DAD and results on bioactive compounds are summarized in Table 3. The total bioactive compound content (TBCC), expressed as the sum of the most important biologically active molecules detected in the extracts and reported as mg/100 g of fresh weight, showed a mean value of 413.64 ± 39.96 mg/100 g FW, considerably lower than commercial berries such as goji [39], but close to the value of cornelian cherry [33]. The analysis revealed the presence of 23 compounds, grouped in three different classes to evaluate each class contribution. Polyphenols, with a percentage of 65.56%, were the largest class, followed by monoterpenes (27.40%) and vitamin C (7.04%).

Table 3. Phytochemical fingerprint of autumn olive berries.

Bioactive Class	Compound	Mean Value	SD
Monoterpenes	limonene	34.34	1.91
	phellandrene	8.33	0.07
	sabinene	26.16	0.03
	γ-terpinene	28.90	1.40
	terpinolene	15.59	0.03
Vitamin C	ascorbic acid	5.66	0.70
	dehydroascorbic acid	23.46	2.75
Cinnamic acids	caffeic acid	0.78	0.02
	chlorogenic acid	10.93	0.13
	coumaric acid	5.82	0.02
	ferulic acid	1.32	0.19
Flavonols	hyperoside	7.20	0.49
	isoquercitrin	0.10	0.03
	quercetin	8.95	0.72
	quercitrin	0.15	0.09
	rutin	0.76	0.08
Benzoic acids	ellagic acid	5.50	1.17
	gallic acid	0.16	0.12
Catechins	catechin	1.62	1.35
	epicatechin	3.38	0.99
Tannins	castalagin	5.00	1.07
	vescalagin	24.54	3.34
Anthocyanins		194.99	0.817

The results are reported as mg/100 g FW (FW = fresh weight). Mean value and standard deviation are given for each sample ($n = 3$).

Polyphenols are compounds derived from secondary plant metabolism, present at high levels in several edible species. They perform many essential roles in plant physiology and as health-promoting compounds. Their healthy properties in humans were first linked to their antioxidant activity. In the last few years, recent findings have challenged this view, through the investigation of more complex actions [40]. As discussed above, very little is known about the polyphenolic composition of autumn olive berries. Among polyphenols, anthocyanins represent the most important compounds (71.9%), followed by tannins (10.9%), cinnamic acids (6.9%), flavonols (6.3%), benzoic acids (2.1%), and catechins (1.8%). Recently, a strong interest has been paid to the anthocyanins class, which may be among the principal polyphenols responsible for health benefits [41]. Indeed, they show strong anti-oxidant activity that helps to prevent several diseases such as cardiovascular illnesses, diabetes, cancer, and inflammation [42].

Monoterpenes, a class of volatile chemicals found in many fruits, were the second class of bioactive compounds in terms of quantity detected (27.40% of TBCC). Among them, limonene was the most represented compound found in autumn olive berries (34.34 mg/100 g FW). Many studies had focused on the anticancer properties of limonene, highlighting the positive role of monoterpenes in fighting the course of breast cancer [43].

The amount of vitamin C in *E. umbellata* berries was assayed as the sum of ascorbic and dehydroascorbic acids, shown as the average value of 29.12 ± 3.46 mg/100 g FW. This was in line with the findings of a previous study [27], but rather higher than previous research on *E. umbellate* [4,7]. Considering the ascorbic acid, berries recorded significantly lower values (5.66 ± 0.70 mg/100 g FW) compared to other super fruits (strawberry 90.13 ± 2.24 mg/100 g FW, blueberry 73.21 ± 0.35 mg/100 g FW, blackberry 52.41 ± 11.31 mg/100 g FW) [28]. However, autumn olive represents a good source of vitamin C. The consumption of 100 g of berries may cover from 30% to 50% of the recommended daily intake (60–90 mg/d) [44].

4. Conclusions

The preliminary results of this work allowed to contribute to the knowledge of *E. umbellata* fruits, especially concerning their nutraceutical aspects. Little information is yet available on the properties of this underutilized fruit. In addition, several factors make it difficult to recognize the different species and genotypes of *Elaeagnus*.

Concerning the results of phytochemical traits, phenolic is the larger class, mainly represented by anthocyanins. Although no comparable values are recorded yet for this species, studies on the Russian olive (*Elaeagnus angustifolia* L.) confirm the high content of anthocyanins. The importance of anthocyanins as health-promoting compounds is also represented by the positive correlation between total anthocyanin content (TAC) and antioxidant capacity (r = 0.929). The total polyphenolic content (TPC) is higher if compared to other studies on the same species, and similar to the values recorded for other known superfruits such as red raspberry, blueberry, and cherry. The autumn olive berries also contain a high percentage of organic acids, monoterpenes, and vitamin C.

To conclude, this work contributes to highlighting the potential of autumn olive as a source of valuable bioactive compounds, both for fresh consumption and fruit-derived products. However, further studies on *E. umbellata* will be fundamental to improve the knowledge of important aspects such as phytochemical fingerprint, health benefits, and antioxidant activity.

Author Contributions: Conceptualization, G.G. and G.L.B.; data curation, G.G.; formal analysis, G.G. and D.D.; investigation, G.G.; methodology, G.G. and D.D.; resources, D.D., I.R., and M.D.B.; supervision, G.L.B.; validation, D.D. and M.G.M.; writing—original draft, G.G.; writing—review and editing, G.G., D.R., and G.L.B. All authors have read and agreed to the published version of the manuscript.

Acknowledgments: Thanks are due to Mauro Caviglione and Marco D'Oria. Indeed, they managed all the cultivation aspects and provided the fruits for the analysis.

References

1. VVAA. The Plant List. Available online: http://www.theplantlist.org/ (accessed on 10 January 2020).
2. Fordham, I.M.; Zimmerman, R.H.; Black, B.L.; Clevidence, B.M.; Wiley, E.R. Autumn olive: A potential alternative crop. In Proceedings of the XXVI International Horticultural Congress: Berry Crop Breeding, Production and Utilization for a New Century 626, Toronto, ON, Canada, 1 November 2003; pp. 429–431.

3. Patel, S. Plant genus Elaeagnus: Underutilized lycopene and linoleic acid reserve with permaculture potential. *Fruits* **2015**, *70*, 191–199. [CrossRef]
4. Ahmad, S.; Sabir, S.; Zubair, M. Ecotypes diversity in autumn olive (Elaeagnus umbellata Thunb): A single plant with multiple micronutrient genes. *Chem. Ecol.* **2006**, *22*, 509–521. [CrossRef]
5. Wang, S.Y.; Fordham, I.M. Differences in chemical composition and antioxidant capacity among different genotypes of Autumn Olive (Elaeagnus umbellate Thunb.). *Food Technol. Biotechnol.* **2007**, *45*, 402.
6. Wu, M.-C.; Hu, H.-T.; Yang, L.; Yang, L. Proteomic analysis of up-accumulated proteins associated with fruit quality during autumn olive (Elaeagnus umbellata) fruit ripening. *J. Agric. Food Chem.* **2010**, *59*, 577–583. [CrossRef] [PubMed]
7. Shahidi, F.; Shi, J.; Ho, C.-T. *Functional Foods of the East*; CRC Press: Boca Raton, FL, USA, 2010.
8. Sabir, M.S.; Ahmad, D.S.; Hussain, I.M.; Tahir, K.M. Antibacterial activity of Elaeagnus umbellata (Thunb.) a medicinal plant from Pakistan. *Saudi Med. J.* **2007**, *28*, 259–263.
9. Ri-Lei, S.; Tao, W.; Hai-Tao, H.; Ling, Y. Research Situation about Elaeagnus umbellate Thunb. *J. Shanxi Agric. Sci.* **2012**, *9*, 26.
10. Dittberner, P.L.; Dietz, D.R.; Wasser, C.H. Autumn Olive (*Eleagnus umbellata*). *US Army Corps Eng. Wildl. Resour. Manag. Man.* **1992**, *7.5.7*, 1–25.
11. Dirr, A. Manual of Landscape Plants: Their Identification. In *Ornamental Characteristics, Culture, Propagation and Uses*, 5th ed.; University of Georgia, Department of Horticulture: Athens, GA, USA, 1998; ISBN 0-87563-795-7.
12. De Leo, M.; Camangi, F.; Muscatello, B.; Iannuzzi, A.; Giacomelli, C.; Graziani, F.; Trincavelli, M.; Martini, C.; Braca, A. Phytochemical analysis and antisenescence activity of Sorbus torminalis (L.) Crantz and Elaeagnus umbellata Thunb fruits. In Proceedings of the 113° Congresso della Società Botanica Italiana V International Plant Science Conference, Fisciano, Italy, 12–15 September 2018; p. 51.
13. Fordham, I.M.; Clevidence, B.A.; Wiley, E.R.; Zimmerman, R.H. Fruit of autumn olive: A rich source of lycopene. *HortScience* **2001**, *36*, 1136–1137. [CrossRef]
14. Pei, R.; Yu, M.; Bruno, R.; Bolling, B.W. Phenolic and tocopherol content of autumn olive (*Elaeagnus umbellate*) berries. *J. Funct. Foods* **2015**, *16*, 305–314. [CrossRef]
15. Slinkard, K.; Singleton, V.L. Total phenol analysis: Automation and comparison with manual methods. *Am. J. Enol. Vitic.* **1977**, *28*, 49–55.
16. Giusti, M.M.; Wrolstad, R.E. Characterization and measurement of anthocyanins by UV-visible spectroscopy. *Curr. Protoc. Food Anal. Chem.* **2001**, *1*, F1.2.1–F1.2.13. [CrossRef]
17. Lee, J.; Durst, R.W.; Wrolstad, R.E. Determination of total monomeric anthocyanin pigment content of fruit juices, beverages, natural colorants, and wines by the pH differential method: Collaborative study. *J. AOAC Int.* **2005**, *88*, 1269–1278. [CrossRef] [PubMed]
18. Benzie, I.F.; Strain, J. Ferric reducing/antioxidant power assay: Direct measure of total antioxidant activity of biological fluids and modified version for simultaneous measurement of total antioxidant power and ascorbic acid concentration. In *Methods in Enzymology*; Elsevier: Amsterdam, The Netherlands, 1999; Volume 299, pp. 15–27.
19. Donno, D.; Mellano, M.G.; De Biaggi, M.; Riondato, I.; Rakotoniaina, E.N.; Beccaro, G.L. New findings in Prunus padus L. fruits as a source of natural compounds: Characterization of metabolite profiles and preliminary evaluation of antioxidant activity. *Molecules* **2018**, *23*, 725. [CrossRef]
20. De Biaggi, M.; Donno, D.; Mellano, M.G.; Gamba, G.; Riondato, I.; Rakotoniaina, E.N.; Beccaro, G.L. Emerging species with nutraceutical properties: Bioactive compounds from Hovenia dulcis pseudofruits. *Food Chem.* **2020**, *310*, 125816. [CrossRef] [PubMed]
21. González-Molina, E.; Moreno, D.A.; García-Viguera, C. Genotype and harvest time influence the phytochemical quality of Fino lemon juice (Citrus limon (L.) Burm. F.) for industrial use. *J. Agric. Food Chem.* **2008**, *56*, 1669–1675. [CrossRef] [PubMed]
22. Donno, D.; Mellano, M.G.; Prgomet, Ž.; Cerutti, A.K.; Beccaro, G.L. Phytochemical characterization and antioxidant activity evaluation of Mediterranean medlar fruit (Crataegus azarolus L.): Preliminary study of underutilized genetic resources as a potential source of health-promoting compound for food supplements. *J. Food Nutr. Res.* **2017**, *56*, 18–31.
23. Hussain, I. Physiochemical and sensory characteristics of Elaeagnus umbellata (Thunb) fruit from Rawalakot (Azad Kashmir) Pakistan. *Afr. J. Food Sci.* **2011**, *2*, 151–156.

24. Ayaz, F.A.; Kadioğlu, A.; Doğru, A. Soluble Sugar Composition of Elaeagnus angustifoliaL. var. orientalis (L.) Kuntze (Russian olive) Fruits. *Turk. J. Bot.* **1999**, *23*, 349–354.
25. Doty, T. Fructose sweetness: A new dimension. *Cereal Foods World* **1976**, *21*, 62–63.
26. Sakamura, F.; Suga, T. Changes in chemical components of ripening oleaster fruits. *Phytochemistry* **1987**, *26*, 2481–2484. [CrossRef]
27. Khattak, K.F. Free radical scavenging activity, phytochemical composition and nutrient analysis of Elaeagnus umbellata berry. *J. Med. Plants Res.* **2012**, *6*, 5196–5203.
28. De Souza, V.R.; Pereira, P.A.P.; da Silva, T.L.T.; de Oliveira, L.C.; Pio, R.; Queiroz, F. Determination of the bioactive compounds, antioxidant activity and chemical composition of Brazilian blackberry, red raspberry, strawberry, blueberry and sweet cherry fruits. *Food Chem.* **2014**, *156*, 362–368. [CrossRef] [PubMed]
29. Donno, D.; Cavanna, M.; Beccaro, G.L.; Mellano, M.; Torello Marinoni, D.; Cerutti, A.K.; Bounous, G. Currants and strawberries as bioactive compound sources: Determination of antioxidant profi les with HPLC-DAD/MS. *J. Appl. Bot. Food Qual.* **2013**, *86*, 1–10.
30. Benvenuti, S.; Pellati, F.; Melegari, M.a.; Bertelli, D. Polyphenols, anthocyanins, ascorbic acid, and radical scavenging activity of Rubus, Ribes, and Aronia. *J. Food Sci.* **2004**, *69*, FCT164–FCT169. [CrossRef]
31. Hassanzadeh, Z.; Hassanpour, H. Evaluation of physicochemical characteristics and antioxidant properties of Elaeagnus angustifolia L. *Sci. Hortic.* **2018**, *238*, 83–90. [CrossRef]
32. Raj, A.; Ahmad, F. Evaluation of anthocyanin content in the fruits of different Russian olive (Elaeagnus angustifolia) genotypes of Ladakh. *Progress. Hortic.* **2013**, *45*, 298–301.
33. De Biaggi, M.; Donno, D.; Mellano, M.G.; Riondato, I.; Rakotoniaina, E.N.; Beccaro, G.L. Cornus mas (L.) fruit as a potential source of natural health-promoting compounds: Physico-chemical characterisation of bioactive components. *Plant Foods Hum. Nutr.* **2018**, *73*, 89–94. [CrossRef]
34. Donno, D.; Mellano, M.; Prgomet, Z.; Beccaro, G. Advances in Ribes x nidigrolaria Rud. Bauer & A. Bauer fruits as potential source of natural molecules: A preliminary study on physico-chemical traits of an underutilized berry. *Sci. Hortic.* **2018**, *237*, 20–27.
35. Tang, X.; Kälviäinen, N.; Tuorila, H. Sensory and hedonic characteristics of juice of sea buckthorn (Hippophae rhamnoides L.) origins and hybrids. *LWT Food Sci. Technol.* **2001**, *34*, 102–110. [CrossRef]
36. Ayaz, F.; Kadioglu, A.; Bertoft, E.; Acar, C.; Turna, I. Effect of fruit maturation on sugar and organic acid composition in two blueberries (Vaccinium arctostaphylos and V. myrtillus) native to Turkey. *N. Z. J. Crop. Hortic. Sci.* **2001**, *29*, 137–141. [CrossRef]
37. Liu, R.H. Potential synergy of phytochemicals in cancer prevention: Mechanism of action. *J. Nutr.* **2004**, *134*, 3479S–3485S. [CrossRef] [PubMed]
38. Robards, K.; Prenzler, P.D.; Tucker, G.; Swatsitang, P.; Glover, W. Phenolic compounds and their role in oxidative processes in fruits. *Food Chem.* **1999**, *66*, 401–436. [CrossRef]
39. Donno, D.; Beccaro, G.L.; Mellano, M.G.; Cerutti, A.; Bounous, G. Goji berry fruit (Lycium spp.): Antioxidant compound fingerprint and bioactivity evaluation. *J. Funct. Foods* **2015**, *18*, 1070–1085. [CrossRef]
40. Yadav, B.S.; Yadav, R.; Yadav, R.B.; Garg, M. Antioxidant activity of various extracts of selected gourd vegetables. *J. Food Sci. Technol.* **2016**, *53*, 1823–1833. [CrossRef] [PubMed]
41. Veberic, R.; Slatnar, A.; Bizjak, J.; Stampar, F.; Mikulic-Petkovsek, M. Anthocyanin composition of different wild and cultivated berry species. *LWT Food Sci. Technol.* **2015**, *60*, 509–517. [CrossRef]
42. Yousuf, B.; Gul, K.; Wani, A.A.; Singh, P. Health benefits of anthocyanins and their encapsulation for potential use in food systems: A review. *Crit. Rev. Food Sci. Nutr.* **2016**, *56*, 2223–2230. [CrossRef]
43. Kunnumakkara, A.B. *Anticancer Properties of Fruits and Vegetables: A Scientific Review*; World Scientific: Singapore, 2014.
44. Monsen, E.R. Dietary reference intakes for the antioxidant nutrients: Vitamin C, vitamin E, selenium, and carotenoids. *J. Acad. Nutr. Diet.* **2000**, *100*, 637.

13

Traditional Decoction and PUAE Aqueous Extracts of Pomegranate Peels as Potential Low-Cost Anti-Tyrosinase Ingredients

Federica Turrini *, Paola Malaspina, Paolo Giordani, Silvia Catena, Paola Zunin and Raffaella Boggia

Department of Pharmacy, University of Genoa, Viale Cembrano 4, 16148 Genoa, Italy; malaspina@difar.unige.it (P.M.); giordani@difar.unige.it (P.G.); catena@difar.unige.it (S.C.); zunin@difar.unige.it (P.Z.); boggia@difar.unige.it (R.B.)

* Correspondence: turrini@difar.unige.it

Featured Application: The recycling of the external peels of pomegranate represents an important goal for pomegranate juice manufacturers, since their disposal is expensive and not eco-friendly. Traditional decoction and an innovative ultrasound-assisted method of extraction of pomegranate peels using just water have both led to obtaining aqueous extracts rich in polyphenolic compounds and endowed with anti-tyrosinase activity. Although these aqueous extracts may require a further formulation step for preservation, these findings suggest the possibility of using them as low-cost lightening and/or anti-browning agents, even extemporarily.

Abstract: The aim of the study is to evaluate the anti-tyrosinase activity of different aqueous extracts obtained from pomegranate juice processing by-products. External pomegranate peels of two certified cultivars (Akko and Wonderful), were extracted using only water as the extraction solvent. A traditional decoction and a pulsed ultrasound-assisted extraction (PUAE), both 10 min long, were performed and compared. All the aqueous extracts proved to be rich in bioactive compounds. In particular, the total phenolic content (TPC) ranged from 148 to 237 mg gallic acid equivalent (GAE)/g of dried peels (DW), the radical-scavenging ability (RSA) ranged from 307 to 472 mg ascorbic acid equivalent (AAE)/g DW, the free ellagic acid content (EA) ranged from 49 to 94 μg/mL, and the ellagitannins (ETs) ranged from 242 to 340 μg/mL. For both cultivars, PUAE extracts had higher ET content and a lower EC50, while the decoctions had slightly higher TPC, RSA, and free EA amounts. Principal component analysis (PCA) highlighted the direct correlation between the ET content and the tyrosinase enzyme inhibition (lower values of EC50). These findings suggest the potential use of both these natural extracts as low-cost lightening and/or anti-browning ingredients exploitable in several formulations (e.g., cosmetics) or extemporarily usable.

Keywords: pomegranate peels; anti-tyrosinase activity; waste recovery; green extraction

---

1. Introduction

Pomegranate (*Punica granatum* L.) is one of the oldest edible fruits. Mentioned in the Bible, the Koran and Egyptian texts, the first pomegranate crops date back to 3000–4000 BC. [1].

Native to the Middle East and North Africa, today pomegranate is spread globally due to its high longevity, drought and salinity resistance, and adaptability to different climatic conditions [2]. In particular, pomegranate is widely cultivated in Iran, India, China, USA, several countries of the former USSR, South Africa, and in Mediterranean countries such as Spain, Turkey, Egypt, Israel, Morocco and Tunisia [3]. In Italy, this resilient and rustic crop recently has shown a growing diffusion, especially in central and southern areas, in response to increasing market demand for pomegranate and, at the same time, with the aim of valorizing marginal land facing climatic change.

Pomegranate juice is the main industrial product obtained from this fruit. In addition to direct consumption, fresh arils (marketed as ready-to-eat products) and pomegranate seed oil have also recently gained an important industrial relevance [3].

One drawback in pomegranate juice industrial production is the large amount of waste, since juice represents about only 30% of the pomegranate fruit fresh weight. External peels are the most abundant by-products (about 50% of the total fruit weight) [4,5]. Even if they represent an expensive disposal problem, they are at the same time a promising source of phenolic compounds for exploitation. Ellagic acid (EA), in its free form or in the form of ellagitannins (ETs), is considered the main phenolic compound responsible for the numerous health properties of pomegranate, and is mainly concentrated in the peels with respect to the juice [6,7]. The functional properties of EA are largely reported in the literature [8,9]. Among the described healthy properties of pomegranate peel extracts, a previous study indicated that its methanolic peel extracts also inhibit tyrosinase activity [10,11].

The tyrosinase metallo-enzyme, widely distributed in nature, is fundamental in melanogenesis and enzymatic browning. It can be reversibly or irreversibly inhibited by several molecules that block the melanogenesis process in animals, as well as causing the undesired browning in fruits and vegetables [12]. Anti-tyrosinase compounds can be useful both as lightening and anti-browning ingredients in several commodities, such as cosmetics, pharmaceutics, and agri-food products. The color of skin, as well as hair and eyes, is determined by the melanin pigment [13]. In human beings, physiological changes in the normal production of melanin may lead to the appearance of freckles, skin spots or, in the worst case, to the development of melanomas [14–16]. Melanin is synthesized starting from a series of reactions controlled mainly by the activity of the tyrosinase enzyme, a monophenol monooxygenase capable of enclosing a single oxygen atom in the phenolic substrate, oxidizing it to *o*-diphenol and then transforming it into o-quinone [17,18].

EA is a cosmetic ingredient classified as a skin conditioner (CAS number: 476-66-4) [19]. In particular, it is considered an anti-aging, antiwrinkle, antimicrobial, antioxidant, astringent, moisturizing, and lightening/whitening agent [20]. Several authors have described the action of EA on skin pigmentation [21,22]. EA inhibits tyrosinase activity by chelation of the copper atoms present in the active site of the enzyme itself and, for this reason, it has been approved as a lightening ingredient in cosmetic formulations [21]. Nevertheless, there is a large interest in finding low-cost natural extracts with efficiency and safety features as recently reported by Zolghadri et al. [12].

In previous papers, the authors described different extraction strategies to valorize both the external peels (major waste) and the squeezing marcs (internal by-products), exploiting the cavitation of ultrasound extraction in order to increase the mass transfer rate between the peels and the extraction solvent in order to enhance the bioactive compounds recovery useful for a nutraceutical use [4,23].

In this paper, a simple, rapid, and low-cost strategy in the form of traditional decoction and the more innovative pulsed ultrasound-assisted extraction (PUAE) of oven-dried pomegranate peels were applied for the same time period, with the aim to obtain potential low-cost anti-tyrosinase ingredients from these by-products. Water, which is a basic element of both a greener and safer chemistry approach compared to methanol or other organic solvents [24,25], was employed alone as the extraction solvent. PUAE is an example of 'green' extraction technology, widely used for the extraction of food and natural products, and able to considerably reduce the extraction times and increase the extraction yield maintaining high reproducibility [26].

Akko and Wonderful, corresponding to an early and a late pomegranate variety, respectively, are some of the most wide-spread commercial pomegranate cultivars, in virtue of their soft seeds and welcome organoleptic features [4]. Wonderful is the most cultivated commercial cultivar in the Mediterranean region. However, the Akko cultivar, due to its early availability, has recently been introduced in these areas to ensure a continuous offer for the market [27].

To the best of our knowledge, no studies of the aqueous extracts of the Akko and Wonderful varieties of pomegranate as sources of anti-tyrosinase compounds have been conducted, and this is the object of our investigation.

2. Materials and Methods

2.1. Pomegranate Samples

Pomegranate fruits of Akko and Wonderful certified cultivars were harvested at Masseria FruttiRossi (https://lomesuperfruit.com/it/home) in Castellaneta Taranto (Italy), which includes 250 hectares of crops and represents the major Italian pomegranate producer.

Fruits were collected at full maturity (Maturity Index, MI = 14.5 ± 2.5), during September and November 2018, respectively, for Akko and Wonderful cultivars, and immediately processed to obtain the corresponding juice. Peels, manually separated during the juice processing, were dried using a traditional heating oven (Binder FED53, Goettingen, Germany) for 48 h at 40 °C. Before the extraction process, dried peels were finely ground by a Grindomi × 200 M (Retsch, Haan, Germany) for 20 s at 5000 rpm and finally sieved by a 150 μm sieve to obtain a fine and homogeneous material.

2.2. Standards and Reagents

All standards and reagents used were analytical grade. DPPH (1,1-diphenyl-2-picrylhydrazyl) and Folin-Ciocalteu reagents, gallic acid, ascorbic acid, ellagic acid, cyanidine-3-*O*-glucoside chloride, and methanol were supplied by SIGMA (Steinheim, Germany). Ethanol, acetic acid, hydrochloric acid, and sodium hydroxide were purchased from VWR Chemical (Radnor, PA, USA). L-tyrosine, kojic acid, and mushroom tyrosinase for tyrosinase inhibition assay were supplied by SIGMA (Steinheim, Germany). High purity water (HPW) produced with a Millipore Milli-Q system (Millipore, Bedford, MA, USA) was used throughout. All solvents used for chromatographic purposes were HPLC grade.

2.3. Pomegranate Peel Extraction

Peel extraction, both by traditional decoction and by 'green' extraction exploiting the ultrasound action, was performed. Only water was used as the extraction solvent under both methods. The same extraction time (10 min) and the same solvent/solid ratio (40/1, considering the dried peel weight) were used for both extraction processes. Each extraction was performed in duplicate and all the obtained extracts were analytically analyzed.

2.3.1. Traditional Decoction (D)

The decoction of pomegranate peels was carried out by adding the milled dried materials to 40 mL of Milli-Q water in a beaker. This suspension was heated and kept boiling for 10 min. Then, it was filtered by Buchner, using Whatman n. 1 paper, and centrifuged at relative centrifugation force (RCF or G-force) equal to 2016 for 10 min. The final extracts (AK_D and WO_D) were kept at −20 °C until further analysis.

2.3.2. Green Extraction: Pulsed Ultrasound-Assisted Extraction (PUAE)

Ultrasonication was applied directly by an Hielscher UP200St (Teltow, Germany) in pulsed modality (PUAE). Maximum nominal output power of 200W, frequency of 26 kHz, and a titanium probe (7 mm diameter) were employed for the sonication. The pulse duration and pulse interval refer to "on" time and "off" time of the sonicator. The pulse duration/pulse interval ratio was 4/1 (duty cycle 80%). The amplitude level was set to 50%. During the extraction process, temperature was controlled to be below 65 °C (temperature variation during the extraction period was lower than 40°C). The obtained extracts (AK_PUAE and WO_PUAE), similarly to the decoction described in the previous paragraph, were filtered, centrifuged and stored frozen until analysis.

2.4. *Characterization of the Peel Aqueous Extracts*

pH was evaluated by electrochemical measurements using a pHmeter (Jenway 3510, Stone, UK). The total soluble content (TSS), expressed in °Brix, was determined at 20 °C by a digital refractometer (Hanna Instruments, Milano, Italy) (Table 1). The total polyphenol content (TPC) and the Radical Scavenging Activity (RAS) of all the aqueous peel extracts (D and PUAE) were determined spectrophotometrically. The total anthocyanin content (TAC) and the EA and ET amounts were quantified by chromatography.

Table 1. pH, TSS, and TAC values of Akko and Wonderful pomegranate peel aqueous extracts obtained by the traditional (D) and innovative extraction technique (PUAE). Results are reported as mean ± SE.

	Cultivar	Extraction Method	pH	TSS (°Brix)	*TAC (mg Cyanidin-3-O-Glucoside/* g DW)
AK_D	Akko	Decoction	3.92 ± 0.04	3.10 ± 0.10	0.14 ± 0.01
AK_PUAE	Akko	PUAE	4.04 ± 0.03	1.95 ± 0.05	0.06 ± 0
WO_D	Wonderful	Decoction	3.56 ± 0.02	2.05 ± 0.05	0.08 ± 0
WO_PUAE	Wonderful	PUAE	3.65 ± 0.03	1.80 ± 0	0.05 ± 0.02

2.4.1. Determination of Total Polyphenols

TPC was determined by an UV-Vis Agilent 8453 spectrometer (Waldbronn, Germany) following the Folin-Ciocalteu method previously reported by Singleton et al. [28]. TPC was determined in the peel aqueous extracts as milligrams of gallic acid equivalent in 100 mL of extract (mg GAE/100 mL) using an appropriate gallic acid calibration curve (R^2 = 0.9887) as the reference standard. Then, the results were transformed in mg GAE/g of pomegranate peel dry weight (DW). Each sample was analyzed in duplicate and the results were reported as mean values ± standard error (SE).

2.4.2. Determination of the Radical Scavenging Activity

RSA of the achieved extracts was spectrophotometrically determined by DPPH• (1,1-diphenyl–2-picryl-hydrazyl) in vitro assay [29]. This method, widely used for food matrices, allowed the detection of the antiradical activity colorimetrically based on the discoloration of the stable colored DPPH• recorded at 515 nm. Ascorbic acid was used as the reference standard and the recorded absorbances of the extracts were compared with the absorbance of solutions of ascorbic acid (AA) at known concentration ($y = 0.5824x - 0.0036$; $R^2 = 0.9975$; range of linearity 0.1–1 mM). The antiradical activity was obtained as mg ascorbic acid equivalent in 100 mL of extract (mg AAE/100 mL) and then converted as mg AAE/g of pomegranate peel DW. Two replicated determinations were performed for each sample and data were reported as mean values ± SE.

2.5. *HPLC Analysis*

2.5.1. Determination of EA and ETs

The HPLC determination of EA and ETs was realized using an Agilent 1100 LC-DAD (Agilent Technologies, Palo Alto, USA) [4]. A C-18 Kromasil 100® (Akzo-Nobel, Amsterdam, NL) column (250 × 4 mm, 5 μm), thermostat-controlled at 30 °C, was used for the chromatographic separations. Gradient elution of acetic acid/methanol/water (2:400:598) (solvent A) and methanol (solvent B), with a 1 mL/min flow rate was employed as follows: 100% A at 0 min, 0% A at 20 min, 100% A reset in 10 min and held for 5 min. The injection volume was 10 μL, and the detection wavelengths were set between 220 and 600 nm. Free EA in the extracts was quantified at 245 nm by external standard, using an appropriate 4-point calibration line ($y = 251.58x - 204.41$; $R^2 > 0.999$; range of linearity 2.5–200 μg/mL; LOD = 0.78 μg/mL; LOQ = 2.36 μg/mL). The total ET content was determined after the preliminary acid hydrolysis (performed in replicate) of extracts in order to hydrolyze ETs in EA [4,30]. A quantity of

2 mL of each extract, added to 2 mL HCl 2 M, was heated at 100 °C for 1 h in a boiling water bath. After the cooling time, 1 mL of NaOH 2M and 6 mL of methanol were added. The final solution was vortexed and filtered before the injection. Two replicated determinations of EA and ETs were performed for each sample analyzed and data were reported as mean values ± SE. The EA chromatogram of one pomegranate peel aqueous extract is reported in the Supplementary Materials Figure S1.

2.5.2. Determination of Total Anthocyanins

TAC identification and quantification was conducted using an HPLC–DAD method [31]. Analysis were carried out on a C-18 core-shell column (Agilent Poroshell 120 EC, 3 mm × 150 mm, 2.7 μm particle size) thermostat-controlled at 30 °C. Gradient elution of water acidified at pH 2.14 by formic acid (solvent A) and acetonitrile (solvent B), with a 0.4 mL/min flow rate, was employed as follows: 95% A at 0 min, 70% A at 25 min, 45% A at 35 min, and 0% A at 42 min, held for 3 min. Anthocyanins were quantified at 515 nm by external standard, using an appropriate 4-point cyanidin-3-*O*-glucoside calibration line ($y = 71.52x - 12.54$; $R^2 > 0.999$; range of linearity 1.5-150 μg/mL; LOD = 0.39 μg/mL; LOQ = 1.17 μg/mL). Each sample was analyzed in duplicate and the results, expressed as μg cyanidin-3-*O*-glucoside/g DW, were reported as mean values ± SE. The anthocyanin profile of one pomegranate peel aqueous extract is reported in the Supplementary Materials Figure S2.

2.6. *Tyrosinase Inhibition Property*

A 25 mg/mL stock solution of each cultivar and treatment, prepared as described in the previous paragraph, was diluted in water to obtain a series of test solutions with final concentrations of 10, 50, 100, 250, 350, and 500 μg/mL. Components of the reaction mix were added to each well of 96-well plates in the following order: 70 μL of phosphate buffer, 60 μL of extract solutions (water for controls), 10 μL of mushroom tyrosinase (Sigma-Aldrich, T3824, 25 kU, 125 U/mL in phosphate buffer, pH 6.8), and 70 μL L-tyrosine (0.3 mg/mL in water). Kojic acid was used instead of pomegranate solutions as a positive control. Blank samples without enzyme were also included for all conditions. Plates were then incubated at 30 °C for 60 min, and absorbance was read at 505 nm in a microplate reader (Spectra Max 340PC). Percent inhibitory activity (I%) was calculated according to the formula:

$$I\% = \left[1 - \frac{(A_{ex/en} - A_{ex})}{(A_{en} - A_{bk})}\right] \times 100$$

where Aex/en = absorbance of sample mixture with extract and enzyme; Aex = absorbance of sample mixture with extract and without enzyme; Aen = absorbance of sample mixture with enzyme and without extract; Abk = absorbance of sample mixture without enzyme and extract (blank).

2.7. *Statistical Analysis*

All the measurements performed were replicated and the results are expressed as mean value ± SE. Analysis of variance (ANOVA) was performed using the Excel Data Analysis Tool (Microsoft Corporation, Seattle, WA, USA). A *p*-value lower than 0.05 was statistically significant. Principal component analysis (PCA), based on the NIPALS algorithm [32], was performed by CAT (Chemometric Agile Tool) [33]. This chemometric software, based on R, was developed by the Chemistry Group of the Italian Chemical Society.

3. Results and Discussion

It is known that bioactive compounds are variable in pomegranate, and generally in plant material, according to genetic factors, different collection stages, pedoclimatic conditions of the sampling sites (growing wild or cultivation), application of agricultural practices, and post-harvest handling [34,35].

For this investigation, pomegranates of Akko and Wonderful cultivars were grown in the same cultivation area in Southern Italy, under the same pedoclimatic conditions, and using the same agro-techniques. These samples, coming from one of the biggest Italian producers, are representative of the commercial cultivars most widespread and marketed in Italy. Fruits were harvested in different collection periods according to the cultivar maturity but at the same maturity status.

pH, TSS, and TAC of both the aqueous extracts (D and PUAE) of Akko and Wonderful cultivar are reported in Table 1.

One-way ANOVA, analyzing the mean differences of the pH values, showed significant differences ($p < 0.05$) between the cultivars (Akko and Wonderful), but no significant differences are highlighted between the two different extraction methods (D and PUAE) for the same cultivar (Table 2).

Table 2. One-way ANOVA results.

Variable	ANOVA Data	AK_D/AK_PUAE	WO_D/WO_PUAE	AK_D/ WO_D	AK_PUAE/ WO_PUAE
pH	F	7.353	8.022	89.379	84.5
	p value	0.113	0.105	0.011	0.012
TSS	F	105.8	25	88.2	9
	p value	0.009	0.038	0.011	0.095
RSA	F	3.038	17.838	12.012	9.064
	p value	0.223	0.052	0.074	0.095
TPC	F	51.789	5.184	43.586	0.798
	p value	0.019	0.151	0.022	0.466
TAC	F	64	5.444	36	1
	p value	0.015	0.145	0.027	0.423
EA	F	17.323	5.758	57.772	9.221
	p value	0.053	0.138	0.017	0.093
ETS	F	3.959	9.755	0.542	0.236
	p value	0.185	0.089	0.538	0.675

As regards TSS, one-way ANOVA highlighted significant differences ($p < 0.05$) between D and PUAE extracts for both the cultivars. In particular, D extracts (AK_D and WO_D) showed higher TSS with respect to the corresponding PUAE extracts (AK_PUAE and WO_PUAE). This is likely because the higher boiling temperature of decoction compared to sonication allowed the partial hydrolysis of glucosides and the release of sugar moieties [36]. No significant difference between AK_PUAE and WO_PUAE was observed, probably because the extraction temperature was similarly maintained under control (<65 °C). According to previous studies [37], extraction temperature in the range of 60–70 °C was optimal for the UAE of EA from pomegranate peels.

For both the extraction methods the obtained extracts can be considered almost sugar-free if compared with the corresponding pomegranate juice (Akko: TSS = 15.20 ± 0.42; Wonderful: TSS = 17.01 ± 0.57), as previously studied by the authors [23].

Previous studies have shown that cultivar, maturity stage, and environmental factors could significantly influence the TAC of pomegranate peel extracts [5,38,39]. Cyanidin and pelargonidin derivatives are the most abundant anthocyanin pigments isolated from the peels. In particular, cyanidin 3-*O*-glucoside was considered one of the major anthocyanins detected in these by-products [38]. In all the extracts the TAC was slightly lower compared to those reported in literature for other pomegranate cultivars [40] even if the cited authors used methanol as an extraction solvent. One-way ANOVA, analyzing the mean differences of the TAC, showed significant differences ($p < 0.05$) between the cultivars when extracts were obtained by decoction. On the contrary, no significant differences between AK_PUAE and WO_PUAE were observed. Different results were shown for the two cultivars by comparing the two extraction methods (D and PUAE).

Figure 1 reports the TPC and the RSA results of the peel aqueous extracts (D and PUAE) belonging to the two cultivars investigated.

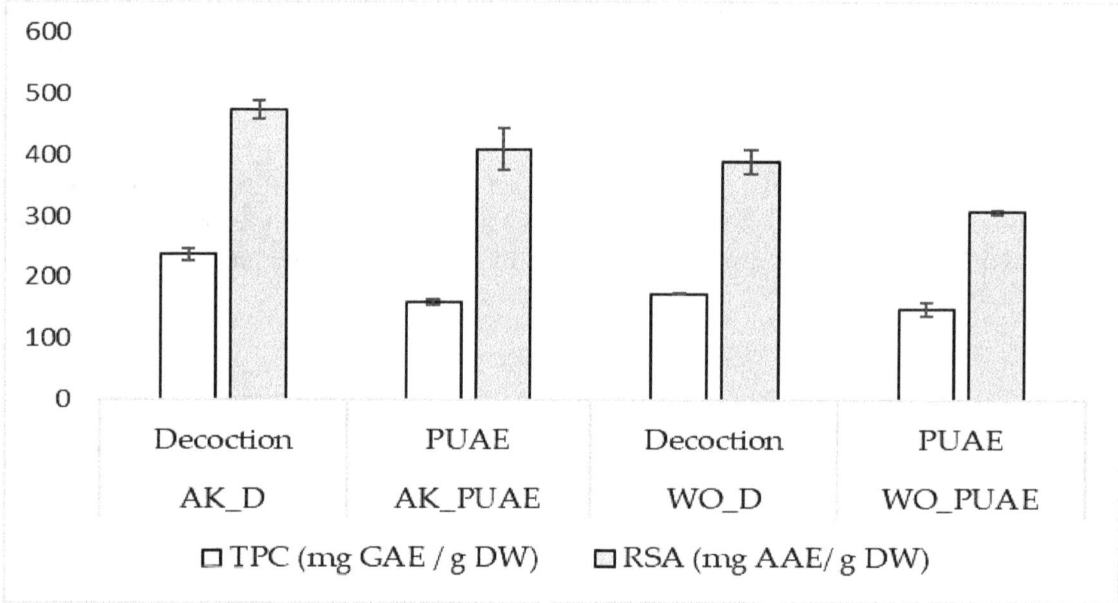

Figure 1. TPC and RSA of Akko and Wonderful pomegranate peel aqueous extracts obtained by the traditional (D) and innovative extraction technique (PUAE). Bars show mean values and SE of the replicated data.

TPC and RSA values were moderately correlated ($R^2 = 0.7304$). The decoction demonstrated higher TPC compared to the extract obtained by sonication (PUAE) in both cultivars. In fact, one-way ANOVA, analyzing the mean differences of the TPCs, showed significant differences ($p < 0.05$) between the extraction methods (D and PUAE) for both cultivars. Analyzing the two different cultivars, there is a significant difference between AK_D and W_D, with a higher value for Akko. On the contrary, no significant differences in TPC were observed between the cultivars when the extraction was performed by PUAE.

As regards RSA, no significant differences were observed by ANOVA in Akko and Wonderful cultivars extracted both by decoction and PUAE, although the statistical significance was very low (Table 2).

Some previous studies, which considered aqueous extracts of pomegranate peels starting from different cultivars, showed an extraction efficiency, expressed as TPC, lower than that obtained in the present work; for example, El-Said et al. 2014 [41] reported a TPC equal to 16.343 mg GAE/g for aqueous extracts obtained from similarly oven-dried peels, which is more than 10 times less than those reported in Figure 1. Rahja et al. 2019 [24] described different 'green' extraction methods using just water as a solvent to efficiently extract the bioactive fraction of pomegranate peels. From a comparison of different aqueous extraction methods applied to pomegranate peels, such as ultrasound (UAE), infrared, pulsed electric fields, and high-voltage electrical discharges (HVED), HVED-assisted extraction, applied for 7 min., yielded a maximal concentration of phenolics equal to 46 mg GAE/g DW. After the same period, the UAE method yielded phenolic recovery equal to 14.5 mg of GAE/g DW, which is approximately 10–16 times lower than the TPCs of those reported in Figure 1. Recently, Kaderides et al. 2019 [42], exploiting the action of ultrasound and microwave to extract the phenolic compounds from pomegranate peels, described TPCs equal to 119.82 mg GAE/g dry peel and 199.4 mg GAE/g dry peel, respectively, which are more in accordance with the values described in this study (148–237 mg GAE/g DW).

Figure 2 reports the free EA and ET amounts of the peel aqueous extracts (D and PUAE) belonging to the two different cultivars investigated.

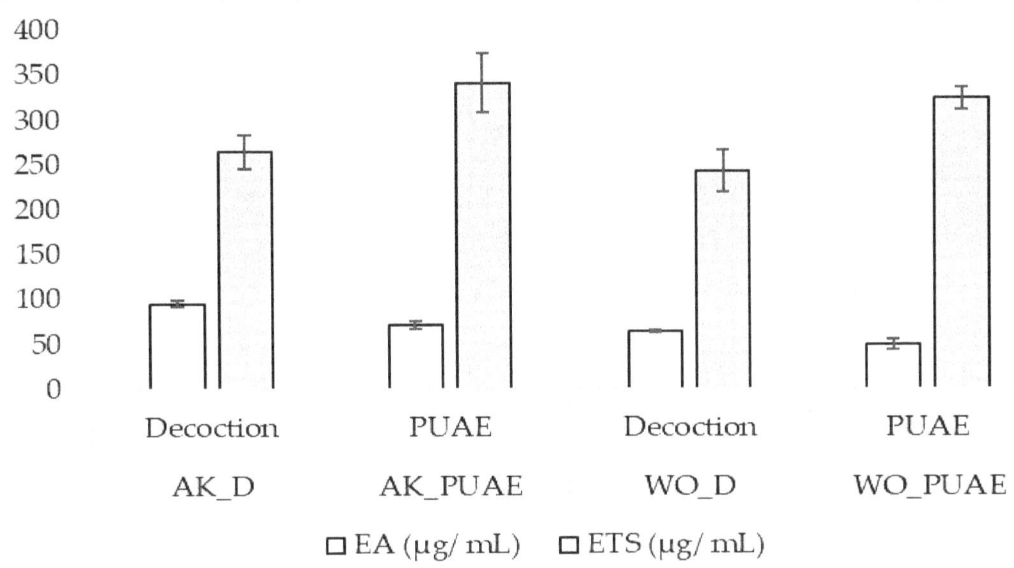

Figure 2. EA and ET amounts of Akko and Wonderful pomegranate peel aqueous extracts obtained by the traditional (D) and innovative extraction technique (PUAE). Bars show mean values and SE of the replicated data.

Free EA and ET contents were not correlated. In particular, for both cultivars, the decoction (AK_D and WO_D) showed higher EA and lower ET contents compared to the PUAE extracts (AK_PUAE and WO_PUAE). The PUAE extract, according to several other green strategies reported in the literature [42–44], confirms its superiority in terms of ET recovery, even if the simplest decoction is endowed with a higher free EA content, probably due to the highest boiling temperature, which allows the partial hydrolysis of ETs with the consequent release of the common aglycone (EA) and some sugar moieties [36]. The aim of this investigation was the comparison between the innovative PUAE and the traditional decoction. For this reason, the same experimental conditions (extraction time, liquid/solid ratio, extraction solvent) were maintained for both of the extraction strategies with the exception of the temperature, which was the only variable that changed (PUAE < 65 °C and D = 100 °C). ETs are stable in acidic conditions (pH = 2–4), which is their natural condition; nevertheless, they rapidly degrade in neutral and mildly basic media, especially at higher temperatures [36]. In acidic conditions, as in the pomegranate extracts, ETs show high stability in the range of temperature 20–60 °C but at 80 °C they gradually degrade [36].

One-way ANOVA, analyzing the mean differences of the free EA content, showed significant differences ($p < 0.05$) only between AK_D and WO_D. On the contrary, as regards the mean differences of the ET content, one-way ANOVA did not reveal significant differences between the studied couples as reported in Table 2.

Figure 3 reports the percentage of tyrosinase inhibition of the peel aqueous extracts (Akko and Wonderful) obtained by the innovative (a) and the traditional (b) extraction techniques.

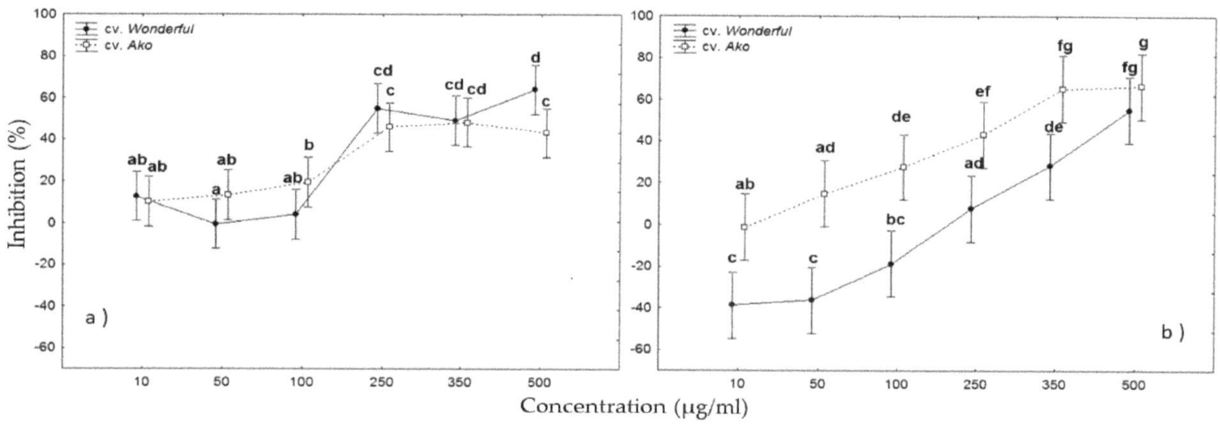

Figure 3. Percentage of tyrosinase inhibition of Akko and Wonderful pomegranate peel aqueous extracts obtained by innovative (**a**) and the traditional (**b**) extraction techniques. Bars show mean values and SE of the replicated data as a function of concentration. The letters represent homogeneous groups with $p > 0.05$ (LSD Fisher post-hoc test). Same letters denote groups that are not statistically different.

The PUAE extracts of the two cultivars showed inhibition values not significantly different at the different concentrations tested, except for those observed at 500 μg/mL. More relevant differences were found for traditional decoctions: in these extracts the Akko cultivar showed greater inhibitions at all concentrations except the highest one considered. From the inhibition values obtained from the various concentrations tested, it was possible to calculate the EC50. In general, the extracts obtained from the innovative extraction technique had better EC50 values (AK_PUAE = 117.73 μg/mL; WO_PUAE = 159.04 μg/mL) compared to traditional extracts (AK_D = 147.38 μg/mL; WO_D = 365.91 μg/mL).

In order to analyze the data using a multivariate approach, principal component analysis (PCA), an unsupervised pattern recognition technique, was applied to the data matrix $D_{8,8}$, whose rows are the extracts and the columns are all the determined experimental variables. In detail, the eight extracts are those obtained by PUAE and decoction for both cultivars, in duplicate, and correspondingly categorized. PCA was performed on the autoscaled data matrix, since autoscaling, which consists of mean-centering followed by division of each column (variable) by its standard deviation, allows elaboration of multivariate data characterized by different scales and units. Figure 4 a-b shows the PCA results obtained from the above-mentioned data matrix $D_{8,8}$.

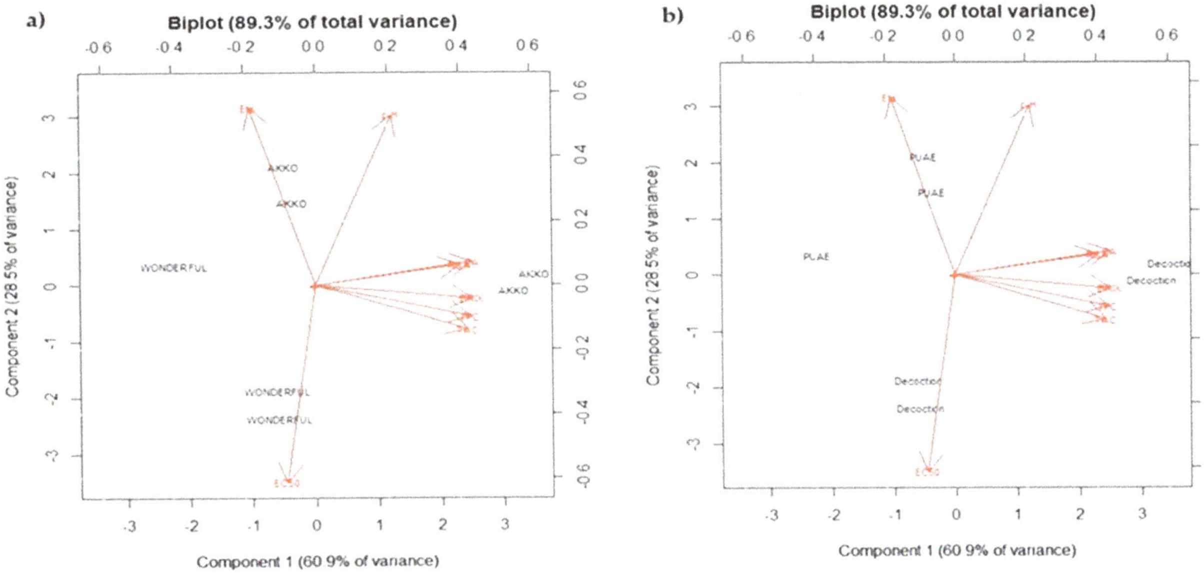

Figure 4. Biplot (score and loading plot) on PC1–PC2 obtained by principal component analysis (PCA). (**a**): extracts are categorized by the different cultivar (Akko and Wonderful); (**b**): data are categorized by the different extraction techniques (D and PUAE).

The first two principal components (PCs) together explain almost 90% of the total information of the whole data set since they visualize almost 90% of the total variance of the dataset. Figure 4a,b shows the biplot PC1 vs. PC2, which represents the scores and loadings plot, on the first two PCs, highlighting the different categorization of the extracts (a—the extracts are categorized by the different cultivar; and b—the data are categorized by the different extraction techniques).

PC1, the direction of maximum variance (60.9%), for both cultivars, discriminates the PUAE extracts from decoctions which have more positive scores on the first PC (Figure 4b). Decoction could be associated with higher °Brix, RSA, TPC, TAC, and EA (highest loadings on PC1). Nevertheless, as far as anti-tyrosinase activity is concerned, PC2, whose variance is about 29%, is the most important component, highlighting the indirect correlation between the ET content (highest loadings on PC2) and the EC50 (lowest loading on PC2). For both cultivars, PUAE extracts could be associated with the highest ET content (highest loading on PC2) and the highest anti-tyrosinase activity. AK_PUAE, which represents the extract with the highest content of ETs, is the one endowed with the highest anti-tyrosinase activity (lowest EC50). Since PCs are mathematically uncorrelated (orthogonal) variables, it seems that ET content, among all the determined variables, is the most important to determine the anti-tyrosinase activity, together with pH, whose highest value in the Akko cultivar could further positively influence the anti-tyrosinase activity [10,11]. The remaining variables, having high loadings on the PC1, do not seem correlated with the anti-tyrosinase activity.

Water was employed as an extraction solvent with the dual aim of achieving a greener and safer chemistry approach compared to methanol or other organic solvents, and developing a low-cost recovery strategy of these by-products. The aqueous decoction of pomegranate peels represents the simplest and cheapest strategy to rapidly obtain extracts, and has widely been used as a folk remedy in traditional medicine. In fact, due to its high concentration of tannins, which gives the peel a strong astringency, the peel decoction has been used to treat dysentery and other gastro-intestinal disorders [45]. Moreover, another advantage of decoction is that, being an extemporaneous preparation, there is no need to stabilize the extract. This is particularly relevant in the case of the extract obtained with ultrasound, since the stability over time of aqueous extracts is very limited.

Ultrasound-assisted extraction (UAE) is a green and energy-saving technology which is being increasingly employed in the extraction of natural products as a simple and efficient alternative to conventional extraction techniques. Substantial shortening of extraction time, reduction of reagent consumption, increase of extraction yield, and faster kinetics are the most important advantages of

UAE [4–26]. The sonication used in pulsed mode (PUAE) drastically reduces the operating temperature, allowing the extraction of thermolabile compounds. The superiority of PUAE to produce antioxidants from pomegranate peels has been previously demonstrated [46]. Longer times of extraction have not been tested in the present paper in order to minimize the potential degradation of the aqueous extracts. In fact, during the sonication process of vegetal material in water, a small amount of active oxidizing species (i.e., HO· and hydrogen atoms) are generated, and this process is time-dependent [47]. Although these aqueous extracts may require a further formulation step for preservation over time [48], we did not tackle this point, since our priority was to emphasize whether or not they deserve further formulative investigations.

4. Conclusions

The results of this research highlighted that water, as an extraction solvent, was able to extract, in a limited extraction time (10 min), significant amounts of bioactive compounds, particularly ETs, from pomegranate peels of the commercial cultivars most widespread in Italy: Akko and Wonderful. This is of great importance considering the need for 'greener' and safer extractions of natural compounds.

Compared to PUAE, traditional decoction has the advantages of being easily and extemporaneously obtainable and leads to extracts endowed with higher values of EA, TPC, RSA, and TAC for both the cultivars investigated. Nevertheless, PUAE has the advantage of yielding extracts endowed with a higher content of ETs, whose content is directly correlated with enzymatic activity.

Based on the results obtained, both of the 'green' extraction strategies proposed proved to be promising methods to produce low-cost anti-tyrosinase ingredients. EA is already approved as a lightening/whitening agent in cosmetic formulations; however, considering these results, the cheaper natural extract rich in ETs could represent a potential new cosmetic ingredient. Stabilization to preserve the polyphenolic compounds over time and formulation of a hydrophilic gel containing the pomegranate peel extract, as well as the tests necessary to evaluate their in vivo lightening properties, are currently under study.

These findings represent an important aim for pomegranate juice manufacturers, since peels are the major form of processing waste, and their disposal is expensive and not eco-friendly.

Author Contributions: Conceptualization, R.B. and P.Z.; methodology, R.B., F.T., P.G., P.M.; software, F.T., R.B., P.G.; investigation, F.T., P.M., S.C.; writing—original draft preparation, R.B., F.T.; writing—review and editing, R.B., P.G.; supervision, R.B., P.Z., P.G. All authors have read and agreed to the published version of the manuscript.

Acknowledgments: The authors are grateful to LOME SuperFruit for providing the pomegranate samples.

References

1. Chandra, R.; Babu, D.K.; Jadhav, V.T.; Teixeira da Silva, J.A. Origin, history and domestication of pomegranate. *Fruit Veg. Cereal Sci. Biotechnol.* **2010**, *4*, 1–6.
2. Zarfeshany, A.; Asgary, S.; Javanmard, S. Potent health effects of pomegranate. *Adv. Biomed. Res.* **2014**, *3*, 100. [CrossRef] [PubMed]
3. Teixeira da Silva, J.A.; Rana, T.S.; Narzary, D.; Verma, N.; Meshram, D.T.; Ranade, S.A. Pomegranate biology and biotechnology: A review. *Sci. Hortic.* **2013**, *160*, 85–107. [CrossRef]
4. Turrini, F.; Zunin, P.; Catena, S.; Villa, C.; Alfei, S.; Boggia, R. Traditional or hydro-diffusion and gravity microwave coupled with ultrasound as green technologies for the valorization of pomegranate external peels. *Food Bioprod. Process.* **2019**, *117*, 30–37. [CrossRef]
5. Bar-Ya'akov, I.; Tian, L.; Amir, R.; Holland, D. Primary Metabolites, Anthocyanins, and Hydrolyzable Tannins in the Pomegranate Fruit. *Front. Plant Sci.* **2019**, *10*, 620. [CrossRef]

6. Akhtar, S.; Ismail, T.; Fraternale, D.; Sestili, P. Pomegranate peel and peel extracts: Chemistry and food features. *Food Chem.* **2015**, *174*, 417–425. [CrossRef]
7. Šavikin, K.; Živković, J.; Alimpić, A.; Zdunić, G.; Janković, T.; Duletić-Laušević, S.; Menković, N. Activity guided fractionation of pomegranate extract and its antioxidant, antidiabetic and antineurodegenerative properties. *Ind. Crop. Prod.* **2018**, *113*, 142–149. [CrossRef]
8. Alfei, S.; Turrini, F.; Catena, S.; Zunin, P.; Grilli, M.; Pittaluga, A.; Boggia, R. Ellagic Acid a multi-target bioactive compound for drug discovery in CNS? A narrative review. *Eur. J. Med. Chem.* **2019**, *183*, 111724. [CrossRef]
9. Tomás-Barberán, F.A.; González-Sarrías, A.; García-Villalba, R.; Núñez-Sánchez, M.A.; Selma, M.V.; García-Conesa, M.T.; Espín, J.C. Urolithins, the rescue of "old" metabolites to understand a "new" concept: Metabotypes as a nexus among phenolic metabolism, microbiota dysbiosis, and host health status. *Mol. Nutr. Food Res.* **2017**, *61*, 1500901. [CrossRef]
10. Fawole, O.A.; Makunga, N.P.; Opara, U.L. Antibacterial, antioxidant and tyrosinase-inhibition activities of pomegranate fruit peel methanolic extract. *BMC Complement. Altern. Med.* **2012**, *12*, 200. [CrossRef]
11. Mphahlele, R.R.; Fawole, O.A.; Makunga, N.P.; Opara, U.L. Effect of drying on the bioactive compounds, antioxidant, antibacterial and antityrosinase activities of pomegranate peel. *BMC Complement. Altern. Med.* **2016**, *16*, 143. [CrossRef] [PubMed]
12. Zolghadri, S.; Bahrami, A.; Hassan Khan, M.T.; Munoz-Munoz, J.; Garcia-Molina, F.; Garcia-Canovas, F.; Saboury, A.A. A comprehensive review on tyrosinase inhibitors. *J. Enzym. Inhib. Med. Chem.* **2019**, *34*, 279–309. [CrossRef] [PubMed]
13. Jablonski, N.G.; Chaplin, G. The colours of humanity: The evolution of pigmentation in the human lineage. *Philos. Trans. R. Soc. B Biol. Sci.* **2017**, *372*, 20160349. [CrossRef] [PubMed]
14. Ito, S.; Wakamatsu, K. Chemistry of melanins. In *The Pigmentary System. Physiology and Pathophysiology*, 2nd ed.; Nordlund, J.J., Boissy, R.E., Hearing, V.J., King, R.A., Ortonne, J.P., Eds.; Blackwell Publishing: Oxford, UK, 2006; pp. 282–310.
15. Lee, S.J.; Hann, S.K.; Im, S. Mixed Epidermal and Dermal Hypermelanoses and Hyperchromias. In *The Pigmentary System. Physiology and Pathophysiology*, 2nd ed.; Nordlund, J.J., Boissy, R.E., Hearing, V.J., King, R.A., Ortonne, J.P., Eds.; Blackwell Publishing: Oxford, UK, 2006; pp. 1020–1025.
16. Won, Y.K.; Loy, C.J.; Randhawa, M.; Southall, M.D. Clinical efficacy and safety of 4-hexyl-1,3-phenylenediol for improving skin hyperpigmentation. *Arch. Dermatol. Res.* **2014**, *306*, 455–465. [CrossRef] [PubMed]
17. Solano, F. On the Metal Cofactor in the Tyrosinase Family. *Int. J. Mol. Sci.* **2018**, *19*, 633. [CrossRef]
18. Mason, H.S.; Fowlks, W.L.; Peterson, E. Oxygen transfer and electron transport by the phenolase complex. *J. Am. Chem. Soc.* **1955**, *107*, 4015–4027. [CrossRef]
19. Cosmetic Ingredient Database. Available online: https://ec.europa.eu/growth/toolsdatabases/cosing/index.cfm?fuseaction=search.details_v2&id=56131 (accessed on 22 January 2020).
20. Special Chem INCI Database Directory (International Nomenclature of Cosmetic Ingredients Database). Available online: https://cosmetics.specialchem.com/searchsites/searchproducts?q=ellagic%20 (accessed on 22 January 2020).
21. Shimogaki, H.; Tanaka, Y.; Tamai, H.; Masuda, M. In vitro and in vivo evaluation of ellagic acid on melanogenesis inhibition. *Int. J. Cosmet. Sci.* **2000**, *22*, 291–303. [CrossRef]
22. Özer, Ö.; Mutlu, B.; Kıvçak, B. Antityrosinase Activity of Some Plant Extracts and Formulations Containing Ellagic Acid. *Pharm. Biol.* **2007**, *45*, 519–524. [CrossRef]
23. Turrini, F.; Boggia, R.; Donno, D.; Parodi, B.; Beccaro, G.; Baldassari, S.; Signorello, M.G.; Catena, S.; Alfei, S.; Zunin, P. From pomegranate marcs to a potential bioactive ingredient: A recycling proposal for pomegranate squeezed-marcs. *Eur. Food Res. Technol.* **2020**, *246*, 273–285. [CrossRef]
24. Rajha, H.N.; Abi-Khattar, A.M.; El Kantar, S.; Boussetta, N.; Lebovka, N.; Maroun, R.G.; Louka, N.; Vorobien, E. Comparison of aqueous extraction efficiency and biological activities of polyphenols from pomegranate peels assisted by infrared, ultrasound, pulsed electric fields and high-voltage electrical discharges. *Innov. Food Sci. Emerg.* **2019**, *58*, 102212. [CrossRef]
25. Panda, D.; Manickam, S. Cavitation Technology—The Future of Greener Extraction Method: A Review on the Extraction of Natural Products and Process Intensification Mechanism and Perspectives. *Appl. Sci.* **2019**, *9*, 766. [CrossRef]

26. Chemat, F.; Rombaut, N.; Sicaire, A.G.; Meullemiestre, A.; Fabiano-Tixier, A.S.; Abert-Vian, M. Ultrasound assisted extraction of food and natural products. Mechanisms, techniques, combinations, protocols and applications. A review. *Ultrason. Sonochem.* **2017**, *34*, 540–560. [CrossRef] [PubMed]
27. Passafiume, R.; Perrone, A.; Sortino, G.; Gianguzzi, G.; Saletta, F.; Gentile, C.; Farina, V. Chemical–Physical characteristics, polyphenolic content and total antioxidant activity of three Italian-grown pomegranate cultivars. *NFS J.* **2019**, *16*, 9–14. [CrossRef]
28. Singleton, V.L.; Rossi, J.A., Jr. Colorimetry of total phenolics with phosphomolybdic-phosphotungstic acid reagents. *Am. J. Enol. Viticult.* **1965**, *16*, 144–158.
29. Brand-Williams, W.; Cuvelier, M.E.; Berset, C. Use of a free radical method to evaluate antioxidant activity. *LWT Food Sci. Technol.* **1995**, *28*, 25–30. [CrossRef]
30. Huerga-González, V.; Lage-Yusty, M.A.; Lago-Crespo, M.; López-Hernández, J. Comparison of methods for the study of ellagic acid in pomegranate juice beverages. *Food Anal. Method* **2005**, *8*, 2286–2293. [CrossRef]
31. Turrini, F.; Boggia, R.; Leardi, R.; Borriello, M.; Zunin, P. Optimization of the Ultrasonic-Assisted Extraction of Phenolic Compounds from Oryza Sativa, L. 'Violet Nori' and Determination of the Antioxidant Properties of its Caryopses and Leaves. *Molecules* **2018**, *23*, 844. [CrossRef]
32. Barnes, R.J.; Dhanoa, M.S.; Lister, S.J. Standard normal variate transformation and de-trending of near-infrared diffuse reflectance spectra. *Appl. Spectrosc.* **1989**, *43*, 772–777. [CrossRef]
33. Italian Chemical Society. Division of Analytical Chemistry-Group of Chemometrics. CAT Chemometric Agile Tool. Available online: http://www.gruppochemiometria.it/index.php/software (accessed on 10 January 2020).
34. Višnjevec, A.M.; Ota, A.; Skrt, M.; Butinar, B.; Možina, S.S.; Cimerman, N.G.; Nečemer, M.; Arbeiter, A.B.; Hladnik, M.; Krapac, M.; et al. Genetic, Biochemical, Nutritional and Antimicrobial Characteristics of Pomegranate (Punica granatum L.) Grown in Istria. *Food Technol. Biotechnol.* **2017**, *55*, 151–163. [CrossRef]
35. Fawole, A.M.; Opara, U.L. Developmental changes in maturity indices of pomegranate fruit: A descriptive review. *Sci. Hortic.* **2013**, *159*, 152–161. [CrossRef]
36. Sójka, M.; Janowski, M.; Grzelak-Błaszczyk, K. Stability and transformations of raspberry (Rubus idaeus L.) ellagitannins in aqueous solutions. *Eur. Food Res. Technol.* **2019**, *245*, 1113–1122. [CrossRef]
37. Živković, J.; Šavikin, K.; Janković, T.; Ćujić, N.; Menković, N. Optimization of ultrasound-assisted extraction of polyphenolic compounds from pomegranate peel using response surface methodology. *Sep. Purif. Technol.* **2018**, *194*, 40–47. [CrossRef]
38. Zhao, X.; Yuan, Z.; Fang, Y.; Yin, Y.; Feng, L. Characterization and evaluation of major anthocyanins in pomegranate (Punica granatum L.) peel of different cultivars and their development phases. *Eur. Food Res. Technol.* **2013**, *236*, 109–117. [CrossRef]
39. Fischer, U.A.; Carle, R.; Kammerer, D.R. Identification and quantification of phenolic compounds from pomegranate (Punica granatum L.) peel, mesocarp, aril and differently produced juices by HPLC-DAD-ESI/MSn. *Food Chem.* **2011**, *127*, 807–821. [CrossRef] [PubMed]
40. Zhu, F.; Yuan, Z.; Zhao, X.; Yin, Y.; Feng, L. Composition and contents of anthocyanins in different pomegranate cultivars. *Acta Hortic.* **2015**, *1089*, 35–42. [CrossRef]
41. El-Said, M.M.; Haggag, H.F.; Fakhr El-Din, H.M.; Gad, A.S.; Farahat, A.M. Antioxidant Activities and Physical Properties of Stirred Yoghurt Fortified with Pomegranate Peel Extracts. *Ann. Agric. Sci.* **2014**, *59*, 207–212. [CrossRef]
42. Kaderides, K.; Papaoikonomou, L.; Serafim, M.; Goula, A.M. Microwave-assisted extraction of phenolics from pomegranate peels: Optimization, kinetics, and comparison with ultrasounds extraction. *Chem. Eng. Process. Process Intensif.* **2019**, *137*, 1–11. [CrossRef]
43. Çam, M.; Hışıl, Y. Pressurised water extraction of polyphenols from pomegranate peels. *Food Chem.* **2010**, *123*, 878–885. [CrossRef]
44. Kaderides, K.; Goula, A.M.; Adamopoulos, K.G. A process for turning pomegranate peels into a valuable food ingredient using ultrasound-assisted extraction and encapsulation. *Innov. Food Sci. Emerg.* **2015**, *31*, 204–215. [CrossRef]
45. Bhowmik, D.; Gopinath, H.; Kumar, B.P.; Duraivel, S.; Aravind, G.; Kumar, K.P.S. Medicinal Uses of Punica granatum and Its Health Benefits. *J. Pharmacog. Phytochem.* **2013**, *1*, 28–35.

46. Pan, Z.; Qu, W.; Ma, H.; Atungulu, G.G.; McHugh, T.H. Continuous and pulsed ultrasound-assisted extractions of antioxidants from pomegranate peel. *Ultrason. Sonochem.* **2011**, *18*, 1249–1257. [CrossRef] [PubMed]
47. Vinatoru, M.; Mason, T.J.; Calinescu, I. Ultrasonically assisted extraction (UAE) and microwave assisted extraction (MAE) of functional compounds from plant materials. *Trend Anal. Chem.* **2017**, *97*, 159–178. [CrossRef]
48. Panichayupakaranant, P.; Itsuriya, A.; Sirikatitham, A. Preparation method and stability of ellagic acid-rich pomegranate fruit peel extract. *Pharm. Biol.* **2010**, *48*, 201–205. [CrossRef] [PubMed]

14

Cucurbita Plants: From Farm to Industry

Bahare Salehi [1], Javad Sharifi-Rad [2,*], Esra Capanoglu [3], Nabil Adrar [3,4], Gizem Catalkaya [3], Shabnum Shaheen [5], Mehwish Jaffer [5], Lalit Giri [6], Renu Suyal [6], Arun K Jugran [7], Daniela Calina [8], Anca Oana Docea [9], Senem Kamiloglu [10], Dorota Kregiel [11], Hubert Antolak [12], Ewelina Pawlikowska [11], Surjit Sen [12,13], Krishnendu Acharya [12], Moein Bashiry [14], Zeliha Selamoglu [15], Miquel Martorell [16,17,*], Farukh Sharopov [18], Natália Martins [19,20,*], Jacek Namiesnik [21,*] and William C. Cho [22,*]

1 Student Research Committee, School of Medicine, Bam University of Medical Sciences, Bam 44340847, Iran
2 Zabol Medicinal Plants Research Center, Zabol University of Medical Sciences, Zabol 61615-585, Iran
3 Istanbul Technical University, Faculty of Chemical & Metallurgical Engineering, Food Engineering Department, Maslak 34469, Istanbul, Turkey
4 Laboratoire de Biotechnologie Végétale et d'Ethnobotanique, Faculté des Sciences de la Nature et de la Vie, Université de Bejaia, Bejaia 06000, Algérie
5 Department of Plant Sciences, LCWU, Lahore 54000, Pakistan
6 G.B. Pant National Institute of Himalayan Environment & Sustainable Development Kosi-Katarmal, Almora 263 643, Uttarakhand, India
7 G.B. Pant National Institute of Himalayan Environment & Sustainable Development Garhwal Regional Centre, Srinagar 246174, Uttarakhand, India
8 Department of Clinical Pharmacy, University of Medicine and Pharmacy of Craiova, 200349 Craiova, Romania
9 Department of Toxicology, University of Medicine and Pharmacy of Craiova, 200349 Craiova, Romania
10 Mevsim Gida Sanayi ve Soguk Depo Ticaret A.S. (MVSM Foods), Turankoy, Kestel, Bursa 16540, Turkey
11 Institute of Fermentation Technology and Microbiology, Lodz University of Technology, Wolczanska 171/173, 90-924 Lodz, Poland
12 Molecular and Applied Mycology and Plant Pathology Laboratory, Department of Botany, University of Calcutta, Kolkata 700019, India
13 Department of Botany, Fakir Chand College, Diamond Harbour, West Bengal 743331, India
14 Department of Food Science and Technology, Nutrition and Food Sciences Faculty, Kermanshah University of Medical Sciences, Kermanshah 6719851351, Iran
15 Department of Medical Biology, Faculty of Medicine, Nigde Ömer Halisdemir University, Campus, Nigde 51240, Turkey
16 Department of Nutrition and Dietetics, Faculty of Pharmacy, University of Concepcion, Concepcion 4070386, Chile
17 Universidad de Concepción, Unidad de Desarrollo Tecnológico, UDT, Concepcion 4070386, Chile
18 Department of Pharmaceutical Technology, Avicenna Tajik State Medical University, Rudaki 139, 734003 Dushanbe, Tajikistan
19 Faculty of Medicine, University of Porto, Alameda Prof. Hernâni Monteiro, 4200-319 Porto, Portugal
20 Institute for Research and Innovation in Health (i3S), University of Porto, 4200-135 Porto, Portugal
21 Department of Analytical Chemistry, Faculty of Chemistry, Gdańsk University of Technology, 80-233 Gdańsk, Poland
22 Department of Clinical Oncology, Queen Elizabeth Hospital, Hong Kong, China
* Correspondence: javad.sharifirad@gmail.com (J.S.-R.); martorellpons@gmail.com (M.M.); ncmartins@med.up.pt (N.M.); chemanal@pg.edu.pl (J.N.); chocs@ha.org.hk (W.C.C.)

Abstract: The *Cucurbita* genus, a member of Cucurbitaceae family, also known as cucurbits, is native to the Americas. Genus members, like *Cucurbita pepo* and *Cucurbita maxima*, have been used for centuries in folk medicine for treating gastrointestinal diseases and intestinal parasites. These pharmacological effects are mainly attributed to their phytochemical composition. Indeed, *Cucurbita* species are a natural source of carotenoids, tocopherols, phenols, terpenoids, saponins, sterols, fatty acids, functional carbohydrates, and polysaccharides, that beyond exerting remarkable biological effects, have also been increasingly exploited for biotechnological applications. In this article, we specifically cover the habitat, cultivation, phytochemical composition, and food preservative abilities of *Cucurbita* plants.

Keywords: *Cucurbita* plants; cucurbits; pumpkin; phytochemical composition; food industry

---

1. Introduction

Natural products are a rich source of chemical diversity that has boosted pharmaceutical industry over the centuries [1,2]. Plants and herbs have been applied in both prevention and treatment of human disorders since ancient times [3–5]. Indeed, many investigations on herbs and plants have been conducted, and their efficacy proved as a compelling source of antioxidant, antimicrobial, anti-inflammatory [6], anticancer and neuroprotective agents [7,8].

The Cucurbitaceae (pumpkin) family contains many species as human foods. This family frames a huge gathering with roughly 130 genera and 800 species. Cucurbitaceae plants are commonly known as cucurbits, extensively cultivated in tropical and subtropical countries. Cucurbit species include pumpkins, squashes, gourds and melons [9]. In addition, it is an economically important family with a rootage of various valuable products, such as edible vegetables, fruits, seed, seed oils, and drugs. Indeed, they include a large variety of vegetables, often used through various forms for cooking, pickling, salad, dessert fruits, candied, confectionary, etc. In addition, *Cucurbita* products have a high nutritional value, being also an important source of vitamins, and widely used in culinary for biscuits, bread, desserts, soup and beverages production [10–12].

Overall, this article aims to provide an update on the *Cucurbita* plants sources, as well as historical culinary usage, habitat and cultivation, phytochemical composition and industrial purposes.

2. *Cucurbita* Plants: An Historical Culinary Usage

Cucurbita plants were first explained by Linnaeus in the middle of the eighteen century and are among the earliest known plants that have been grown by mankind. Primarily, they are classified by their shape or harvest season (summer or winter), although there are both female and male types. The male flowers produce pollen and the female ones produce the fruit. *Cucurbita* species have bristly and prickly stems and leaves. Broadly, leaves are large, occasionally lobed or spotted, and spiraled clinging tendrils are frequently given at the leaf axils. Both leaves and stems can be rough or prickly. Yellow or orange trumpet shaped flowers develop into variously shaped, sized, marked, and colored fruits [13]. However, these plants are also cultivated for their edible and ornamental fruit, also having therapeutic and wholesome advantages. The juvenile natural products are often expended as a vegetable, but some assortments of natural products are used with beautiful purposes in the Halloween party. They can be consumed as raw or cooked, and also for animal feed, but due to their high nutraceutical value, *Cucurbita* plants have been widely used in many countries as constituents of many commercial products. For instance, in Indian cuisine, squashes (ghia) are traditionally cooked with seafood, such as prawns. French people use marrows (courges) as a gratin. In Italy, many of regional dishes are prepared from squashes. Japanese people use *Cucurbita moschata* Duchesne pumpkins (kabocha) for preparation of different Japanese foods. *C. moschata* fruits can be round, oblate, oval, oblong, or pear-shaped, variously ribbed, 15–60 cm in diameter, and weigh up to 45 kg. In African countries soup is prepared from squash, and soft alcoholic drinks are made from *Cucurbita ficifolia* Bouché. *C. ficifolia* fruits are oblong with a diameter of 20 cm, weighs 5 kg to 6 kg, and its skin can vary from light or dark green to cream-colored.

Specifically, the commercially produced pumpkin is mainly used for production of pumpkin pie, bread, biscuits, cheesecake, desserts, donuts, granola, ice cream, lasagna dishes, pancakes, pudding, pumpkin butter, salads, soups, and stuffing. The seeds, wealthy in oil, likewise are used in Mexico, with nectar to make pastries, known as palanquetas. Blossom buds and blooms are used in Mexico to cook quesadillas. Indeed, *Cucurbita* products contain carbohydrates, protein and are also rich in vitamin C, pyridoxin (B6) and riboflavin (B2). The content of fat is negligible. Fruit and root of *Cucurbita foetidissima* Kunth is also rich in saponin, which can be used as soap, shampoo and bleach [10–12,14].

3. Habitat and Cultivation of *Cucurbita* Plants

3.1. Habitat

The *Cucurbita* genus is native to the Americas. Archaeological observations have explained that, for more than 8000 years, *Cucurbita* domestication has moved from the southern parts of Canada to Argentina and Chile [10–12,14]. Five species of the genus, namely *Cucurbita argyrosperma* C.Huber, *C. ficifolia*, *C. moschata*, *Cucurbita maxima* Duchesne, and *Cucurbita pepo* L. were habituated and cultivated in several areas of North and South America [15–17]. *C. pepo* is considered as one of the most seasoned and developed varieties, by Mexican archeological evidence of 7000 BC. Along these lines, it was extensively developed through aboriginal people through Central, North America and Mexico, earlier the landing of Europeans. *C. pepo* is local to Northern Mexico and Southwestern and eastern USA [18]. *C. pepo* fruits can be oval, cylindrical, flattened, globular, scalloped, fusiform, and/or tapering to a curved or straight neck on one or both ends. They can be up to 5 times longer than wide and their weight varies from 30 g to 50 kg. The skin can be smooth, warty, wrinkled, furrowed, or/and have shallow to deep longitudinal ridges. Often there is more than one color to the soft to hard skin: white, yellow, light to dark green, nearly black, cream, and/or orange. Subsequently, *Cucurbita* species were cultivated in all tropical, subtropical and temperate regions of the planet and are now considered as one of the valuable foods for most of the world's inhabitants [12,19].

Cucurbita species also show diverse habitat use, growing in terrestrial and wetland environments, as monoecious climbers or annuals; they may be found in meadows, fields, and on the shores of rivers or lakes [20].

3.2. Cultivation

3.2.1. Climate

In general, *Cucurbita* species prefer warm weather. Temperatures of 18–27 °C are ideal for maximum crop production. So, a long warm season is important to obtain a quality production. For seed germination, soil temperatures above 16 °C are essential and it takes about 14 days for the crop to leaves at this temperature, and it was also reported that when soil temperature rises to 20 °C seed emerge within a week [21]. *Cucurbita* species requires a continuous water supply, but overwatering also lead to crop spoiling. Uniform moisture supply is, therefore, important during the growing season of the crop. *C. argyrosperma* is generally cultivated in regions with little arid climate with proper watering or in regions with a distinct rainy season [22]. *C. ficifolia* grows in specific environmental parameters, such as not in a high frost condition, but it prefers heavy rain agricultural systems [23]. *C. maxima* are mainly grown in regions with temperate climate, and exceptionally grown in warm and moist area [24]. The shape of *C. maxima* fruit can be an elongated cylinder, oval, flattened, globular, heart-shaped, and/or tapering to a curved neck on one or both ends. The length (from 5.8 cm to 71.6 cm), width (from 11.2 cm to 48.6 cm) and weight (usually ranging from 0.3 kg to 50 kg, some pumpkins can grow over 90 kg) is very variable. The skin can be smooth, warty, wrinkled, or/and have shallow to deep longitudinal ridges. Often there is more than one color on the soft to hard skin: red, white, gray, black, green, cream, and/or orange. *C. moschata* is reported mainly from regions with low altitude, hot climate and high humidity [25,26]. *C. pepo* can adapt to different ecological conditions, but prefers low altitude and warm/humid places [27].

3.2.2. Soil

Cucurbita spp. can be grown in a wide range of soil varieties, but favors well-drained fertile ground [22]. A well-drained soil is preferred, and the crop roots can penetrate up to a meter deep into the soil. The ideal soil pH is in the range of 6.0 to 6.5, but the crop can withstand both slightly acidic and alkaline soils. In areas with low soil pH, the application of lime or dolomite is essential to allow better uptake of nutrients. Well-drained loamy fertile soils or sandy loam soils are good for commercial cultivation. However, heavier soils (clay) can also be used as long as drainage is adequate.

3.2.3. Propagation and Planting Method

Cultivated *Cucurbita* spp. are usually propagated by planting seeds in the ground. Sometimes, seeds are germinated in small pots and seedlings are transplanted to the field when climatic and edaphic factors are favorable [22]. Transplant seedling are often used to establish an early season crop or when using permanent beds [21]. It has been reported that *Cucurbita* species that are developed from transplanted seedling have luxuriant growth, larger fruit size and significantly higher seed yield compared to direct sowing method [28,29]. Commercially cultivated varieties are sometimes grown with traditional crops, like maize, beans or even in vegetable gardens along with other species. Plant density affects fruit size, yield and its number per plant. Napier [21] reported that in *C. maxima* and *C. moschata* higher plant densities resulted in smaller fruit size, higher total yield and fewer fruit per plant.

3.2.4. Irrigation

The first irrigation is important just after planting, and subsequent irrigation is given at a weekly basis or depending upon growth of the plant and soil condition. Waterlogging should be avoided throughout the cultivation process. However, in the absence of rain, the crop should be regularly watered. Irrigation is vital during flowering, fruit set and fruit fill, but should be minimized at the time of fruit maturity. Various types of irrigation methods are practiced in *Cucurbita* species cultivation, such as furrow, drip and overhead irrigation. Furrow irrigation needs the type of soil which passes water to reach laterally, without penetrating very deep into the soil, and drip irrigation is practiced in permanent bed systems which help to minimize weeds in the field [21].

3.2.5. Fertilizer

Proper fertilizer application is essential for *Cucurbita* species cultivation, but the excessive use of nitrogen fertilizer, early in the growing period, results in huge foliage growth, delayed fruit set and lower crop yield [21,30–32]. For *C. maxima* production, mineral fertilizers are used, which consists of NPK-nitrogen (N), phosphorous (P) and potassium (K)-applied either manually or with sub-soiled in a row. A nitrogen side-dressing in the form of urea, is also applied about two weeks after crop emergence [33]. In case of *C. maxima*, the recommended amounts of fertilizers are about 150 kg nitrogen/ha, 95 kg phosphorus/ha, 80 kg potassium/ha and 10 kg gypsum/ha [33]. Bannayan et al. [34] reported that, in *C. pepo*, the optimum nitrogen rate not only can increase crop growth, but can also boost up its resistance to higher temperatures.

3.2.6. Pest and Disease Management

Cucurbita species are very prone to pests and diseases, and some pathogens attack this economically important crop. Thus, it is important to protect them to obtain a good quality and high commercial yield *Cucurbita*. Several notorious fungal pathogens are associated with *Cucurbita* species, e.g., *Cladosporium cucumerinum* which causes a scab or gummosis [35], while *Choanephora cucurbitarum* causes fruit rot of *C. pepo* [36]. This disease, also known as "wet rot" and "blossom end rot", can spoil many blossoms and fruit during prolonged damp weather. *Pseudoperonospora cubensis* is an unusual organism of downy mildew *Cucurbita* species, mainly cucumbers, melons, squashes, gourds and watermelons [37]. *Phytophthora capsici* causes blight and mostly infect the seedlings, vines, leaves, and fruits of *Cucurbita* plants [38]. Cucurbits powdery mildew, caused by *Erysiphe cichoracearum*, is the most critical disease of cultivated *Cucurbita* spp. [39,40]. *Fusarium oxysporum* is a soil borne fungal pathogen that causes a damping off and wilt disorder [41]. Powdery mildew is caused by *Sphaerotheca fuliginea*, which forms pads of whitish mycelium on upper and under leaf sides, petioles, and stems [42]. Important bacterial diseases of *Cucurbita* species are across leaf spot evoked by *Pseudomonas syringae* pv. *Lachrymans* [43,44]. Bacterial wilt occurs in *Cucurbita* species infected with *Erwinia tracheiphila*. This pathogenic bacterium is imparted with striped (*Acalymma vittatum*) and spotted (*Diabrotica undecimpunctata*) cucumber beetles [45]. Several viral variants have also been identified, causing many problems to the crops due to the rate of disease expansion, asperity of infection and difficulty in controlling the diseases. The most important viral variants are *clover yellow vein virus* (CYVV), *papaya ringspot virus Type W* (PRSV), *squash mosaic virus* (SqMV), *tobacco tingspot virus* (TRSV), *tomato ringspot virus* (ToRSV), *watermelon mosaic virus* (WMV), and *zucchini yellow mosaic virus* (ZYMV) [22,46,47]. Many insects invade *Cucurbita* species, e.g., aphid species (*Myzus persicae* and *Aphis gossypii*) and beetle species (*A. vittatum* and *D. undecimpunctata*), which causes significant crop losses. Proper crop rotation is the best way to minimize pests and diseases. Thus, the application of appropriate fungicide, like copper oxychloride, bravo, cupravit, dithane, and dichlorophen, at specific doses can control fungal pathogens of *Cucurbita* species. However, the control of viral diseases is difficult. The breeding of disease resistant varieties by the hybridization technique or the application of innovative methods to promote resistant varieties is an additional way to control viral diseases. *C. pepo* cultivar contains unique transgenic forms that show resistance to viruses like WMV and ZYMV [22].

4. *Cucurbita* Plants Phytochemical Composition

Twenty-eight *Cucurbita* species are named in the literature [48,49], but some of them could just be hybrids or synonyms [49]. The relative lack of studies on some *Cucurbita* species may be linked to their rarity and endemic aspect, as is the case of *Cucurbita okeechobeensis* (Small) L.H.Bailey [50], also considered as an endangered species that must be protected [50,51]. The potential toxicity of the wild species may also be a limiting factor [52].

Edible kinds of pumpkins and squashes, like *C. ficifolia, C. maxima, C. moschata* and *C. pepo* can be a natural source of some bioactive components. Indeed, these species are rich in tocopherols and carotenoids, especially the seeds and the fruit peel, respectively [53]. Generally, it is complicated to make a straight qualitative or quantitative distinction between the species, because of the high variability within a single species depending either on their subsequent varieties or environmental effects and ripening stage. This aspect is also true for other phytochemicals. Depending on the edible part, *Cucurbita* species are found to be very rich in compounds with nutritious value, especially carbohydrates, proteins, minerals (Table 1), fatty acids (Table 2) and amino acids [53].

Table 1. Proximate composition of some common *Cucurbita* spp. *.

Percentage (%)	*Cucurbita moschata*			*Cucurbita pepo*			*Cucurbita maxima*			References
	Flesh	Peel	Seed	Flesh	Peel	Seed	Flesh	Peel	Seed	
Carbohydrate	4.34	9.63	14.02	2.62–48.40	4.37–19.45	6.37–37.9	13.35	20.68	12.90–24.45	[53–62]
Protein	0.30–1.89	1.13–4.45	29.81	0.20–15.50	0.92–23.95	27.48–38.0	1.13	1.65	14.31–27.48	
Lipid/Oil	0.04–0.13	0.31–0.66	28.7–45.67	0.055–0.18	0.47–6.57	21.9–54.9	0.42	0.87	30.7–52.43	
Fiber	0.74–1.24	0.13–33.92	10.85	0.37–11.25	1.23–29.62	1.00–14.84	1.09	2.23	2.55–16.15	
Ash	0.70–1.09	1.13–1.39	5.31	0.34–06.64	0.63–10.65	3.0–5.50	1.05	1.12	3.60–4.42	
Moisture	89.61–94.23	80.04–88.47	5.18	18.03–96.77	9.76–93.59	1.80–7.40	84.04	75.67	2.75–3.08	
Minerals (µg/g)										
Macroelements										[54–57,61, 63]
K	30,170.31–49,416.70	17,860.27–30,765.8	NQ	160		2372.4	NQ	NQ	358.67	
P	2046.99–3553.36	6065.97–11,312.84	NQ	11.38		476.8	NQ	NQ	2241.45	
Ca	3113.37–9854.33	4350.13–6865.78	NQ	3662.0	5571.0	97.8–420.5	NQ	NQ	294.74	
Mg	1214.01–1615.07	2518.87–4927.18	NQ	190		674.1	NQ	NQ	348.71	
Microelements										
Na	532.11–785.91	616.67–772.32	NQ	159		1703.5	NQ	NQ	296.90	
Fe	29.69–33.48	53.18–84.09	NQ	91.33		247.30	37.5–149.64	NQ	NQ	
Zn	18.65–26.92	18.82–49.01	NQ	320.50	42.92	89.29–141.4	NQ	NQ	39.85	
Cu	7.40–10.42	2.78–8.15	NQ	16.25	12.91	24.49	NQ	NQ	ND	
Se	NQ	NQ	NQ	0.0140	0.0127	12.40	NQ	NQ	NQ	
Co	NQ	NQ	NQ	NQ	NQ	21.7	NQ	NQ	ND	
Mn	0.51–6.90	2.35–14.8	NQ	0.5		0.6	NQ	NQ	17.93	
Ni	NQ	NQ	NQ	0.5		NQ	NQ	NQ	NQ	
Pb	NQ	NQ	NQ	0.29		NQ	NQ	NQ	NQ	
Nitrate	NQ	NQ	NQ	NQ	NQ	22.7	NQ	NQ	NQ	

* Results expressed in dry basis; ND: Not detected; NQ: Not quantified.

Table 2. Seed fatty acid composition of some common *Cucurbita* spp. *.

Fatty acid (%)	*Cucurbita moschata*	*Cucurbita pepo*	*Cucurbita maxima*	References
Myristic acid (C14:0)	ND	0.1–0.23	0.16	
Palmitic acid (C16:0)	12.78–20.74	9.5–14.5	10.84–15.97	
Palmitoleic (C16:1n7)	NQ	0.58	NQ	
Heptadecanoic acid (C17:0)	ND	ND	0.18	
Stearic acid (C18:0)	7.33–7.47	03.1–8.67	4.68–11.2	
Vaccenic acid (C18:1n7)	NQ	01.8	NQ	
Oleic acid (C18:1n9)	22.66–31.34	21.0–46.9	14.83–44.11	
Linoleic acid (C18:2)	35.72–48.52	0.17–60.8	34.77–56.60	
Linolenic (C18:3)	ND	ND–0.68	0.24	[53,55,58–62,64]
Arachidic acid (C20:0)	ND	0.39	0.36	
Gadoleic acid (C20:1n–9)	ND	00.1–1.14	0.07	
Arachidonic acid (C20:4)	NQ	00.5	0.41	
Behenic acid (C22:00)	ND	0.37	0.09	
Saturated	20.11	18.69–19.35	17.47–21.07	
Mono-unsaturated	31.34	32.40	14.90–44.12	
Poly-unsaturated	35.72	36.40	34.78–56.84	
Total unsaturated	67.06	7.6–80.65	71.74–78.90	

* Results expressed in dry base of seeds; ND: Not detected; NQ: Not quantified.

The content of carbohydrates is highly variable within each species and edible parts, starting from 2.62% to 48.40% on dry basis. In general, the seeds and peels are richer than flesh, and *C. maxima* and *C. pepo* were described as containing higher levels of carbohydrates when compared to *C. moschata*. The mineral contents of *Cucurbita* fit the recommended daily intake values of FAO in various essential elements. In addition, it seems to be far from the upper limits [65], when the values are converted on a fresh matter basis. Seeds contain high amount of proteins and fats, ranging from 14.3% to 38.0% and 21.9% to 54.9%, respectively. In contrast, fruit seems to have relatively low and variable levels of proteins (0.20% to 23.95%), and a very low content of lipids (0.04% to 6.57%). *Cucurbita*, especially the seed parts, can also be a good source of amino acids [53]. Indeed, among the 20 amino acids which constitute the human proteins, 17 are present in *Cucurbita*, including the 8 + 1 essential amino acids [53,55]. In addition, Fang, Li, Niu, and Tseng [66] discovered for the first time a new amino acid in *C. moschata*, named as cucurbitine.

4.1. Carotenoids and Tocopherols in Cucurbita

Carotenoids are present in high amount in the fruit of these plants and their hybrids, α- and β- carotene; ζ-carotene; neoxanthin; violaxanthin; lutein; zeaxanthin; taraxanthin; luteoxanthin; auroxanthine; neurosporene; flavoxanthin; 5,6,5′,6′-diepoxy-β-carotene; phytofluene; α-cryptoxanthin; and β-cryptoxanthin [53,67–70]. The total carotenoid content varies in range from 234.21 μg/g to 404.98 μg/g in *C. moschata* fruit [71], and 171.9 μg/g to 461.9 μg/g in *C. pepo* fruit [61]. The concentration of carotenoids is much higher (10 fold higher) in the peel of *C. moschata* than flesh [57]. Azizah et al. [72] investigated the effect of different baking procedure on β-carotene and lycopene contents of *C. moschata*. It was observed that boiling led to a 4 and 40-fold increase in β-carotene and lycopene contents, respectively. There are also several reports on carotenoid content of several *Cucurbita* plants, such as landrace pumpkins (*C. moschata*) [71], *C. moschata* and *C. pepo* [73,74], and *C. maxima* [75]. A summary of the major carotenoids found in *Cucurbita* species is given in Table 3.

Table 3. Content of major carotenoid present in the edible flesh of *Cucurbita* spp. varieties *.

Cucurbita Species	Variety	α-Carotene (mg/100 g)	β-Carotene (mg/100 g)	Lutein+ Zeaxanthin (mg/100 g)	References
Cucurbita pepo	Acorn Table	0.15	2.1	1.8	[70]
	Acorn Tay Bell	0.17	0.94	0.37	
	Tonda Padana (Americano)	0.12	2.3	1.5	
	Carneval di Venezia	0.03	0.06	ND	
	Melonette Jaspée Vende	0.05	1.3	0.43	
	Acorn Table	ND	0.36	0.09	[74]
	Table King Bush	ND	0.09	0.02	
	Thelma Sander's Sweet Potato	ND	0.06	0.01	
	Fordhook Acorn	ND	0.04	0.01	
	PI 314806	ND	ND	ND	
	Sweet Lightning	NQ	0.7	0.13	[76]
Cucurbita maxima	Uchiki Kuri	1.4	2.5	3	[70]
	Flat White Boer	7.5	6.2	7.5	
	Umber Cup	0.79	3.7	11	
	Hyvita	0.99	2.5	17	
	Buen Gusto	1	3.3	6.3	
	Gelber Zentner	ND	2.2	0.8	
	Mini Green Hubbard	0.42	1.4	5.6	
	Autumn Cup	0.8	5.2	2.7	
	Imperial Elite	1.1	7.4	7.1	
	Snow Delite	1.5	6.4	1.6	
	Walfish	0.9	4.3	3.9	
	Japan 117	1	7.2	1.8	
	Bambino	NQ	4.2	NQ	[77]
	Amazonka	NQ	13.1	NQ	
	Justynka F1	NQ	13.1	NQ	
	Karowita	NQ	4.2	NQ	
	Otylia F1	NQ	0.6	NQ	
	Bischofsmütze	NQ	0.5	0.03	[76]
	Golden Nuggets	NQ	1.9	2.6	
	Halloween	NQ	0.8	0.87	
	Hokkaido I	NQ	0.27	3.6	
	Hokkaido II	NQ	7.1	6.1	
Cucurbita moschata	Burpee Butterbush	0.98	3.1	0.08	[70]
	Long Island Cheese	5.9	7	0.14	
	Mousquée de Provence	2.8	4.9	1.1	
	Martinica	1.6	5.4	0.41	
	Butterbush	1.5	1.5	0.09	[74]
	Ponca Butternut	0.21	0.03	0.06	
	Waltham Butternut	0.3	0.38	0.12	
	Sucrine DuBerry	0.26	0.21	0.03	
	PI 458728	0.04	0.06	0.03	
	Tennessee Sweet Potato	ND	0.2	0.03	
	Muscade de Provence	1.1	0.9	NQ	[76]
	Butternuts	0.06	1.14	0.14	

* Results expressed in dry base of edible flesh part; NQ: Not quantified; ND: Not detected.

Edible *Cucurbita* seeds are also rich in vitamin E (49.49 μg/g to 92.59 μg/g); γ-tocopherol is more abundant than α-tocopherol [53,62]. The amounts of α-, β-, γ- and δ-tocopherol from the cold pressed oil extracted from six samples of pumpkin seeds (*C. pepo*) from Serbia were reported by Rabrenović et al. [78], which were in the range of 38.03 to 64.11 mg/100 g oil. *C. maxima* var. *béjaoui* seed oil was found as a rich source of tocopherols, where δ-tocopherol was the dominant tocopherol with 42% of the total [64]. However, for *C. pepo* seed oils, γ-tocopherol was stated as the remarkably abundant tocopherol (13–21%) compared to α- and δ-tocopherols [79].

4.2. *Phenolic Compounds in Cucurbita*

Table 4 presents the main phenolic compounds found in *Cucurbita* species and their structures. *C. moschata* fruit seems to have a low total phenolic content in comparison with other fruits [57]. No flavonoids were found in either the fruit nor seeds of *C. moschata* in the study of Eleiwa et al. [80]. However, Li et al. [81] have previously discovered five novel phenolic glycosides from *C. moschata* seeds, named cucurbitosides A–E. Other new phenolic glycosides were discovered later from the same source [81,82]. In another work, Li et al. [83] isolated eight different cucurbitoside compounds (F–M).

Table 4. Chemical structures of phenolic compounds found in the *Cucurbita* spp. *.

Compound Name	Synonym(s)	Empirical Formula	Structure
Protocatechuic acid	3,4-Dihydroxybenzoic acid	$C_7H_6O_4$	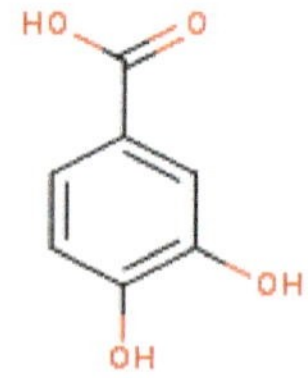
p-Hydroxybenzoic acid	4-Hydroxybenzoic acid	$C_7H_6O_3$	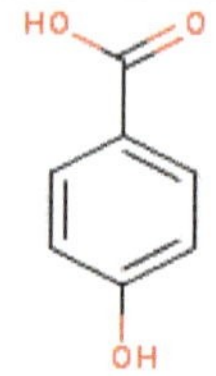
p-Hydroxybenzaldehyde	4-Hydroxybenzaldehyde	$C_7H_6O_2$	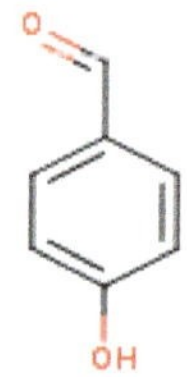
Vanillic acid	4-Hydroxy-3-methoxybenzoic acid; p-Vanillic acid	$C_8H_8O_4$	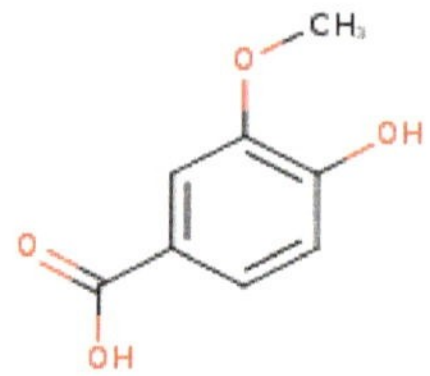
Caffeic acid	3,4-Dihydroxycinnamic acid	$C_9H_8O_4$	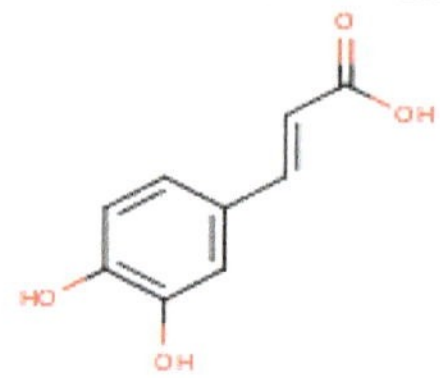
Syringic acid	3,5-Dimethoxy-4-hydroxybenzoic acid	$C_9H_{10}O_5$	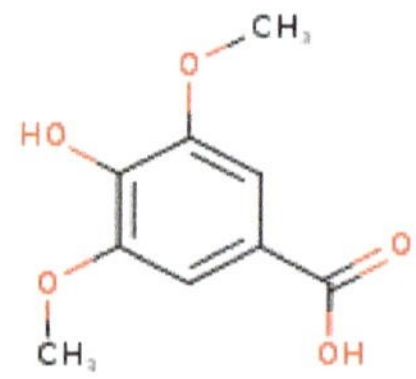
Trans-p-coumaric acid	trans-4-Hydroxycinnamic acid	$C_9H_8O_3$	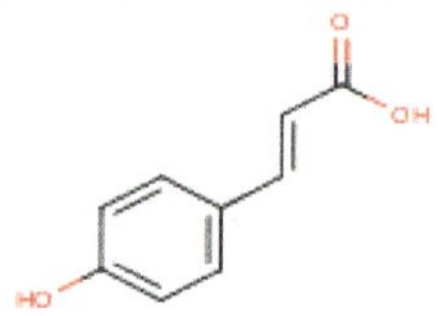
Ferulic acid	3-Methoxy-4-Hydroxycinnamic acid; 3-Methylcaffeic acid; Coniferic acid	$C_{10}H_{10}O_4$	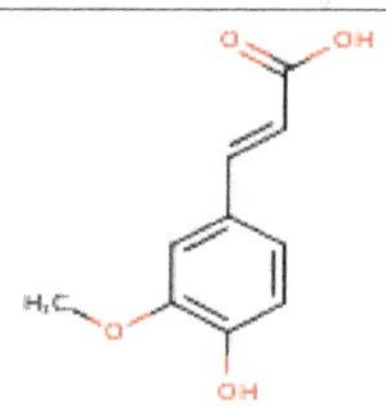

Table 4. *Cont.*

Compound Name	Synonym(s)	Empirical Formula	Structure
Trans-sinapic acid	trans-4-Hydroxy-3,5-dimethoxy-cinnamic acid; trans-Sinapinic acid	$C_{11}H_{12}O_5$	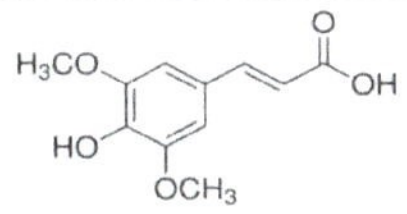
Tyrosol	p-HPEA; 4-(2-Hydroxyethyl)phenol; 2-(4-Hydroxyphenyl)ethanol; 2,4-Hydroxyphenyl-ethyl-alcohol; 4-Hydroxyphenylethanol	$C_8H_{10}O_2$	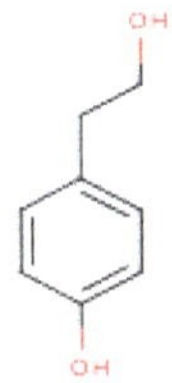
Vanillin	4-Hydroxy-3-methoxy-benzoic aldehyde; Methylprotocatechuic aldehyde; Vanillic aldehyde; p-Vanillin	$C_8H_8O_3$	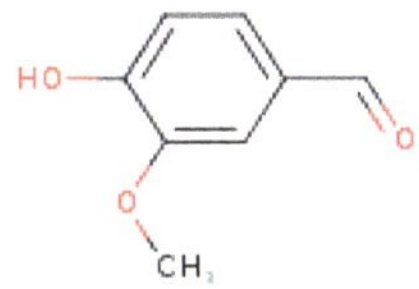
Luteolin	5,7,3′,4′-Tetrahydroxyflavone	$C_{15}H_{10}O_6$	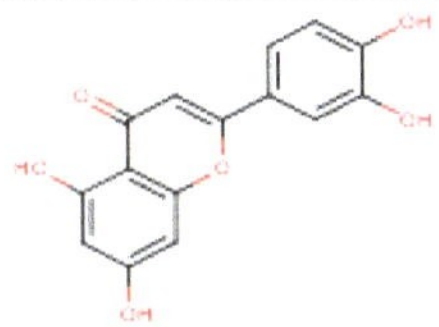
Kaempferol	3,5,7,4′-Tetrahydroxyflavone	$C_{15}H_{10}O_6$	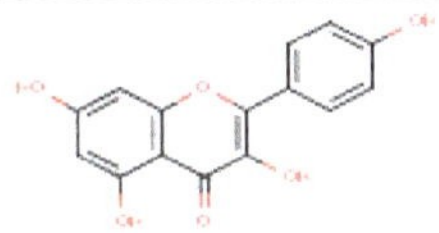

* The data were collected from the Phenol-Explorer database which is an online comprehensive database on polyphenol contents in foods, http://phenol-explorer.eu/ (Accessed on 09.12.2018).

A study by Yang et al. [84] showed no flavonoid content (detection limit: 0.05 mg/100 g) in either the immature or mature fruits of *C. maxima*. Only the shoots and buds showed positive results. However, in accordance with [85], the total flavonoid and phenolic contents of this species were determined as approximately 2.7 mg quercetin equivalent/g extract and 8.8 mg gallic acid equivalent (GAE)/g extract, respectively. Sreeramulu and Raghunath [86] reported that average total phenolic content of *C. maxima* was 46.43 mg GAE/100 g. In another study, *C. maxima* was analyzed for its flavonoid content, and kaempferol was found to be the only flavonoid present in this species at a concentration of 371.0 mg/kg of dry weight [87].

C. pepo was also found to have low polyphenol content. However, Iswaldi et al. [88] have reported for the first time a list of 34 polyphenols, including a variety of flavonoids in the *C. pepo* fruit, in addition to other unknown polar compounds. Also, the *C. pepo* flowers may contain considerable amounts of phenolic compounds. A total polyphenol content ranging from 0.054 to 0.297 μg GAE/μg dry biomass has been reported to be dependent on the extraction conditions and flower sex [89]. Andjelkovic et al. [90] studied the phenolic content of six pumpkin (*C. pepo*) seed oils and identified the following compounds: tyrosol, luteolin, ferulic acid, vanillic acid, and vanillin. Among them, tyrosol was the most abundant compound, ranging from 1.58 mg/kg to 17.69 mg/kg.

Five major compounds in *C. ficifolia* fruit aqueous extract were identified by Jessica et al. [91] as: *p*-coumaric acid, *p*-hydroxybenzoic acid, salicin, stigmast-7,2,2-dien-3-ol and stigmast-7-en-3-ol. On the other hand, Peričin et al. [92] assessed the phenolic acids content of *C. pepo* seeds. *p*-Hydroxybenzoic acid was found to be the prevailing phenolic acid, with 34.72%, 51.80%, and 67.38% of the total phenolic acids content in whole dehulled seed, hulls, and kernels, respectively. Aside from *p*-hydroxybenzoic acid, the most dominant phenolic substances can be listed in a decreasing order of quantity as follows: caffeic, ferulic, and vanillic acids in whole dehulled seeds. *Trans*-sinapic and protocatechuic acids, and *p*-hydroxybenzaldehyde were the abundant phenolic acids presented in kernels of hulled pumpkin variety; the hulls comprised *p*-hydroxybenzaldehyde, vanillic, and protocatechuic acids with considerable amounts.

4.3. Terpenoids, Saponins and Sterols in Cucurbita

Badr et al. [55] have demonstrated the existence of calotropoleanly ester and cholesterol in *C. pepo* fruit, and Younis et al. [62] also represented the cholesterol content in seeds (<0.2 to 3 mg/100 g). These plant parts were also reported as containing more β-sitosterol (383.89 mg/kg fresh weight) than those of *C. moschata* and *C. maxima* (277.58 mg/kg and 235.16 mg/kg fresh weight, respectively) [53]. Dubois et al. [93] have reported that, besides cucurbitacins, a new triterpenoid saponin, foetidissimoside A (3,28-bidesmosidic triterpenoid saponin) is also present in *C. foetidissima* roots. Ten years later, Gaidi et al. [94] discovered the foetidissimoside B in the same source. Also, Matus et al. [95] extracted sterols from seeds, and the most abundant were Δ7.22.25-stigmastatrienol, β-sitosterol, spinasterol and Δ7.25-stigmastadienol [61].

Cucurbitacin is a triterpenoid [96] with a bitter taste, isolated from members of the Cucurbitaceae family, and there are more than 18 types of cucurbitacin in the nature. Cucurbitacins are a group of distinctive highly oxygenated triterpenoid substances, having tetracyclic triterpenes with a cucurbitane skeleton. Figure 1 details the structure of 19-(10→9β)-abeo-10α-lanost-5-ene. They are cucurbitane triterpenes with double bonds between C4 and C5, a hydroxyl at C16, C20 and C25 and a ketone at C11 and C22 [20]. These compounds are well-recognized for their bitterness and toxicity [97].

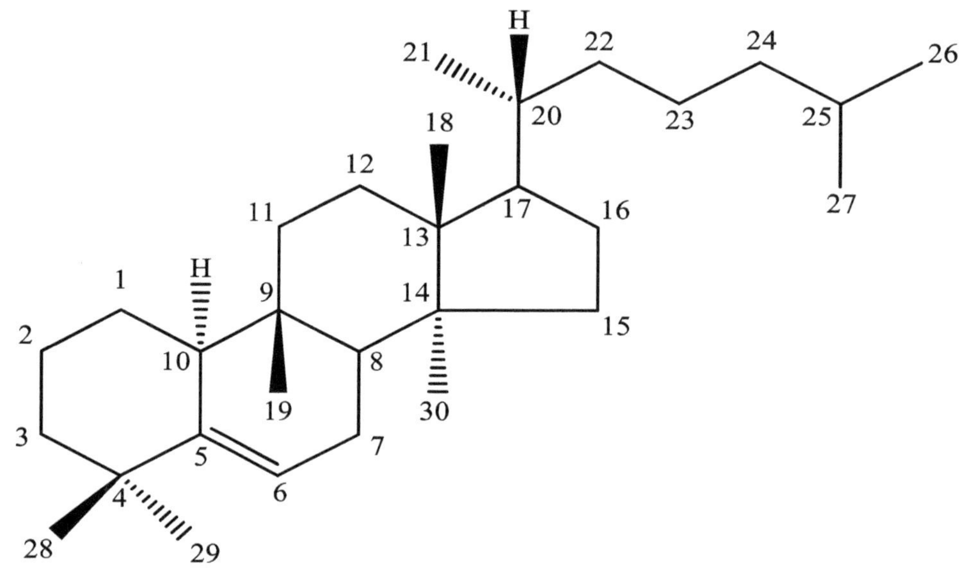

Figure 1. Principal structure of cucurbitacins (19-(10→9β)-abeo-10α-lanost-5-ene).

Cucurbitacins are randomly divided into 12 groups, specifically cucurbitacins A–T, varying in their oxygen functionalities at different positions. The chemical structures of a few cucurbitacins (A, B, C, and D) are presented in Figure 2, and the cucurbitacin composition in different *Cucurbita* species is summarized in Table 5.

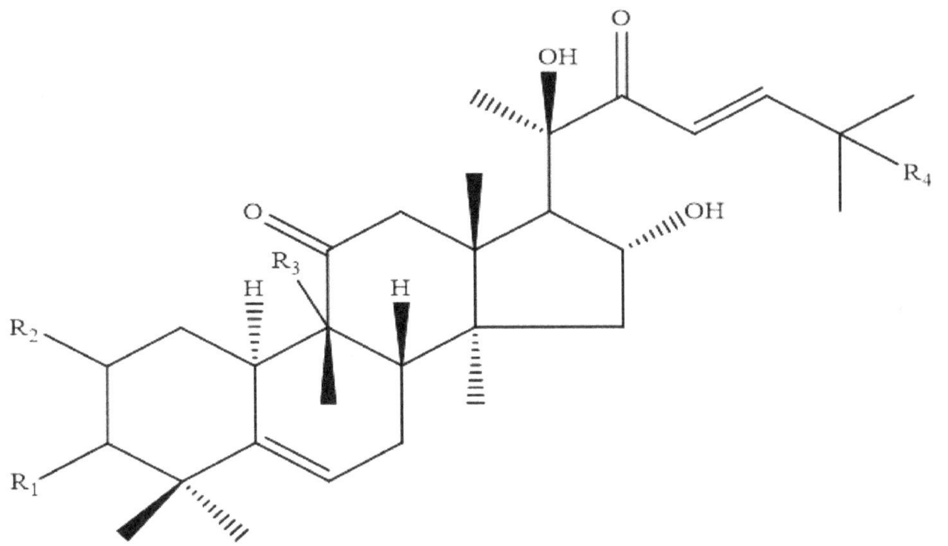

(**a**) R_1: =O R_2: OH R_3: CH_2OH R_4: $OCOCH_3$
(**b**) R_1: =O R_2: OH R_3: H R_4: $OCOCH_3$
(**c**) R_1: OH R_2: H R_3: CH_2OH R_4: $OCOCH_3$
(**d**) R_1: =O R_2: OH R_3: H R_4: OH

Figure 2. Structure of different cucurbitacin: (**a**) Cucurbitacin A, (**b**) Cucurbitacin B, (**c**) Cucurbitacin C and (**d**) Cucurbitacin D.

Table 5. Cucurbitacin content of *Cucurbita* spp. (mg/g fresh weight) *.

Species	Plant Part	B	D	E	I	References
Cucurbita maxima	Radicles	0.1–1	Tr	0.01–0.1	ND	[98]
	Cotyledons	0.1–1	0.01–0.1	0.01–0.1	ND	
	Leaf, fruit, root	<0.02	<0.02	<0.02	<0.02	[48]
Cucurbita andreana	Leaf	0.15	0.12	ND	ND	[48]
	Fruit	2.78	0.42	ND	ND	
	Root	0.58	0.51	ND	ND	
Cucurbita. andreana × *C. maxima*	Fruit	1.17	0.09	ND	ND	[99]
Cucurbita mixta Pang.	Cotyledons	0.01–0.1	ND	ND	ND	[98]
Cucurbita pepo	Radicles	Tr	ND	0.1–1	Tr	[98]
	Cotyledons	0.1–1	0.01–0.1	0.01–0.1	ND	
	Fruits	ND	ND	3.1	ND	[52]
	Flesh at the stem end	ND	ND	7.2	ND	
	Fruit—central portion	ND	ND	2.7	ND	
	Fruit	ND	ND	0.6	ND	[100]
	Fruit	ND	ND	1.12	ND	[101]
Cucurbita texana Gray	Leaf	ND	ND	Tr	Tr	[48]
	Fruit	ND	ND	0.07	0.367	
	Root	ND	ND	0.18	0.08	
Cucurbita texana × *C. pepo*	Fruit	ND	ND	0.23	0.09	[99]
Cucurbita martinezii Bailey	Leaf	ND	ND	0.42	0.25	[48]
	Fruit	ND	ND	0.36	0.45	
	Root	ND	ND	0.23	0.65	
Cucurbita lundelliana Bailey	Leaf	0.47	0.12	ND	ND	[48]
	Fruit	0.63	0.15	ND	ND	
	Root	0.53	0.29	ND	ND	
Cucurbita foetidissima	Root	ND	ND	0.28	1.72	[99]

* Tr.: Trace, ND: Not detected.

Seedlings of the pumpkin *C. maxima* have been reported to involve high amounts of cucurbitacin B and small amounts of cucurbitacin D and E in radicles and cotyledons [98]. Eighteen *Cucurbita* plants species were analyzed for their cucurbitacin contents. Bitter species having comparatively high contents of cucurbitacins B and D and no detectable cucurbitacins E and I were identified as *Cucurbita andreana* Naudin, *Cucurbita ecuadorensis* Cutler & Whitaker, *Cucurbita radicans* Naudin, *Cucurbita lundelliana* L.H.Bailey, *C. argyrosperma* and *Cucurbita pedatifolia* L.H.Bailey. The other group of wild, bitter species having relatively large amounts of cucurbitacins E and I were *Cucurbita cylindrata* L.H.Bailey, *C. foetidissima*, *C. martinezii*, *C. okeechobeensis*, and *Cucurbita palmata* S.Watson, *Cucurbita pepo* var. *texana (Scheele) D.S.Decker* was found to contain nearly all cucurbitacins as cucurbitacin E-glycoside. However, no cucurbitacin could be identified in domesticated and sweet species, including *C. ficifolia*, *C. maxima*, *C. moschata*, and *C. pepo* [48]. The same group of investigators also determined the cucurbitacin and cucurbitacin glycoside content in fruits of two *Cucurbita* plant hybrids (*C. andreana* × *C. maxima* and *C. texana* × *C. pepo*), as well as in *C. foetidissima* roots. As a result, *C. andreana* × *C. maxima* fruits contained cucurbitacins B and D, whereas *C. texana* × *C. pepo* fruits and *C. foetidissima* roots presented cucurbitacins E and I [99]. With regards to *C. andreana* fruits extract, it was chromatographically fractionated, and cucurbitacins B, D, E and I, as well as cucurbitacin E and I aglycones and cucurbitacin B, E, and I glucosides were detected in this species [102]. *C. pepo* comprises the most investigated *Cucurbita* plant for its cucurbitacin content. In an earlier study, cucurbitacin E was detected as a primary bitter component in seedling *C. pepo* radicles, whereas cucurbitacins B and I were found in trace amounts in the same tissue. On the other hand, cotyledons of this species were found to include cucurbitacin D and E in moderate and low concentrations, respectively [103]. Freeze-dried samples of Blackjack cultivar of *C. pepo* were analyzed by two research teams in different years. Ferguson et al. [101] found 1.12 mg cucurbitacin E-glycoside/g fresh weight, whereas Hutt and Herrington [100] detected 0.6 mg cucurbitacin E-glycoside/g fresh weight. Wang et al. [104] investigated *C. pepo* cv dayangua for its phytochemical content, and cucurbitacin L and cucurbitacin K were isolated at concentrations of 2.13 mg/kg dry matter and 2.67 mg/kg dry matter, respectively. In a very recent study, cucurbitacin C and E glycosides in *C. pepo* fruit were reported for the first time. The corresponding concentrations of compounds were 105 μg/g fresh fruit for cucurbitacin C and 438 μg/g fresh fruit cucurbitacin E. The authors also demonstrated that gamma irradiation did not affect the cucurbitacins concentration, when compared to non-irradiated control group [105].

From a biological point of view, it has been demonstrated that cucurbitacins exert several bioactivities, such as antitumor, anti-inflammatory, anti-atherosclerotic, antidiabetic effects [106]. There is a large body of evidence suggesting that cucurbitacins hold very high orders of cytotoxicity towards a vast quantity of malignancies. Seed and fruit portions of few cucurbits are found to exhibit purgative, emetic and anthelmintic activities due to presence of cucurbitacin triterpenoids [107,108]. Jayaprakasam et al.[109] isolated cucurbitacins B, D, E, and I from *C. andreana* fruits and evaluated their effects at a level of growth suppression of human breast (MCF-7), colon (HCT-116), lung (NCI-H460), and central nervous system (CNS) (SF-268) tumor cell lines; cyclooxygenase-1 (COX-1) and cyclooxygenase-2 (COX-2) enzymes; and even on lipid peroxidation. All isolated cucurbitacins were able to abate the proliferation of investigated cancer cell lines in varying percentages. Among them, cucurbitacin B exhibited more than 80% proliferation inhibitory activity. Additionally, cucurbitacins B, D, E, and I inhibited COX-2 enzyme, an enzyme responsible for inflammation, by 32%, 29%, 35%, and 27%, respectively, at a concentration of 100 mg/mL. A cucurbitacin derivative, with a cucurbitacin D-like structure, was separated from the methanolic extract of *C. pepo* seeds and revealed to have antiulcer activity in a dose-dependent manner [110].

In contrast to their biological activities, cucurbitacins have toxic effects in mammalians. According to Le Roux et al. [111], 353 poisoning cases linked to *C. pepo* cucurbitacins were reported to French Poison Control Centers between 1 January 2012 and 12 December 2016. In 1980s, various human poisoning cases were stated due to the consumption of commercially produced zucchini (*C. pepo*) in Australia. The most common developed characteristic symptoms evidenced by exposed individuals include a bitter taste in the mouth, abdominal pain, diarrhea and rarely, collapse [101]. Pfab et al. [112] reported that, 81 symptomatic cases were registered to Poison Information Centre (PIC) Munich between 2002 to 2015. The primary symptom was colitis with bloody diarrhea after zucchini (*C. pepo*) consumption. As the authors stated, cucurbitacins, the responsible toxins of poisonings, are not often identified in cultivated fruits, but some fruits spontaneously produced them. In an in vivo experiment, mice were fed with *C. pepo* fruit of two cultivars, 'Blackjack' and 'Straightneck', and an accession of the bitter species, *C. texana*. As a result, mice having the diet with 1% *C. texana*, containing cucurbitacins E glycoside and I, exhibited poor growth, severe diarrhea, anemia and 40% mortality. When the *C. texana* percentage increased to 10 or 20%, mortality rate reached 100% within a few days. However, no detectable cucurbitacins in *C. pepo* cultivars were identified and, animals fed up to 20% freeze-dried squash in their diets displayed no toxicity-related symptoms [113].

4.4. Functional Carbohydrates and Polysaccharides in Cucurbita

C. moschata fruit is a rich source of polysaccharides, with a useful biological benefit, i.e., cytoprotective and antioxidative activities [114,115], that can reach 16.2% in dry matter, under optimised conditions [116]. Xia and Wang [117] reported high amounts of D-chiro-inositol, a hypoglycaemic molecule, in *C. ficifolia* fruit (without seeds). In addition to D-chiro-inositol, the plant was found to be rich in other carbohydrates, like myo-inositol, fagopyritols and sucrose [117].

4.5. Fatty Acids of the Oil of Cucurbita Seeds

Seeds of *Cucurbita* species are also rich in fat (around 45%) and a variety of fatty acids, such as saturated, unsaturated (around 55% of the oil), and conjugated fatty acids (CFA) [118,119], therefore, may be considered as a source of molecules with high pharmacological potential and health benefits. Specifically, CFA are polyunsaturated fatty acids containing conjugated double bonds with positional and geometric isomers, and have several beneficial effects [120].

4.6. Other

C. ficifolia can also be considered a safe source of proteinases, with a high potential to be used for bioactive peptides production [121,122]. Other enzymes, like peroxidases can be obtained from *C. moschata* [123]. No alkaloids were found in neither the fruit nor seeds of *C. moschata* [80]. In contrast, Chonoko and Rufai [124] have represented alkaloid contents both in the back peels and seeds of *C. pepo*. Elinge et al. [56] also reported the presence of phytate (35.06 mg/100 g), oxalate (0.02 mg/100 g), hydrocyanic acid (0.22 mg/100 g) and nitrate (2.27 mg/100 g) as antinutrient compounds in *C. pepo* seeds.

5. *Cucurbita* Plants for Industrial Purposes: Key Role as a Food Preservative

Three main pumpkin varieties, including *C. pepo*, *C. maxima*, and *C. moschata*, are considered both as nutritional and medicinal foods in many countries [125]. Some biological activities are reported in pumpkins, among them antimicrobial activity [126,127]. The reason why this plant show antimicrobial applications is related to its high vitamins content (mainly A and C), phenolic compounds, minerals, dietary fiber, amino acids and other advantageous compounds to humans. Indeed, antioxidant, antibacterial and intestinal antiparasitic activities are also part of the active function of this crop [125,128]. Pumpkin extracts are rich in steroids, flavonoids, tannins, alkaloids and saponins, showing momentous antimicrobial and antifungal activity against some microorganisms [124,129]. Based on Muruganantham et al. [130] study, the ethyl acetate extract of *C. maxima* flowers has meaningful antifungal and antibacterial activity against some microorganisms, like *Escherichia coli*, *Salmonella typhi*, *Bacillus cereus*, *Enterobacter faecalis*, *Candida albicans*, and *Curvularia lunata*. Nonetheless, the antioxidant and antimicrobial effects of pumpkin seeds have also been reported. The extracted oil from pumpkin seeds chiefly contains fatty acids, among them linoleic, oleic, palmitic and stearic acids. In addition, the oil is also full of tocopherols (δ-tocopherol, γ-tocopherol, β-tocopherol and carotenoids, like lutein and β-carotene), characterized by displaying strong antioxidant effects. It is worth noting that pumpkin seeds oil can preserve lipids by having selenium, tocopherol, enzymes, hormones and vitamins. Adeel et al. [126] stated that pumpkin seed oil exhibits high antibacterial activity against *Staphylococcus aureus*, and pumpkin seeds are also able to markedly inhibit *Rhodotorula rubra* and *C. albicans* growth at 0.5 mg/mL and 1.0 mg/mL, respectively [129]. Other research showed that *Bacillus subtilis*, *S. aureus*, *E. coli* and *Klebsiella pneumonia* are easily affected by the antibacterial properties of the methanolic extract from seed oil at 1.0 mg/mL, 2.0 mg/mL, 2.0 mg/mL and 3.0 mg/mL, respectively [127]. Moreover, the authors stated that the antibacterial activity is not the only property of the oil, since it also exerts a remarkable antifungal activity against *R. rubra* and *C. albicans*, at concentrations of 0.5 mg/mL and 1.0 mg/mL, respectively. It has even been stated that there is a high susceptibility of *R. rubra* to the seeds' oil. Still, researchers have stressed that 1.0 mg/mL of pumpkin oil seeds was effective against *Penicillium chrysogenum* and *Aspergillus parasiticus*, and 2.0 mg/mL against *A. flavus* [127].

Pumpkin rinds and leaves contain some special bioactive proteins, which have shown preservative effects. For example, pumpkin leaves contain the PR-5 antifungal protein [131], highly homologous to thaumatin. In addition, the antimicrobial activity of this protein, besides the synergistic effect of nikkomycin against *C. albicans* development, has been proved. Moreover, the growth and survival of the phytopathogenic bacteria *Erwinia amylovora*, *Phytophthora infestans* and *Pseudomonas solanacearum* is prohibited by a ribosome-inactivating protein purified from *C. moschata* [132]. Black pumpkin seeds have another component, named cucurmoschin and identified as an antifungal peptide abundant in glycine, arginine, and glutamate residues. Additionally, Park and et al. [133] found two novel antifungal proteins (Pr-1 and Pr-2) from pumpkin rinds that showed strong in vitro antifungal activity against *Botrytis cinerea*, *Colletotrichum coccodes*, *Fusarium solani*, *F. oxysporum*, and *Trichoderma harzianum* at 10–20 μM.

6. Conclusions and Future Perspectives

Overall, *Cucurbita* species have chemical components with an intriguing impact in health promotion. Several squash and pumpkin species are a natural and rich source of potential bioactive compounds, such as carotenoids, tocopherols, phenols, terpenoids, saponins, sterols, fatty acids, functional carbohydrates and polysaccharides. Of these triterpenoids, cucurbitacins are particularly noteworthy for their multiple marked abilities. The presence of active phytochemicals in Cucurbitaceae species makes them a great matrix to be further exploited for both preventive and therapeutic purposes, beyond biotechnological applications. For an emphasis on *Cucurbita* plants' pharmacological potential, please refer to other review [134].

Author Contributions: All authors contributed significantly to this work. In addition, J.S.-R., M.M., N.M., W.C.C., and J.N., critically reviewed the manuscript. All the authors read and approved the final manuscript.

Acknowledgments: This work was supported by CONICYT PIA/APOYO CCTE AFB170007. N. Martins would like to thank the Portuguese Foundation for Science and Technology (FCT-Portugal) for the Strategic project ref. UID/BIM/04293/2013 and "NORTE2020-Northern Regional Operational Program" (NORTE-01-0145-FEDER-000012).

References

1. Sharifi-Rad, M.; Nazaruk, J.; Polito, L.; Morais-Braga, M.F.B.; Rocha, J.E.; Coutinho, H.D.M.; Salehi, B.; Tabanelli, G.; Montanari, C.; Contreras, M.D.M.; et al. *Matricaria* genus as a source of antimicrobial agents: From farm to pharmacy and food applications. *Microbiol. Res.* **2018**, *215*, 76–88. [CrossRef] [PubMed]
2. Sharifi-Rad, J.; Sharifi-Rad, M.; Salehi, B.; Iriti, M.; Roointan, A.; Mnayer, D.; Soltani-Nejad, A.; Afshari, A. In vitro and in vivo assessment of free radical scavenging and antioxidant activities of *Veronica persica* Poir. *Cell. Mol. Biol.* **2018**, *64*, 57–64. [CrossRef] [PubMed]

3. Mishra, A.P.; Saklani, S.; Salehi, B.; Parcha, V.; Sharifi-Rad, M.; Milella, L.; Iriti, M.; Sharifi-Rad, J.; Srivastava, M. *Satyrium nepalense*, a high altitude medicinal orchid of Indian Himalayan region: Chemical profile and biological activities of tuber extracts. *Cell. Mol. Biol.* **2018**, *64*, 35–43. [CrossRef] [PubMed]
4. Mishra, A.P.; Sharifi-Rad, M.; Shariati, M.A.; Mabkhot, Y.N.; Al-Showiman, S.S.; Rauf, A.; Salehi, B.; Župunski, M.; Sharifi-Rad, M.; Gusain, P.; et al. Bioactive compounds and health benefits of edible *Rumex* species-A review. *Cell. Mol. Biol.* **2018**, *64*, 27–34. [CrossRef]
5. Sharifi-Rad, M.; Fokou, P.V.T.; Sharopov, F.; Martorell, M.; Ademiluyi, A.O.; Rajkovic, J.; Salehi, B.; Martins, N.; Iriti, M.; Sharifi-Rad, J. Antiulcer Agents: From Plant Extracts to Phytochemicals in Healing Promotion. *Molecules* **2018**, *23*, 1751. [CrossRef]
6. Denev, P.; Kratchanova, M.; Ciz, M.; Lojek, A.; Vasicek, O.; Blazheva, D.; Nedelcheva, P.; Vojtek, L.; Hyrsl, P. Antioxidant, antimicrobial and neutrophil-modulating activities of herb extracts. *Acta Biochim. Pol.* **2014**, *61*, 359–367. [CrossRef]
7. Selamoglu, Z. The natural products and healthy life. *J. Tradit. Med. Clin. Naturop.* **2018**, *7*, e146.
8. Selamoğlu, Z. Polyphenolic Compounds in Human Health with Pharmacological Properties. *J. Tradit. Med. Clin. Naturop.* **2017**, *6*, e138. [CrossRef]
9. Shah, B.N.; Seth, A.K.; Desai, R.V. Phytophannacological profile of lagenaria siceraria, a review. *Asian J. Plant Sci.* **2010**, *9*, 152–157.
10. Andolfo, G.; Di Donato, A.; Darrudi, R.; Errico, A.; Cigliano, R.A.; Ercolano, M.R. Draft of zucchini (*Cucurbita pepo* L.) proteome: A resource for genetic and genomic studies. *Front. Genet.* **2017**, *8*. [CrossRef]
11. Dubey, S.D.; Dubey, S.D. Overview on *Cucurbita maxima*. *Int. J. Phytopharm.* **2012**, 2. [CrossRef]
12. Paris, H.S. Historical records, origins, and development of the edible cultivar groups of *Cucurbita pepo* (Cucurbitaceae). *Econ. Bot.* **1989**, *43*, 423–443. [CrossRef]
13. Neelamma, G.; Swamy, B.D.; Dhamodaran, P. Phytochemical and pharmacological overview of *Cucurbita maxima* and future perspective as potential phytotherapeutic agent. *Eur. J. Pharm. Med. Res.* **2016**, *3*, 277–287.
14. Adnan, M.; Gul, S.; Batool, S.; Fatima, B.; Rehman, A.; Yaqoob, S.; Shabir, H.; Yousaf, T.; Mussarat, S.; Ali, N.; et al. A review on the ethnobotany, phytochemistry, pharmacology and nutritional composition of *Cucurbita pepo* L. *J. Phytopharm.* **2017**, *6*, 133–139.
15. Jeffrey, C. Systematics of the cucurbitaceae: An overview. In *Biology and Utilization of the Cucurbitaceae*; Bates, D.M., Robinson, R.W., Jeffrey, C., Eds.; Cornell University Press: Ithaca, NY, USA, 1990; pp. 449–463.
16. Sanjur, O.I.; Piperno, D.R.; Andres, T.C.; Wessel-Beaver, L. Phylogenetic relationships among domesticated and wild species of Cucurbita (Cucurbitaceae) inferred from a mitochondrial gene: Implications for crop plant evolution and areas of origin. *Proc. Natl. Acad. Sci. USA* **2002**, *99*, 535–540. [CrossRef] [PubMed]
17. Smith, B.D. Documenting plant domestication: The consilience of biological and archaeological approaches. *Proc. Natl. Acad. Sci. USA* **2001**, *98*, 1324–1326. [CrossRef] [PubMed]
18. Smith, B.D. The initial domestication of *Cucurbita pepo* in the americas 10,000 years ago. *Science* **1997**, *276*, 932–934. [CrossRef]
19. FAOSTAT. Available online: http://www.fao.org/statistics/en/ (accessed on 16 August 2019).
20. Wiart, C. Terpenes. In *Lead Compounds from Medicinal Plants for the Treatment of Cancer*; Wiart, C., Ed.; Academic Press: Cambridge, MA, USA, 2013; pp. 97–265.
21. Napier, T. Pumpkin production. *Primefacts* **2009**, *964*, 1–8.
22. OECD. Squashes, pumkins, zucchinis and gourds (*Cucurbita* species). In *Safety Assessment of Transgenic Organisms in the Environment*; OECD Publishing: Paris, France, 2016.
23. Andres, T.C. Biosystematics, theories on the origin, and breeding potential of *Cucurbita ficifolia* (cucurbitaceae). In *Biology and Utilization of the Cucurbitaceae*; Bates, D.M., Robinson, R.W., Jeffrey, C., Eds.; Cornell University Press: Ithaca, NY, USA, 1990; pp. 102–118.
24. Funt, R.C.; Hall, H.K. *Raspberries (Crop Production Science in Horticulture)*; CAB International: Cambridge, UK, 2013.
25. Esquinas-Alcazar, J.T.; Gulick, P.J. *Genetic Resources of Cucurbitaceae: A Global Report*; International Board for Plant Genetic Research: Rome, Italy, 1983.
26. Whitaker, T.W. Ecological aspects of the cultivated cucurbita. *HortScience* **1968**, *3*, 9–11.
27. Azurdia-Pérez, C.A.; González-Salán, M. *Informe Final del Proyecto de Recolección de Algunos Cultivos Nativos de Guatemala*; Facultad de Agronomía; Universidad de San Carlos de Guatemala (USAC), Instituto de Ciencia y

Technología Agrícolas (ICTA) and Consejo Internacional de Recursos Fitogenétic, International Board for Plant Genetic Resources (IBPGR): Guatemala, 1986.

28. Bahlgerdi, M. The Study of Plant Density and Planting Methods on Some Growth Characteristics, Seed and Oil Yield of Medicinal Pumpkin (*Cucurbita pepo* Var. Styriaca, Cv. Kaki). *Am. J. Life Sci.* **2014**, *2*, 319. [CrossRef]
29. Bavec, F.; Gril, L.; Grobelnik-Mlakar, S.; Bavec, M. Seedlings of oil pumpkins as an alternative to seed sowing: Yield and production costs. *Bodenkultur* **2002**, *53*, 39–43.
30. Buwalda, J.; Freeman, R. Hybrid squash: Responses to nitrogen, potassium, and phosphorus fertilisers on a soil of moderate fertility. *N. Z. J. Exp. Agric.* **1986**, *14*, 339–345. [CrossRef]
31. Reiners, S.; Riggs, D.I. Plant Spacing and Variety Affect Pumpkin Yield and Fruit Size, but Supplemental Nitrogen Does Not. *HortScience* **1997**, *32*, 1037–1039. [CrossRef]
32. Swiader, J.M.; Sipp, S.K.; Brown, R.E. Pumpkin Growth, Flowering, and Fruiting Response to Nitrogen and Potassium Sprinkler Fertigation in Sandy Soil. *J. Am. Soc. Hortic. Sci.* **1994**, *119*, 414–419. [CrossRef]
33. Manu, V.T.; Holo, T.F.; Pole, F.S.; Halavatau, S.; Kanongata'a, S.; Fakalata, O.K. *Conventional Squash Production*; Ministry of Agriculture and Forestry: Nukualofa, Tonga, 1995.
34. Bannayan, M. Growth Analysis of Pumpkin (*Cucurbita pepo* L.) Under Various Management Practices and Temperature Regimes. *Agric. Res. Technol. Open Access J.* **2017**, *11*, 555801. [CrossRef]
35. Zitter, T.A. *Scab of Cucurbits*; Vegetable Crops. Cornell University: Ithaca, NY, USA, 1986; p. 732.50.
36. Nair, P.V.; Thomas, K.G. Hydrazine-Induced Room-Temperature Transformation of CdTe Nanoparticles to Nanowires. *J. Phys. Chem. Lett.* **2010**, *1*, 2094–2098. [CrossRef]
37. Colucci, S.J.; Holmes, G.J. Downy mildew of cucurbits. *Plant Health Instr.* **2010**. [CrossRef]
38. Babadoost, M. Phytophthora blight of cucurbits. *Plant Health Instr.* **2005**. [CrossRef]
39. Leibovich, G.; Cohen, R.; Shtienberg, D.; Paris, H.S. Variability in the reaction of squash (*Cucurbita pepo*) to inoculation with Sphaerotheca fuliginea and methodology of breeding for resistance. *Plant Pathol.* **1993**, *42*, 510–516.
40. Nagy, G.S. Studies on powdery mildews of cucurbits. In *The Powdery Mildews*; Spencer, D.M., Ed.; Academic Press: New York, NY, USA; San Francisco, CA, USA, 1976; Volume 2, pp. 205–210.
41. Egel, D.S.; Martyn, R.D. Fusarium wilt of watermelon and other cucurbits. *Plant Health Instr.* **2007**. [CrossRef]
42. Jahn, M.; Munger, H.M.; McCreight, J.D. Breeding cucurbit crops for powdery mildew resistance. In *The Powdery Mildews: A Comprehensive Treatise*; Bélanger, R., Bushnell, W.R., Dik, A.J., Carver, T.L.W., Eds.; The American Phytopathological Society: Saint Paul, MN, USA, 2002; pp. 239–248.
43. Zitter, T.A.; Hopkins, D.L.; Thomas, C.E. *Compendium of Cucurbit Diseases*; APS Press: Saint Paul, MN, USA, 1996; p. 89054.
44. Bradbury, J.F. *Guide to Plant Pathogenic Bacteria*; CAB International Mycological Institute: London, UK, 1986; p. 334.
45. Rand, R.V. Transmission and control of bacterial wilt of cucurbits. *J. Agric. Res.* **1916**, *6*, 417–434.
46. Brunt, A.A.; Crabtree, K.; Dallwitz, M.J.; Gibbs, A.J.; Watson, L.; Zurcher, E.J. *Plant Viruses Online: Descriptions and Lists from the Vide Database*; CAB International: Wallingford, UK, 1990.
47. Jossey, S.; Babadoost, M. First Report of Tobacco ringspot virus in Pumpkin (*Cucurbita pepo*) in Illinois. *Plant Dis.* **2006**, *90*, 1361. [CrossRef] [PubMed]
48. Metcalf, R.L.; Rhodes, A.M.; Ferguson, J.; Lu, P.-Y. Cucurbitacin Contents and Diabroticite (Coleoptera: Chrysomelidae) Feeding upon *Cucurbita* spp. *Environ. Èntomol.* **1982**, *11*, 931–937. [CrossRef]
49. Nee, M. The domestication of *Cucurbita* (Cucurbitaceae). *Econ. Bot.* **1990**, *44*, 56–68. [CrossRef]
50. Andres, T.C.; Nabhan, G.P. Taxonomic rank and rarity of *Cucurbita okeechobeensis*. *Cucurbit Genet. Coop. Rep.* **1988**, *11*, 83–85.
51. Ward, D.B.; Minno, M.C. Rediscovery of the endangered okeechobee gourd (*Cucurbita okeechobeensis*) along the st. Johns river, florida, where last reported by william bartram in 1774. *Castanea* **2002**, *67*, 201–206.
52. Rymal, K.S.; Chambliss, O.; Bond, M.D.; Smith, D.A. Squash containing toxic cucurbitacin com- pounds occurring in california and alabama. *J. Food Prot.* **1984**, *47*, 270–271. [CrossRef] [PubMed]
53. Mi, Y.K.; Eun, J.K.; Young-Nam, K.; Changsun, C.; Bo-Hieu, L. Comparison of the chemical compositions and nutritive values of various pumpkin (cucurbitaceae) species and parts. *Nutr. Res. Pract.* **2012**, *6*, 21–27.
54. Amoo, I.A.; Eleyinmi, A.F.; Ilelaboye, N.O.A.; Akoja, S.S. Characterisation of oil extracted from gourd (*Cucurbita maxima*) seed. *J. Food Agric. Environ.* **2004**, *2*, 38–39.

55. Badr, S.E.; Shaaban, M.; Elkholy, Y.M.; Helal, M.H.; Hamza, A.S.; Masoud, M.S.; El Safty, M.M. Chemical composition and biological activity of ripe pumpkin fruits (*Cucurbita pepo* L.) cultivated in Egyptian habitats. *Nat. Prod. Res.* **2011**, *25*, 1524–1539. [CrossRef]
56. Elinge, C.; Muhammad, A.; Atiku, F.; Itodo, A.; Peni, I.; Sanni, O.; Mbongo, A. Proximate, mineral and anti-nutrient composition of pumpkin (*Cucurbita pepo* L.) seeds extract. *Int. J. Plant Res.* **2012**, *2*, 146–150.
57. Jacobo-Valenzuela, N.; Zazueta-Morales, J.D.J.; Gallegos-Infante, J.A.; Aguilar-Gutierrez, F.; Camacho-Hernandez, I.L.; Rocha-Guzman, N.E.; Gonzalez-Laredo, R.F. Chemical and physicochemical characterization of winter squash (*Cucurbita moschata* D.). *Not. Bot. Horti Agrobot. Cluj-Napoca* **2015**, *39*, 34–40. [CrossRef]
58. Jarret, R.L.; Levy, I.J.; Potter, T.L.; Cermak, S.C.; Merrick, L.C. Seed oil content and fatty acid composition in a genebank collection of *Cucurbita moschata* Duchesne and C. argyrosperma C. Huber. *Plant Genet. Resour.* **2013**, *11*, 149–157. [CrossRef]
59. Mitra, P.; Ramaswamy, H.S.; Chang, K.S. Pumpkin (*Cucurbita maxima*) seed oil extraction using supercritical carbon dioxide and physicochemical properties of the oil. *J. Food Eng.* **2009**, *95*, 208–213. [CrossRef]
60. Murkovic, M.; Hillebrand, A.; Winkler, J.; Leitner, E.; Pfannhauser, W. Variability of fatty acid content in pumpkin seeds (*Cucurbita pepo* L.). *Eur. Food Res. Technol.* **1996**, *203*, 216–219. [CrossRef]
61. Perez Gutierrez, R.M. Review of *Cucurbita pepo* (Pumpkin) its phytochemistry and pharmacology. *Med. Chem.* **2016**, *6*, 012–021. [CrossRef]
62. Younis, Y.; Ghirmay, S.; Al-Shihry, S. African *Cucurbita pepo* L.: Properties of seed and variability in fatty acid composition of seed oil. *Phytochemistry* **2000**, *54*, 71–75. [CrossRef]
63. Noelia, J.; Roberto, M.M.; Jesús, Z.J.D.; Alberto, G.J. Physicochemical, technological properties, and health-benefits of *Cucurbita moschata* Duchense vs. Cehualca—A review. *Food Res. Int.* **2011**, *44*, 2587–2593.
64. Rezig, L.; Chouaibi, M.; Msaada, K.; Hamdi, S. Chemical composition and profile characterisation of pumpkin (*Cucurbita maxima*) seed oil. *Ind. Crop. Prod.* **2012**, *37*, 82–87. [CrossRef]
65. FAO. *Vitamin and Mineral Requirements in Human Nutrition*; World Health Organization: Geneva, Switzerland, 2005.
66. Fang, S.D.; Li, L.C.; Niu, C.I.; Tseng, K.F. Chemical studies on *Cucurbita moschata* Duch. I. The isolation and structural studies of cucurbitine, a new amino acid. *Sci. Sin.* **1961**, *10*, 845.
67. Azevedo-Meleiro, C.H.; Rodriguez-Amaya, D.B. Qualitative and Quantitative Differences in Carotenoid Composition among *Cucurbita moschata*, *Cucurbita maxima*, and *Cucurbita pepo*. *J. Agric. Food Chem.* **2007**, *55*, 4027–4033. [CrossRef] [PubMed]
68. González, E.; Montenegro, M.A.; Nazareno, M.A.; Mishima, B.A.L.D. Carotenoid composition and vitamin A value of an Argentinian squash (*Cucurbita moschata*). *Arch. Latinoam. Nutr.* **2001**, *51*, 395–399. [PubMed]
69. Hidaka, T.; Anno, T.; Nakatsu, S. The Composition and Vitamin A Value of the Carotenoids of Pumpkins of Different Colors. *J. Food Biochem.* **1987**, *11*, 59–68. [CrossRef]
70. Murkovic, M.; Mülleder, U.; Neunteufl, H. Carotenoid Content in Different Varieties of Pumpkins. *J. Food Compos. Anal.* **2002**, *15*, 633–638. [CrossRef]
71. De Carvalho, L.M.J.; Gomes, P.B.; Godoy, R.L.D.O.; Pacheco, S.; Monte, P.H.F.D.; De Carvalho, J.L.V.; Nutti, M.R.; Neves, A.C.L.; Vieira, A.C.R.A.; Ramos, S.R.R. Total carotenoid content, α-carotene and β-carotene, of landrace pumpkins (*Cucurbita moschata* Duch): A preliminary study. *Food Res. Int.* **2012**, *47*, 337–340. [CrossRef]
72. Azizah, A.; Wee, K.; Azizah, O.; Azizah, M. Effect of boiling and stir frying on total phenolics, carotenoids, and radical scavanging activity of pumpkins (*Cucurbita maschato*). *Int. Food Res. J.* **2009**, *16*, 45–51.
73. Aizawa, K.; Inakuma, T. Quantitation of Carotenoids in Commonly consumed Vegetables in Japan. *Food Sci. Technol. Res.* **2007**, *13*, 247–252. [CrossRef]
74. Itle, R.A.; Kabelka, E.A. Correlation between lab color space values and carotenoid content in pumpkins and squash (*Cucurbita* spp.). *HortScience* **2009**, *44*, 633–637. [CrossRef]
75. Chandrika, U.G.; Basnayake, B.M.L.B.; Athukorala, I.; Colombagama, P.W.N.M.; Goonetilleke, A. Carotenoid Content and In Vitro Bioaccessibility of Lutein in Some Leafy Vegetables Popular in Sri Lanka. *J. Nutr. Sci. Vitaminol.* **2010**, *56*, 203–207. [CrossRef]
76. Kurz, C.; Carle, R.; Schieber, A. Hplc-dad-msncharacterisation of carotenoids from apricots and pumpkins for the evaluation of fruit product authenticity. *Food Chem.* **2008**, *110*, 522–530. [CrossRef]

77. Konopacka, D.; Seroczyńska, A.; Korzeniewska, A.; Jesionkowska, K.; Niemirowicz-Szczytt, K.; Płocharski, W. Studies on the usefulness of *Cucurbita maxima* for the production of ready-to-eat dried vegetable snacks with a high carotenoid content. *LWT* **2010**, *43*, 302–309. [CrossRef]
78. Rabrenović, B.B.; Dimić, E.B.; Novaković, M.M.; Tešević, V.V.; Basić, Z.N. The most important bioactive components of cold pressed oil from different pumpkin (*Cucurbita pepo* L.) seeds. *LWT-Food Sci. Technol.* **2014**, *55*, 521–527. [CrossRef]
79. Nakić, S.N.; Rade, D.; Škevin, D.; Štrucelj, D.; Mokrovčak, Ž.; Bartolić, M. Chemical characteristics of oils from naked and husk seeds of *Cucurbita pepo* L. *Eur. J. Lipid Sci. Technol.* **2006**, *108*, 936–943. [CrossRef]
80. Eleiwa, N.Z.; Bakr, R.O.; Mohamed, S.A. Phytochemical and Pharmacological Screening of Seeds and Fruits Pulp of *Cucurbita moschata* Duchesne Cultivated in Egypt. *Int. J. Pharmacogn. Phytochem.* **2014**, *29*, 1226–1236. [CrossRef]
81. Li, F.-S.; Xu, J.; Dou, D.-Q.; Chi, X.-F.; Kang, T.-G.; Kuang, H.X. Structures of new phenolic glycosides from the seeds of *Cucurbita moschata*. *Nat. Prod. Commun.* **2009**, *4*, 511–512. [PubMed]
82. Li, F.-S.; Dou, D.-Q.; Xu, L.; Chi, X.-F.; Kang, T.-G.; Kuang, H.X. New phenolic glycosides from the seeds of *Cucurbita moschata*. *J. Asian Nat. Prod. Res.* **2009**, *11*, 639–642. [CrossRef] [PubMed]
83. Li, W.; Koike, K.; Tatsuzaki, M.; Koide, A.; Nikaido, T. Cucurbitosides f−m, aaylated phenolic glycosides from the seeds of *Cucurbita pepo*. *J. Nat. Prod.* **2005**, *68*, 1754–1757. [CrossRef]
84. Yang, R.-Y.; Lin, S.; Kuo, G. Content and distribution of flavonoids among 91 edible plant species. *Asia Pac. J. Clin. Nutr.* **2008**, *17*, 275–279.
85. Irshad, M.; Ahmad, I.; Mehdi, S.J.; Goel, H.C.; Rizvi, M.M.A. Antioxidant capacity and phenolic content of the aqueous extract of commonly consumed cucurbits. *Int. J. Food Prop.* **2014**, *17*, 179–186. [CrossRef]
86. Sreeramulu, D.; Raghunath, M. Antioxidant activity and phenolic content of roots, tubers and vegetables commonly consumed in India. *Food Res. Int.* **2010**, *43*, 1017–1020. [CrossRef]
87. Koo, M.H.; Suhaila, M. Flavonoid (myricetin, quercetin, kaempferol, luteolin and apigenin) content of edible tropical plants. *J. Agric. Food Chem.* **2001**, *49*, 3106–3112.
88. Iswaldi, I.; Gómez-Caravaca, A.M.; Lozano-Sánchez, J.; Arráez-Román, D.; Carretero, A.S.; Fernández-Gutiérrez, A. Profiling of phenolic and other polar compounds in Zucchini (*Cucurbita pepo* L.) by reverse-phase high-performance liquid chromatography coupled to quadrupole time-of-flight mass spectrometry. *Food Res. Int.* **2013**, *50*, 77–84. [CrossRef]
89. Tarhan, L.; Kayali, H.A.; Urek, R.O. In Vitro Antioxidant Properties of *Cucurbita pepo* L. Male and Female Flowers Extracts. *Plant Foods Hum. Nutr.* **2007**, *62*, 49–51. [CrossRef] [PubMed]
90. Andjelkovic, M.; Van Camp, J.; Trawka, A.; Verhé, R. Phenolic compounds and some quality parameters of pumpkin seed oil. *Eur. J. Lipid Sci. Technol.* **2010**, *112*, 208–217. [CrossRef]
91. Jessica, G.G.; Mario, G.L.; Alejandro, Z.; Cesar, A.P.J.; Ivan, J.V.E.; Ruben, R.R.; Javier, A.-A.F. Chemical Characterization of a Hypoglycemic Extract from *Cucurbita Ficifolia* Bouche That Induces Liver Glycogen Accumulation in Diabetic Mice. *Afr. J. Tradit. Complement. Altern. Med.* **2017**, *14*, 218–230. [CrossRef] [PubMed]
92. Pericin, D.; Krimer, V.; Trivic, S.; Radulovic, L. The distribution of phenolic acids in pumpkin's hull-less seed, skin, oil cake meal, dehulled kernel and hull. *Food Chem.* **2009**, *113*, 450–456. [CrossRef]
93. Dubois, M.-A.; Bauer, R.; Cagiotti, M.; Wagner, H. Foetidissimoside A, a new 3,28-bidesmosidic triterpenoid saponin, and cucurbitacins from *Cucurbita foetidissima*. *Phytochemistry* **1988**, *27*, 881–885. [CrossRef]
94. Gaidi, G.; Marouf, A.; Hanquet, B.; Bauer, R.; Correia, M.; Chauffert, B.; Lacaille-Dubois, M.-A. A New Major Triterpene Saponin from the Roots of *Cucurbita foetidissima*. *J. Nat. Prod.* **2000**, *63*, 122–124. [CrossRef]
95. Matus, Z.; Molnár, P.; Szabó, L.G. Main carotenoids in pressed seeds (cucurbitae semen) of oil pumpkin (*Cucurbita pepo* convar. *pepo* var. Styriaca). *Acta Pharm. Hung.* **1993**, *63*, 247–256.
96. Chen, J.C.; Chiu, M.H.; Nie, R.L.; Cordell, G.A.; Qiu, S.X. Cucurbitacins and Cucurbitane Glycosides: Structures and Biological Activities. *Nat. Prod. Rep.* **2005**, *22*, 386–399. [CrossRef]
97. Paryzek, Z. Tetracyclic triterpenes. Part A synthetic approach to cucurbitacins. *J. Chem. Soc.* **1979**, *1*, 1222–1227. [CrossRef]
98. Rehm, S.; Wessels, J.H. Bitter principles of the cucurbitaceae. VIII.—Cucurbitacins in seedlings—Occurrence, biochemistry and genetical aspects. *J. Sci. Food Agric.* **1957**, *8*, 687–691. [CrossRef]
99. Metcalf, R.L.; Ferguson, J.E.; Lampman, R.L.; Andersen, J.F. Dry cucubritacin-containing baits for controlling diabroticite beetles (coleoptera chrysomelidae). *J. Econ. Entomol.* **1987**, *80*, 870–875. [CrossRef]

100. Hutt, T.F.; Herrington, M.E. The determination of bitter principles in zucchinis. *J. Sci. Food Agric.* **1985**, *36*, 1107–1112. [CrossRef]
101. Ferguson, J.E.; Fischer, D.C.; Metcalf, M. A report of cucurbitacin poisonings in humans. *Cucurbit Genet. Coop. Rep.* **1983**, *6*, 73–74.
102. Halaweish, F.T.; Tallamy, D.W. A new cucurbitacin profile for *Cucurbita andreana*: A candidate for cucurbitacin tissue culture. *J. Chem. Ecol.* **1993**, *19*, 1135–1141. [CrossRef]
103. Rehm, S.; Enslin, P.R.; Meeuse, A.D.J.; Wessels, J.H. Bitter principles of the cucurbitaceae. VII.—the distribution of bitter principles in this plant family. *J. Sci. Food Agric.* **1957**, *8*, 679–686. [CrossRef]
104. Wang, D.-C.; Pan, H.-Y.; Deng, X.-M.; Xiang, H.; Gao, H.-Y.; Cai, H.; Wu, L.-J. Cucurbitane and hexanorcucurbitane glycosides from the fruits of *Cucurbita pepo* cv Dayangua. *J. Asian Nat. Prod. Res.* **2007**, *9*, 525–529. [CrossRef]
105. Tripathi, J.; Variyar, A.P.; Mishra, P.K.; Variyar, P.S. Impact of radiation processing on the stability of cucurbitacin glycosides in ready-to-cook (RTC) pumpkin during storage. *LWT* **2016**, *73*, 239–242. [CrossRef]
106. Kaushik, U.; Aeri, V.; Mir, S.R. Cucurbitacins—An insight into medicinal leads from nature. *Pharmacogn. Rev.* **2015**, *9*, 12–18.
107. Bisognin, D.A. Origin and evolution of cultivated cucurbits. *Ciência Rural* **2002**, *32*, 715–723. [CrossRef]
108. Rahman, A.H.; Anisuzzaman, M.; Ahmed, F.; Islam, A.K.; Naderuzzaman, A.T. Study of nutritive value and medicinal uses of cultivated cucurbits. *J. Appl. Sci. Res.* **2008**, *4*, 555–558.
109. Jayaprakasam, B.; Seeram, N.P.; Nair, M.G. Anticancer and antiinflammatory activities of cucurbitacins from *Cucurbita andreana*. *Cancer Lett.* **2003**, *189*, 11–16. [CrossRef]
110. Gill, N.S.; Bali, M. Isolation of antiulcer cucurbitane type triterpenoid from the seeds of *Cucurbita pepo*. *Res. J. Phytochem.* **2011**, *5*, 70–79. [CrossRef]
111. Le Roux, G.; Leborgne, I.; Labadie, M.; Garnier, R.; Sinno-Tellier, S.; Bloch, J.; Deguigne, M.; Boels, D. Poisoning by non-edible squash: Retrospective series of 353 patients from French Poison Control Centers. *Clin. Toxicol.* **2018**, *56*, 790–794. [CrossRef] [PubMed]
112. Pfab, R.; Oefele, H.; Pietsch, J.; Kapp, T.; Zellner, T.; Eyer, F. Revenge of the zucchinis—Is this the result of climate change? *Clin. Toxicol.* **2016**, *54*, 501.
113. Stoewsand, G.S.; Jaworski, A.; Shannon, S.; Robinson, R.W. Toxicologic Response in Mice Fed *Cucurbita* Fruit. *J. Food Prot.* **1985**, *48*, 50–51. [CrossRef] [PubMed]
114. Wu, H.; Zhu, J.; Diao, W.; Wang, C. Ultrasound-assisted enzymatic extraction and antioxidant activity of polysaccharides from Pumpkin (*Cucurbita moschata*). *Carbohydr. Polym.* **2014**, *113*, 314–324. [CrossRef]
115. Yang, X.; Zhao, Y.; Lv, Y. Chemical Composition and Antioxidant Activity of an Acidic Polysaccharide Extracted from *Cucurbita moschata* Duchesne ex Poiret. *J. Agric. Food Chem.* **2007**, *55*, 4684–4690. [CrossRef]
116. Pakrokh Ghavi, P. Modeling and optimization of ultrasound-assisted extraction of polysaccharide from the roots of althaea officinalis. *J. Food Process. Preserv.* **2015**, *39*, 2107–2118. [CrossRef]
117. Xia, T.; Wang, Q. D-chiro-Inositol found in *Cucurbita ficifolia* (Cucurbitaceae) fruit extracts plays the hypoglycaemic role in streptozocin-diabetic rats. *J. Pharm. Pharmacol.* **2006**, *58*, 1527–1532. [CrossRef] [PubMed]
118. Rodríguez, R.R.; Valdés, R.M.; Ortiz, G.S. Características agronómicas y calidad nutricional de los frutos y semillas de zapallo *Cucurbita* sp. *Rev. Colomb. Cienc. Anim. RECIA* **2018**, *10*, 86–97. [CrossRef]
119. Wightii, B.S.S. Extraction and characterisation of polysaccharides from leaflets. *Life Sci.* **2012**, *7*, 17–69.
120. Yuan, G.F.; Chen, X.E.; Li, D. Conjugated linolenic acids and their bioactivities: A review. *Food Funct.* **2014**, *5*, 1360–1368. [CrossRef] [PubMed]
121. Pokora, M.; Zambrowicz, A.; Eckert, E.; Pokora, M.; Bobak, Ł.; Da, A. Antioxidant and antidiabetic activities of peptides isolated from a hydrolysate of an egg- yolk protein by-product prepared with a proteinase from Asian pumpkin (*Cucurbita ficifolia*). *RSC Adv.* **2016**, *5*, 10460–10467.
122. Wroc, T.T. Egg-yolk protein by-product as a source of ace-inhibitory peptides obtained with using (*Cucurbita ficifolia*). *J. Proteom.* **2016**, *110*, 107–116.
123. Köksal, E.; Bursal, E.; Aggul, A.G.; Gulcin, I. Purification and Characterization of Peroxidase from Sweet Gourd (*Cucurbita moschata* Lam. Poiret). *Int. J. Food Prop.* **2012**, *15*, 1110–1119. [CrossRef]
124. Chonoko, U.G.; Rufai, A.B. Phytochemical screening and antibacterial activity of curbita pepo (pumpkin) against staphylococcus aureus and salmonella typhi. *J. Pure Appl. Sci.* **2011**, *4*, 145–147.

125. Dinu, M.; Soare, R.; Hoza, G.; Becherescu, A.D. Biochemical Composition of Some Local Pumpkin Population. *Agric. Agric. Sci. Procedia* **2016**, *10*, 185–191. [CrossRef]
126. Adeel, R.; Sohail, A.; Masud, T. Characterization and antibacterial study of pumpkin seed oil (*Cucurbita pepo*). *Life Sci. Leafl.* **2014**, *49*, 53–64.
127. Abed El-Aziz, A.; Abed El-Aziz, H. Antimicrobial proteins and oil seeds from pumpkin. *Nat. Sci.* **2011**, *9*, 105–119.
128. Zhou, C.-L.; Liu, W.; Zhao, J.; Yuan, C.; Song, Y.; Chen, D.; Ni, Y.-Y.; Li, Q.-H. The effect of high hydrostatic pressure on the microbiological quality and physical–chemical characteristics of Pumpkin (*Cucurbita maxima* Duch.) during refrigerated storage. *Innov. Food Sci. Emerg. Technol.* **2014**, *21*, 24–34. [CrossRef]
129. Dar, A.H.; Sofi, S.A. Pumpkin the functional and therapeutic ingredient: A review. *Int. J. Food Sci. Nutr.* **2017**, *2*, 165–170.
130. Muruganantham, N.; Solomon, S.; Senthamilselvi, M.M. Anti-cancer activity of *Cucurbita maxima* flowers (pumpkin) against human liver cancer. *J. Aournal Pharmacogn. Phytochem.* **2016**, *6*, 1356–1359.
131. Cheong, N.E.; Choi, Y.O.; Kim, W.Y.; Bae, I.S.; Cho, M.J.; Hwang, I.; Kim, J.W.; Lee, S.Y. Purification and characterization of an antifungal PR-5 protein from pumpkin leaves. *Mol. Cells* **1997**, *7*, 214–219. [PubMed]
132. Barbieri, L.; Polito, L.; Bolognesi, A.; Ciani, M.; Pelosi, E.; Farini, V.; Jha, A.K.; Sharma, N.; Vivanco, J.M.; Chambery, A.; et al. Ribosome-inactivating proteins in edible plants and purification and characterization of a new ribosome-inactivating protein from *Cucurbita moschata*. *Biochim. Biophys. Acta* **2006**, *1760*, 783–792. [CrossRef] [PubMed]
133. Park, S.-C.; Kim, J.-Y.; Lee, J.-K.; Hwang, I.; Cheong, H.; Nah, J.-W.; Hahm, K.-S.; Park, Y. Antifungal Mechanism of a Novel Antifungal Protein from Pumpkin Rinds against Various Fungal Pathogens. *J. Agric. Food Chem.* **2009**, *57*, 9299–9304. [CrossRef]
134. Salehi, B.; Capanoglu, E.; Adrar, N.; Catalkaya, G.; Shaheen, S.; Jaffer, M.; Giri, L.; Suyal, R.; Jugran, A.K.; Calina, D.; et al. Cucurbits Plants: A Key Emphasis to Its Pharmacological Potential. *Molecules* **2019**, *24*, 1854. [CrossRef]

PERMISSIONS

All chapters in this book were first published by MDPI; hereby published with permission under the Creative Commons Attribution License or equivalent. Every chapter published in this book has been scrutinized by our experts. Their significance has been extensively debated. The topics covered herein carry significant findings which will fuel the growth of the discipline. They may even be implemented as practical applications or may be referred to as a beginning point for another development.

The contributors of this book come from diverse backgrounds, making this book a truly international effort. This book will bring forth new frontiers with its revolutionizing research information and detailed analysis of the nascent developments around the world.

We would like to thank all the contributing authors for lending their expertise to make the book truly unique. They have played a crucial role in the development of this book. Without their invaluable contributions this book wouldn't have been possible. They have made vital efforts to compile up to date information on the varied aspects of this subject to make this book a valuable addition to the collection of many professionals and students.

This book was conceptualized with the vision of imparting up-to-date information and advanced data in this field. To ensure the same, a matchless editorial board was set up. Every individual on the board went through rigorous rounds of assessment to prove their worth. After which they invested a large part of their time researching and compiling the most relevant data for our readers.

The editorial board has been involved in producing this book since its inception. They have spent rigorous hours researching and exploring the diverse topics which have resulted in the successful publishing of this book. They have passed on their knowledge of decades through this book. To expedite this challenging task, the publisher supported the team at every step. A small team of assistant editors was also appointed to further simplify the editing procedure and attain best results for the readers.

Apart from the editorial board, the designing team has also invested a significant amount of their time in understanding the subject and creating the most relevant covers. They scrutinized every image to scout for the most suitable representation of the subject and create an appropriate cover for the book.

The publishing team has been an ardent support to the editorial, designing and production team. Their endless efforts to recruit the best for this project, has resulted in the accomplishment of this book. They are a veteran in the field of academics and their pool of knowledge is as vast as their experience in printing. Their expertise and guidance has proved useful at every step. Their uncompromising quality standards have made this book an exceptional effort. Their encouragement from time to time has been an inspiration for everyone.

The publisher and the editorial board hope that this book will prove to be a valuable piece of knowledge for researchers, students, practitioners and scholars across the globe.

LIST OF CONTRIBUTORS

Gianmaria Fabrizio Ferrazzano
Department of Neurosciences, Reproductive Sciences and Oral Sciences, School of Paediatric Dentistry, University of Naples "Federico II", 80131 Naples, Italy
Unesco Chair on Health Education and Sustainable Development, University of Naples, "Federico II", 80121 Naples, Italy

Cristina Papa, Aniello Ingenito, Giancarla Sangianantoni and Tiziana Cantile
Department of Neurosciences, Reproductive Sciences and Oral Sciences, School of Paediatric Dentistry, University of Naples "Federico II", 80131 Naples, Italy

Antonino Pollio
Department of Biology, University of Naples "Federico II", 80126 Naples, Italy

Su Jin Heo, Ah-Jin Kim, Kimoon Kang and Do Yu Soung
Food Research Institute, CJ Cheil Jedang, 42, Gwanggyo-ro, Yeongtong-gu, Suwon-si, Gyeonggi-do 16495, Korea

Min-Ju Park
BIO Research Institute, CJ Cheil Jedang, 42, Gwanggyo-ro, Yeongtong-gu, Suwon-si, Gyeonggi-do 16495, Korea

Andreia F. R. Silva, Daniela Resende, Mariana Monteiro, Manuel A. Coimbra, Artur M. S. Silva and Susana M. Cardoso
LAQV-REQUIMTE, Department of Chemistry, University of Aveiro, 3810-193 Aveiro, Portugal

Dubravka Vitali Čepo, Kristina Radić, Petra Turčić, Dora Anić, Barbara Komar and Mirela Šalov
Faculty of Pharmacy and Biochemistry, University of Zagreb, Ante Kovačića 1, 10000 Zagreb, Croatia

Lorenzo Zanella and Fabio Vianello
Department of Comparative Biomedicine and Food Science, University of Padua, Viale dell'Università 16, 35020 Legnaro, Italy

Francesca Colombo, Simone Biella and Chiara Di Lorenzo
Department of Pharmacological and Biomolecular Sciences, Università degli Studi di Milano, 20133 Milan, Italy

Patrizia Restani
Department of Pharmacological and Biomolecular Sciences, Università degli Studi di Milano, 20133 Milan, Italy
CRC "Innovation for Well-Being and Environment", Università degli Studi di Milano, 20122 Milan, Italy

Feng Zhao, Meng Li, Lingling Meng, Jinhan Yu and Tiehua Zhang
College of Food Science and Engineering, Jilin University, 5333 Xi'an Road, Changchun 130062, China

Sara M. Fraga and Fernando M. Nunes
CQ-VR, Chemistry Research Centre—Vila Real, Food and Wine Chemistry Lab, Chemistry Department, Universidade de Trás-os-Montes e Alto Douro, Apartado 1013, 5000-801 Vila Real, Portugal

Mohamed Nadjib Boukhatem
The Pharmaceutical Research Institute, Albany College of Pharmacy and Health Sciences, Rensselaer, NY 12144, USA
Département de Biologie et Physiologie Cellulaire, Faculté des Sciences de la Nature et de la Vie, Université-Saad Dahlab-Blida 1, BP 270, Route de Soumaa, Blida 9000, Algeria

Mehdi Rajabi and Shaker A. Mousa
The Pharmaceutical Research Institute, Albany College of Pharmacy and Health Sciences, Rensselaer, NY 12144, USA

Asma Boumaiza
Département de Biologie et Physiologie Cellulaire, Faculté des Sciences de la Nature et de la Vie, Université-Saad Dahlab-Blida 1, BP 270, Route de Soumaa, Blida 9000, Algeria

Hanady G. Nada
The Pharmaceutical Research Institute, Albany College of Pharmacy and Health Sciences, Rensselaer, NY 12144, USA
Drug Radiation Research Department, National Center for Radiation Research and Technology (NCRRT), Atomic Energy Authority (AEA), Cairo 11762, Egypt

Fan Zhang, Chenglong Jin, Shiguang Jiang, Xiuqi Wang, Huichao Yan and Chunqi Gao
College of Animal Science, South China Agricultural University/Guangdong Provincial Key Laboratory of Animal Nutrition Control, Guangzhou 510642, China

Huize Tan
WENS Foodstuff Group Co., Ltd., Guangzhou 527439, China

Guendalina Zuccari, Sara Baldassari, Giorgia Ailuno, Silvana Alfei and Gabriele Caviglioli
Department of Pharmacy, Università di Genova, 16147 Genova, Italy

Giovanni Gamba, Dario Donno, Maria Gabriella Mellano, Isidoro Riondato, Marta De Biaggi and Gabriele Loris Beccaro
Dipartimento di Scienze Agrarie, Forestali e Alimentari, Università degli Studi di Torino, 10095 Grugliasco (TO), Italy

Denis Randriamampionona
Mention Agriculture Tropicale et Développement Durable – Ecole Supérieure des Sciences Agronomiques, Université d'Antananarivo, 101 Antananarivo, Madagascar

Paola Malaspina, Paolo Giordani, Silvia Catena, Paola Zunin and Raffaella Boggia
Department of Pharmacy, University of Genoa, Viale Cembrano 4, 16148 Genoa, Italy

Federica Turrini
Department of Pharmacy, University of Genoa, Viale Cembrano 4, 16148 Genoa, Italy
Department of Pharmacy, Università di Genova, 16147 Genova, Italy

Bahare Salehi
Student Research Committee, School of Medicine, Bam University of Medical Sciences, Bam 44340847, Iran

Javad Sharifi-Rad
Zabol Medicinal Plants Research Center, Zabol University of Medical Sciences, Zabol 61615-585, Iran

Esra Capanoglu and Gizem Catalkaya
Istanbul Technical University, Faculty of Chemical & Metallurgical Engineering, Food Engineering Department, Maslak 34469, Istanbul, Turkey

Nabil Adrar
Istanbul Technical University, Faculty of Chemical & Metallurgical Engineering, Food Engineering Department, Maslak 34469, Istanbul, Turkey
Laboratoire de Biotechnologie Végétale et d'Ethnobotanique, Faculté des Sciences de la Nature et de la Vie, Université de Bejaia, Bejaia 06000, Algérie

Shabnum Shaheen and Mehwish Jaffer
Department of Plant Sciences, LCWU, Lahore 54000, Pakistan

Lalit Giri and Renu Suyal
G.B. Pant National Institute of Himalayan Environment & Sustainable Development Kosi-Katarmal, Almora 263 643, Uttarakhand, India

Arun K Jugran
G.B. Pant National Institute of Himalayan Environment & Sustainable Development Garhwal Regional Centre, Srinagar 246174, Uttarakhand, India

Daniela Calina
Department of Clinical Pharmacy, University of Medicine and Pharmacy of Craiova, 200349 Craiova, Romania

Anca Oana Docea
Department of Toxicology, University of Medicine and Pharmacy of Craiova, 200349 Craiova, Romania

Senem Kamiloglu
Mevsim Gida Sanayi ve Soguk Depo Ticaret A.S. (MVSM Foods), Turankoy, Kestel, Bursa 16540, Turkey

Dorota Kregiel and Ewelina Pawlikowska
Institute of Fermentation Technology and Microbiology, Lodz University of Technology, Wolczanska 171/173, 90-924 Lodz, Poland

Hubert Antolak and Krishnendu Acharya
Molecular and Applied Mycology and Plant Pathology Laboratory, Department of Botany, University of Calcutta, Kolkata 700019, India

Surjit Sen
Molecular and Applied Mycology and Plant Pathology Laboratory, Department of Botany, University of Calcutta, Kolkata 700019, India
Department of Botany, Fakir Chand College, Diamond Harbour, West Bengal 743331, India

Moein Bashiry
Department of Food Science and Technology, Nutrition and Food Sciences Faculty, Kermanshah University of Medical Sciences, Kermanshah 6719851351, Iran

Zeliha Selamoglu
Department of Medical Biology, Faculty of Medicine, Nigde Ömer Halisdemir University, Campus, Nigde 51240, Turkey

Miquel Martorell
Department of Nutrition and Dietetics, Faculty of Pharmacy, University of Concepcion, Concepcion 4070386, Chile
Universidad de Concepción, Unidad de Desarrollo Tecnológico, UDT, Concepcion 4070386, Chile

Farukh Sharopov
Department of Pharmaceutical Technology, Avicenna Tajik State Medical University, Rudaki 139, 734003 Dushanbe, Tajikistan

Natália Martins
Faculty of Medicine, University of Porto, Alameda Prof. Hernâni Monteiro, 4200-319 Porto, Portugal
Institute for Research and Innovation in Health (i3S), University of Porto, 4200-135 Porto, Portugal

Jacek Namiesnik
Department of Analytical Chemistry, Faculty of Chemistry, Gdańsk University of Technology, 80-233 Gdańsk, Poland

William C. Cho
Department of Clinical Oncology, Queen Elizabeth Hospital, Hong Kong, China

Index